OCCUPATIONAL HEALTH SERVICES

A PRACTICAL APPROACH

Tee L. Guidotti, MD, MPH, FACP, FACOM
Professor of Occupational Medicine
University of Alberta

John W.F. Cowell, MD, MSc, FACOM
Vice President Health, Safety and Environment
Nova Corporation of Alberta

Geoffrey G. Jamieson, MD, MSc, FACOM
Consultant in Occupational Medicine
Alberta

With the assistance and contribution of
Alan L. Engelberg, MD, MPH
American Medical Association

American Medical Association

American Medical Association

ISBN: 0-89970-345-3
LC Number: 88-083903

Additional copies may be purchased from:
Order Department OP 328
American Medical Association
P.O. Box 10946
Chicago, Illinois 60610

Comments or inquiries to:
Department of Preventive Medicine
American Medical Association
535 North Dearborn Street
Chicago, Illinois 60610

SCE: 88-057:2M:1/89

CONTENTS

INTRODUCTION   Objectives of This Book / v

SECTION I   **THE OCCUPATIONAL HEALTH CARE SYSTEM**

Chapter 1   The Occupational Health Care System / 3
Chapter 2   The Role of Workers' Compensation / 19
Chapter 3   Occupational Safety and Health Regulation / 37
Chapter 4   Ethics in Occupational Medicine / 49

SECTION II   **OCCUPATIONAL HEALTH CARE DELIVERY**

Chapter 5   The Business Context / 63
Chapter 6   Contract Services / 81
Chapter 7   Preparing for an Occupational Medicine Practice / 95
Chapter 8   Marketing Services / 103

SECTION III   **OFFICE ADMINISTRATION**

Chapter 9   Staffing and Personnel Needs / 123
Chapter 10   Facilities and Equipment / 131
Chapter 11   Office Procedures / 141
Chapter 12   Recordkeeping / 153

SECTION IV   **PROGRAM MANAGEMENT**

Chapter 13   Service Selection and Implementation / 165
Chapter 14   Program Evaluation / 173
Chapter 15   Cost/Benefit Analysis / 183
Chapter 16   Research Management / 191

SECTION V   OCCUPATIONAL HEALTH SERVICES

Chapter 17   Clinical Management / 201
Chapter 18   Fitness-to-Work and Impairment Evaluations / 209
Chapter 19   Equal Access and Opportunity / 237
Chapter 20   Health Monitoring and Surveillance / 243
Chapter 21   AIDS in the Workplace / 263
Chapter 22   Absence Monitoring / 269
Chapter 23   Hazard Evaluation and Control / 279
Chapter 24   Industrial Emergencies Involving Hazardous
                    Substances / 293
Chapter 25   Alcohol and Drug Testing / 301
Chapter 26   Employee Assistance Programs / 323
Chapter 27   Health Promotion / 331

APPENDICES

Appendix 1   An Occupational Health Audit / 341
Appendix 2   Sources of Information for Managing Occupational
                    Health Problems / 361
Appendix 3   Recommended Occupational Medicine Clinic
                    Library / 365
Appendix 4   Survey on Occupational Health Services / 367

OBJECTIVES OF THIS BOOK

The growth of occupational health services is an exciting development in the changing world of health care delivery. Occupational medicine has emerged as a sophisticated and rewarding field of practice that allows health care providers to diversify their practice opportunities while maintaining relative economic stability in uncertain times. Such advantages have spurred interest in the field among practitioners after many years of indifference and even neglect. Private physicians, medical groups, hospitals, and other health professional and institutions now are considering occupational health services as a new frontier.

This frontier is not an uncharted wilderness, however; the field is structured, basic requirements have been identified, and rules for operation are in effect. These structures, requirements, and rules form the subject matter of this book. The purpose behind its writing has been to provide general guidelines for creating, developing, and managing a sound program of high quality occupational health care delivery, with an emphasis on basic medical and nursing services. The authors present it as a reference to consult in case of problems and a road map to follow in entering unfamiliar territory.

This guide is intended for the use of occupational health care providers and managers—physicians in solo or group practice, medical directors of corporations, plant physicians, occupational health nurses, and managers with responsibility for occupational health services in companies, plants, public agencies, and even health care facilities. It thoroughly plots the field of occupational health delivery by:

- Tracing the structure and regulation of occupational health care systems;
- Identifying standards of practice and performance of all occupational health services;
- Explaining the administration of occupational health programs, from staffing and facilities requirements to office procedures and insurance liability;
- Defining the kinds and extent of occupational health services; and
- Delineating the standards by which programs and services should be evaluated.

Like any road map, however, this guide does not detail every house, alley, and country road. Certain generalizations are inevitable and most of the suggested approaches should be adapted, as appropriate, to the local situation. Of course, ethical considerations and basic requirements of occupational health services as discussed here should be uniform in all settings, but the specifics of a particular locale should be weighed in interpreting the sections dealing with the nuts and bolts of program operations.

The authors also note that, while the book serves as a single source for the definition and resolution of common problems, it cannot substitute for first-hand experience. We urge our readers to augment the knowledge gained through this book by touring the facilities of a variety of employers in diverse industries both within and outside their communities. We also suggest that they visit selected clinics to witness in practice the limitations as well as the benefits of different approaches to common problems. In the true spirit of professionalism, problems should be recognized and studied, and the lessons shared with others so that errors will not be repeated blindly.

We would like to acknowledge the assistance of students and colleagues who contributed ideas or reviewed preliminary drafts: Dr. Ron M. Dufresne, Dr. M. Joseph Fedoruk, Dr. Brady C. Hartman, Dr. Phil Jacobs, Dr. David F. Goldsmith, Dr. Colin Soskolne, Dr. D.H. Cordes, Dr. Marc Singer, Dr. W. Prendergast, Dr. J.H. Baillie, Dr. Barry M. Hainer, Dr. Herb Young, Dr. Ernie Mastromatteo, Dr. Joseph Cannella, Dan Horigan, Michael Doering, Joyce F. Zechter, and Carol Jane McNutt. Steffany Tayler put in long hours reworking the text and critiquing it in draft from the standpoint of an adult educator. Linda Fernandez worked tirelessly on organizing and editing the final draft.

We thank those organizations that generously allowed us to use material originally developed for their internal use: Canadian General Electric, the Nova Corporation of Alberta, the Canada Safety Council, the Alberta Federation of Labour Occupational Health Centre, and the Sharp/Rees-Stealy Medical Group. Also, we thank those journals and publishers that allowed the use of figures or tables from our prior publications and that permitted us the opportunity to develop some of these ideas in earlier articles: Annals of Internal Medicine, the Canadian Medical Association Journal, the American Family Physician, the Journal of Occupational Medicine, Occupational Health in Ontario, Seminars in Occupational Medicine, and the American Journal of Industrial Medicine, as well as the American Academy of Family Physicians, the Society for General Internal Medicine, and the Joint Curriculum Development Project in Preventive Medicine of the Association of Teachers of Preventive Medicine and the Center for Educational Development in Health, Boston University. No set of acknowledgments would be complete, however, without extending recognition to two outstanding secretaries, Mrs. Kathy Lasell and Ms. Debbie Sullivan, who worked tirelessly and with dedication on this difficult manuscript.

Tee L. Guidotti, MD, MPH, FACP, FCCP, FCPM, FACOM, CCBOM
John W.F. Cowell, MD, MSc, FACOM, CCFP, CCBOM
Geoffrey G. Jamieson, MD, MSc, FACOM, CCBOM, MFOM

SECTION I
THE OCCUPATIONAL HEALTH CARE SYSTEM

1 THE OCCUPATIONAL HEALTH CARE SYSTEM

Occupational health services are primarily concerned with maintaining the health of people at work or restoring the health and well-being of those who have been injured or exposed to a hazard on the job.

Understanding the place of occupational health services within the context of health care in general requires first understanding the differences between the occupational health care system and the general health care system. Physicians and other clinical health professionals have a working knowledge of the general health care system based on—and to some degree biased by—personal experience and are familiar with the standard elements of the system (health providers, financing, institutions, legal structures, and organizational relationships). At the same time, the general health care system is undergoing rapid and fundamental change in the United States. This pattern of change will continue for many years before a new pattern of stability emerges. By comparison, the occupational health care system is less well known.

In part because it is less familiar but primarily because it is largely driven by workers' compensation, the occupational health care system often appears more stable than it is. In fact, this system also has undergone profound changes in recent years. To appreciate these changes, however, it is first necessary to examine the elements of the system.

The occupational health care system exists in parallel with the larger general health care system in North America. Yet the system is financed separately from and organized around different principles than is general health care, so it is inaccurate to label occupational health care as a subset of the health care system in general. And although to a large extent the two systems share access to practitioners and facilities, they function very differently and often interact poorly, at least in the United States and Canada. In many developing countries, on the other hand, occupational health services function as the basic health care system in newly urbanized or industrialized areas, while in central and eastern Europe, occupational health services commonly are provided through the centralized health care system of neighborhood or workplace clinics.

In North America, medical care is decentralized and individualized, an approach that has resulted in a diffuse and sometimes incomplete network of occupational health care practitioners. These health professionals and the facilities they support primarily serve a centralized workers' compensation system and coexist with medical services sponsored by the larger employers. Large parts of the system, such as the appeals process in workers' compensation cases and the occupational health and safety management efforts within industry, are unknown to the average practitioner. Yet, in order to provide occupational health services effectively, the practitioner must become familiar with the system, know its players, understand the role the physician must play, and become skilled in the services that are provided through the system.

Health Care Delivery in Flux

The vigorous growth of occupational health services is helping to transform the system of health care delivery in North America. In the last decade, primary medical care has been transformed from a "cottage industry" to a "corporate industry"; under the old patterns care was provided to individual patients by physicians in solo practice and payment was primarily through private insurance supplied as a benefit of employment. Now, primary care increasingly is provided for profit by groups of physicians and other health care professionals organized into corporate entities and serving patients grouped according to residence, employer, or other common characteristics. More and more health services are paid for by a capitation allowance that shifts the financial risk from the third-party payer to the provider.

This new approach to providing general health care, combined with a surplus of medical school graduates in many specialities, has directly affected the parallel but distinct system of occupational health care in the United States:

- At the community level of practice, occupational medicine has become mixed with personal health care. Increasingly, directors of occupational health services in industry are called upon to review both individual cases and the employer's total experience with employee health costs, regardless of whether the reasons for care are work-related.
- Because of intensifying competition and financial risk-taking confronting medical practitioners and such health care providers as clinics and hospitals, occupational medical services are being used as a way to attract and "lock-in" large groups of employees and their dependents as a patient base for economic stability.

These outcomes profoundly affect—some might even say distort—the development of occupational health services in the United States. Current trends can be seen in San Diego, which has been studied as a model to aid in understanding changes that are taking place in the occupational health care system. The city serves as an excellent model for health services research. The population of San Diego County is relatively isolated, yet because the city is an affluent and desirable place to live, it already has experienced changes that are just emerging elsewhere in the United States, including a surplus of physicians, centralization of medical care, new methods of financial reimbursement, and empty hospitals. San Diego's responses to these shifts have produced major realignments of the health care system in general and occupational health services in particular.

A recent study by Guidotti and Kuetzing (see "Further Reading" at the end of this chapter) tracked over the period 1974–1984 local trends in San Diego's supply of health services, as reflected by such indicators as facilities and manpower (Table 1.1). The study found out that corporate medical departments had not kept up with rapid industrial growth over the decade, and appeared to be declining as prime providers of health services to employees. By contrast, the numbers of "industrial medicine clinics" had risen swiftly and dramatically, from a single facility to 13 over the period, and had become the dominant form of non-government occupational health care organization in San Diego. These clinics, freestanding ambulatory facilities not associated with a multispecialty group or hospital, now constitute almost half of the facilities providing occupational health care to workers in the city. Yet the industrial medicine clinic is itself under pressure from competitors, particularly freestanding "urgent care centers," which sprang upon the health care market in force in 1981.

Table 1.1. Occupational Health Resources in San Diego County, 1974 and 1984

Occupational health facilities	1974	1984
In-plant services	4	5
University hospital-based clinic	0	1
Hospital-based clinics	0	6
Multispecialty group-associated clinic	1	1
"Industrial medicine clinics"	0	13
"Urgent care clinics" or "medicenters"	0	15*

*Estimated

The study also found that despite a massive overall increase in the numbers of physicians in the San Diego area, occupational physicians with specialty credentials or eligibility remain few and are primarily based in academic or military institutions. At the same time the number of uncertified physicians and of medical groups accepting occupational medicine referrals has increased considerably. University- and HMO-based clinics appear to play only a limited role. Occupational health services in San Diego are obviously in a state of rapid change.

Indeed, it would appear that occupational health is in a free-for-all battle with off-site private health care facilities making great inroads. It is disturbing, however, to realize that most of these facilities lack the specialty expertise and resources required to provide a high level of service. Occupational health services therefore may be in danger of becoming "despecialized" as they become more competitive.

Further studies of occupational health services are urgently needed to assess the significance of these findings. The prominent role of the private practice sector in providing medical care and consulting services has been neglected as have important changes in the relationships between important institutions that affect occupational health care. In particular, the rise of the "industrial medicine clinic" over the last two decades has been almost entirely overlooked until recently. Now the dominant occupational health care provider in many communities, the industrial medicine clinic is itself coming under pressure from competitors, particularly from freestanding urgent care centers. "Industrial medicine clinics" (freestanding ambulatory facilities not associated with a multispecialty group or hospital) now constitute almost half of the facilities providing occupational health care in San Diego.

Part of the reason for this trend is that most routine occupational health services are simple in their execution, however sophisticated they may be in design. Employers are not always aware of differences in quality among potential providers of occupational health services. When faced with selecting a health care provider to take care of simple work-related injuries, many employers do not see any reason to pay a premium for quality when an adequate level will do. They do not perceive such care as specialized or likely to affect their employee's future life or well-being. Also, they are not choosing health services for themselves or their family. This presents a challenge to occupational health professionals and underscores yet another difference between the occupational and the general health care systems.

Foundations of Occupational Health Care

Differences between the two systems of health care—general vs. occupational—spring from the very foundations on which they rest. The basic assumptions of each system may be contrasted in the following respects:

Relationships of the parties. In a traditional fee-for-service setting, the primary relationship is between physician and patient with the insurance carrier or other third-party payer playing a secondary (albeit increasingly more active) role (Figure 1.1). In

---

Figure 1.1. Relationship between the patient and the physician in the general health care system is modified by the insurance carrier or third-party payer but the physician-patient relationship remains primary.

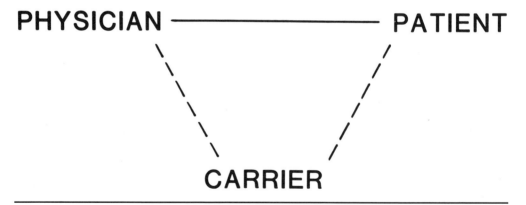

---

occupational health care, the number of players is much greater, including, at a minimum, the physician, the patient, the employer, a government regulatory agency (such as the Occupational Safety and Health Administration), and the workers' compensation carrier (Figure 1.2). The physician's relationship to the patient, while fundamentally the same as in a personal care setting, is modified by the other relationships—it is governed by very explicit rules and procedures designed to protect the legitimate interests of the employer and carrier as well as by government regulation. The physician

Figure 1.2. In the occupational health care system, the physician is one element in a network in which information, responsibility, and authority are shared with others.

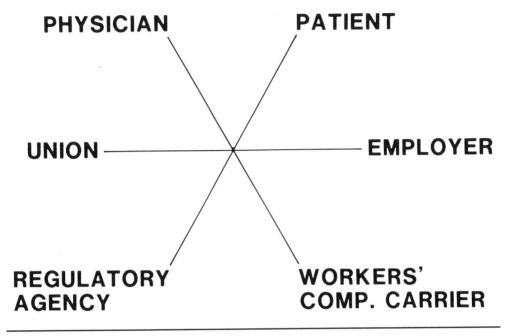

frequently acts as an agent reporting to the employer or to the carrier rather than as the provider of care to the individual patient. The decision-making authority of each player determines how information is circulated, subject to accepted rules of confidentiality, and responsibility for compensation is shared.

Level of utilization generally considered appropriate. In a fee-for-service setting, incentives built into the system tend to favor over-utilization of services because the additional revenue brought in by extra services increases profit margins (or cuts losses). Some third-party carriers have instituted utilization review procedures to rein in this tendency. On the other hand, incentives may favor under-utilization in a prepaid plan, where a fixed sum is paid to cover health care for each patient regardless of actual services performed, precisely because the profit margin increases for each patient whose care does not result in the full expenditure of funds provided. To ensure that needed care is not inadvertently withheld, many health maintenance organizations have introduced quality assurance reviews.

Occupational health care delivery responds to external pressures favoring an intensive utilization of services. Physicians providing workers' compensation services are compensated on a fee-for-service basis according to a fee schedule established by the state. (In Canada, fees are already fixed under the provincial health care plans.) Services provided on behalf of employers usually are determined by contract. In the workers' compensation system, the interests of the employer, insurance carrier, and the patient usually favor a speedy return to work. Thus, frequent return visits to the physician and heavy use of such rehabilitative services as physical therapy, while possibly viewed as overuse of services in a general health care setting, may be quite appropriate here. The test is whether the care contributes to returning the patient to work as soon as he or she is able, effecting a complete recovery or rehabilitation. An additional motivating factor in the system is to reduce the number of appeals and expensive litigation. The intensity of care therefore furthers the interests of reducing losses to the employer due to absence, prompt settlement of claims, and reduction of long-term expenses on the part of the carrier.

Organization of Occupational Health Care Delivery

Occupational health services are delivered through two avenues: "in-plant" and "off-site" facilities and personnel.

In-plant services are provided within the employer's facilities, almost always by a practitioner employed by the organization, typically a "plant physician," a nurse, or a nurse practitioner. Responsibilities of in-plant practitioners may include a variety of services, from simple triage and first aid to fairly comprehensive primary care, but their duties never encompass the setting of corporate policy, which remains the province of a "corporate medical director" and his or her staff. Corporate staff, usually based at the organization's headquarters, have only a limited role in providing patient care but participate in decision-making and in setting policy on health-related matters within the company. In-plant and corporate services are practical only for large enterprises. They are discussed in Chapter 5.

Off-site or commmunity-based health care facilities have displaced in-plant services as the principal means of providing occupational health services. They have established this dominance principally by providing health care for medium-sized and smaller industries.

Many practitioners, especially family physicians, deliver occupational health services out of their own offices. Generally in this type of situation, care is provided on a case-by-case basis although sometimes an employer will negotiate a contractual arrangement with a physician that establishes an ongoing relationship.

The major type of off-site occupational health care delivery, however, is the free-standing "industrial medical clinic." Here a group of medical practitioners devote themselves to providing occupational health services to local industry on a contract or fee-for-service basis. Large multispeciality group practices increasingly are developing occupational medicine services, particularly in the eastern and southwestern sections of the United States. Although they still are not widespread, hospital-based occupational health services are becoming more prominent. (Off-site services are examined in Chapter 6.)

Other, less representative forms of off-site occupational health facilities include clinics sponsored by labor unions for their members, at present confined for the most part to New York and Canada; by government agencies for their employees; and by military services for both active duty and civilian personnel. Off-site care also may be provided by the few private consultants in occupational medicine. Such consultants, who usually are located in major cities, specialize in performing disability evaluations, assessing causation, and reviewing cases being contested or appealed. Consultants typically are drawn from the ranks of practitioners with extensive experience in the field and solid reputations or special or unusual expertise.

Outside of this framework of specialized facilities and practitioners, occupational health services are delivered as a matter of routine by individual medical personnel and hospital emergency rooms, but such care may be best characterized as acute or episodic.

Structures for Occupational Health Care Delivery

Occupational health services may structured in one of four basic ways.

External services serving a single employer commonly are provided by individual physicians or consultants who do part-time work, usually on an as-needed basis, for a particular company or public agency. Usually this activity supplements a private practice, but sometimes it is done because of personal interests, for example, as a way to augment retirement activities, or because of the physician's special relationship with the employer or prior experience in a specialized industry with particular needs, such as aviation. Such arrangements are highly individualized and usually specific to the people involved; they do not transfer easily and tend to fall apart with changes in management. Often they are short-term and temporary in nature, made to resolve a particular problem or case. One danger in extending such arrangements over long periods of time is that cozy relationships may develop between the physician and the employer, leading to bias in the interpretation of cases or even an outright conflict of interest.

Internal services for a single employer, as noted above, are typical of large corporations, large single plants, and public agencies of cities and higher levels of government. This structure encompasses two subgroups:

- The in-plant health service, which may be called the infirmary, dispensary, or as is preferred today, the clinic. It is a facility in which medical care beyond basic first aid can be rendered to ill or injured employees and where programs of medical prevention and health promotion are organized and implemented. The clinic may be supervised by a suitably trained nurse who is on duty full-time or by a physician, typically contracted for designated days and times. The in-plant health service is the first level of care for occupational disorders, providing initial assessment of and treatment for accidents and acute illnesses and evaluations for fitness to work. Unless a plant presents an unusual or particularly serious hazard, such as exist in a shipyard, or is in an unusually isolated location, the clinic should not provide specialized medical or major surgical care.

- The corporate medical department, a unit within the management structure that reports to a high level and participates in forming and making decisions regarding occupational health policy. It is always headed by a physician, usually with an executive title and position, who directs and reviews the provision of health care within the organization and evaluates the medical aspects of employee benefit packages. The corporate department may provide direct medical services to local or headquarters staff or evaluate individual problem cases, but such functions are secondary to the overriding mission of coordinating and advising on policies, procedures, and standards relating to health within the organization.

External services delivering care to multiple employers now predominate in the occupational health care system. Included here are individual physicians, group practices, hospitals, and clinics that accept patients from several local employers on a contract or fee-for-service basis. Because they are external to the employer's organization, these providers often are viewed by employees as neutral or, at least, unswayed by undue influence from management. They are, however, vulnerable to the conflicting pressures described above.

Internal programs providing services to multiple employers are structured as in-plant services open to subsidiaries and affiliates of a larger company (essentially an extended form of the internal, single employer approach); as in-plant services open on a contract or fee-for-service basis to other small companies (a variant of the external, multiple employer approach); or as a contractual arrangement by which an occupational health service provides limited in-plant support services for several employers at the same time. The first two are more common in countries where health care systems are not well developed or where "polyclinics" (health care centers serving the needs of a particular population) are organized by industry or employment, as in eastern Europe. In North America, contractual arrangements to serve multiple employers with in-plant services commonly are embodied by the physician working part-time in more than one plant. Some contractors (usually physicians) have developed systems that place nurses in in-plant facilities and then provide them with supervision and back-up. Given the limited role of in-plant services and the ready availability of medical consultation, these arrangements predictably end with the company hiring the nurse directly as a way of saving money.

The question of whether to develop in-house or contract for occupational health services, as well as ensuing decisions on structuring the services, should be decided with an eye to the realities of the organization and the community of which it is a part. This decision must be guided by specific queries:

- Is qualified medical care from physicians knowledgeable about occupational medicine available in the community and easily accessible?
- Are there any operations within the organization that present particular hazards, use unusual technology, or have the potential for illnesses or injuries the care of which would require special insight or expertise?
- What are the pertinent regulations regarding occupational safety and health?
- What has been the past experience of the organization in terms of occupational health needs and management models and what is its expected future growth?
- Who are the employees, what is their social, ethnic, and economic background, and what patterns of disease are common in their home community?
- How much of an investment is the organization prepared to make in terms of time, personnel, and money?

Finally, the employer must provide for integrating nonmedical functions, such as safety and occupational hygiene, with the medical services. They may be combined into a comprehensive occupational health and safety unit, or they may be organized as separate departments within the organization. Sometimes specific nonmedical services may be obtained by contractual agreement from an outside supplier. Regardless of the form of organization selected, the essential medical and nonmedical function must enjoy clear lines of communication and a close working relationship. Without such rapport, personal or political agendas may subvert the efficient prevention and solution of problems.

Occupational Health and Safety Professionals

"Occupational health and safety" is a broad term encompassing a range of methods and means of protecting workers from hazards on the job and providing care for those injured or adversely affected at work:

- "Safety" usually refers to protection from physical hazards, ranging from mechanical safety devices to procedures for preventing fires or explosions or other traumatic causes of acute injury.
- "Health" generally encompasses means of managing exposure to workplace substances, from toxic chemicals to the more insidious forms of uncontrolled energy, such as radiation, heat, or noise.

The dividing line that distinguishes safety concerns from health concerns is somewhat arbitrary. Generally, health effects are considered to be more gradual in onset, although in some instances, such as heat stress or acute toxicity, they can be as acute as those rendered by lapses in safety. In practice, then, most safety professionals concern themselves at least to some degree with controlling chemical hazards, and health professionals often deal with prevention of repetitive motion trauma and other insidious causes of physical injury.

The occupational physician is a medical doctor who has been trained in and who predominantly or exclusively practices occupational medicine. Evidence of such training includes board certification in occupational medicine by the American Board of Preventive Medicine in the United States or by either the Royal College of Physicians and Surgeons or the Canadian Board of Occupational Medicine in Canada. The majority of practicing occupational physicians, however, lack such certification, primarily because most have entered the specialty in mid-career and are reluctant to return to training to meet the certification requirements. (Many physicians practicing occupational medicine but lacking formal training in the field refer to themselves as "industrial medicine physicans" as a way of avoiding the implication of specialist training.) Most occupational physicians are engaged in private practice or in-plant services. Organizations representing these physicians are the American College of Occupational Medicine and the Occupational Medical Association of Canada, as well as the American College of Preventive Medicine.

The occupational health nurse is a registered nurse specializing in occupational health services, usually in an in-plant setting. Since 1972, the American Board for Occupational Health Nurses, the principal organization for nurses in the field, has provided board certification, emphasizing skills in health education, occupational health and disease recognition, rehabilitation, and administration. The specialty is small and not well known, but offers high levels of autonomy and responsibility. Both occupational health nurse practitioners and physician's assistants in occupational health perform mid-level practitioner duties within the workplace.

The industrial (or occupational) hygienist specializes in recognizing, evaluating, and controlling occupational health hazards. Training in industrial hygiene includes extensive study of ventilation, analytical chemistry, mathematics, and toxicology, and frequently is augmented by engineering studies. These professionals are in great demand by industry. The standard credential in the field is certification by the American Board of Industrial Hygiene; the principal organization for professionals is the American

Industrial Hygiene Association. The American Conference of Governmental Industrial Hygienists, another important organization, recommends allowable exposure standards to industry.

The safety engineer is trained to recognize and control safety hazards. Such training generally is pursued through short-term, intensive institutes or seminars rather than at the graduate level. The principal organizations for professionals are the American Society of Safety Engineers and the National Safety Council in the United States and the Canadian Society of Safety Engineers and the Canada Safety Council in Canada.

The audiologist evaluates hearing and identifies hearing disorders. Within the field of audiology, the occupational hearing conservationist identifies hearing loss induced by noise in the workplace. Hearing conservationists are certified by the Council on Accreditation in Occupational Hearing Conservation as to their skills in performing audiometric evaluations of workers exposed to noise.

The work evaluation or rehabilitation counselor is trained at the undergraduate or graduate level to assess the work skills, physical tolerances, specialized training, and motivation of workers. This assessment is used to judge the extent of disability in workers' compensation cases.

The risk (or loss or liability) control officer is charged with minimizing the likelihood of litigation, limiting the employer's exposure to uncontrolled employee health care costs, and holding down the employer's share of workers' compensation assessments. Many of these business professionals, generally employed by large corporations or public agencies, enter their positions from the fields of personnel management or insurance. The insurance industry itself has established an elaborate system of professional education designed to ensure uniformity and equity in claims-processing. For example, the Insurance Institute of America maintains a nationwide system of classes, self-study courses and examinations on such subjects as industrial hygiene and occupational medicine, leading to the degree of Associate in Loss Control Management. Further study may lead to the advanced credential of the insurance industry, Chartered Property Casualty Underwriter, which allows the professional to investigate insurance claims and evaluate employers for workers' compensation coverage.

Working behind the scenes are many other occupational health professionals: toxicologists; epidemiologists; acoustical engineers; ergonomists (specialists in the human factors to be considered in the design of tools, equipment, and work practices); analytical laboratory technicians; health physicists (who study the control of radiation hazards). The occupational physician is unlikely to encounter these professionals in the usual course of practice; generally, they work as consultants to industry on a project-by-project or as-needed basis.

Varieties of Occupational Health Services

There are two basic categories of occupational health services: ameliorative and preventive. Ameliorative services are intended to cure or limit disease or to manage existing problems; preventive services seek to avoid worker exposure to hazards, detect disorders at an early and potentially curable stage, and to limit disability. The principal occupational health services have both ameliorative and preventive components, as shown in Table 1.2.

Acute care of the injured or ill worker is the most common service provided by the primary care physician. Although most occupational injuries are clinically obvious and straightforward, occupational illnesses are often overlooked or their occupational association is not recognized. Proper provision of acute care for occupational disorders requires reporting the case as prescribed by the legal dictates of the Occupational Safety and Health Administration and promptly communicating with the workers' compensation carrier and the employer if the injured worker needs time off the job. Follow-up and referral for rehabilitation and physical therapy is a particularly important aspect of the management of occupational accidents. The appropriate program of treatment usually is worked out in consultation with a physical therapist; the physician continues to file "supplemental" reports with the workers' compensation carrier on the employee's progress. A final report is submitted when the worker either is fit to return to the job or has recovered as much function as can be expected given the nature of the injury.

Table 1.2. Types of Occupational Health Services

Subsets of Services*	Ameliorative	Preventive
"Industrial Medicine"**	Acute and chronic care disability evaluation	Fitness to work evaluations
Hazard Control (teamwork with other professionals required)	Health hazard evaluation Compliance with government regulations and correction of infractions	Consultation Worker education Biological monitoring Compliance with standards
Personal Health Care (individual health)	Employee assistance programs	Health promotion

* "Occupational medicine" is the medical specialty for physicians engaged in these activities.
** "Industrial medicine" is an obsolete term for occupational medicine, now used to indicate a routine level of services.

Fitness-to-work evaluations, a major responsibility of the occupational physician, include preplacement, periodic health, "return to work," and disability evaluations:

- Preplacement evaluations are medical evaluations of newly hired employees to determine suitability for work to be done. In the past, the term "preemployment examination" was used to describe this process; the newer term is now preferred to avoid misunderstanding related to equal employment opportunity issues. To conduct a meaningful placement evaluation, the physician must be knowledgeable about the precise work to be performed, the physical requirements imposed by the job, and the physiological demands placed on the worker.
- Periodic health evaluations usually are given to employees at risk because of exposure to a known health hazard, with the aim of detecting adverse health effects at the earliest possible time (see Chapter 20). This process is called "surveillance"; when required by law, as for workers exposed to lead, asbestos, and noise, it is

referred to as "mandated surveillance." Periodic evaluation of employees without reference to an expected outcome is called "monitoring." A common use of monitoring in industry is the "executive physical," a routine comprehensive medical evaluation for executives and key personnel whose continued good health is believed to be essential to the company's future. "Multiphasic health screening" is a general screening approach in which a battery of selected tests, usually automated, periodically are given to groups of employees.

- Disability evaluations are conducted to determine workers' compensation awards in the event of disabling injuries or illnesses. Physical assessment is only one part of this evaluation; the worker's skills, motivation, and aptitude for employment also are evaluated, as well as the labor market for the worker's skills. The physician's role in disability evaluation is one of confirming and quantifying the degree of impairment, not qualifying the person for workers' compensation payments on narrowly medical grounds. ("Return-to-work evaluations" following an injury or illness and medical "certification" of absence due to illness are other examples of fitness-to-work evaluations. They are discussed in detail in Chapters 18 and 22.)

  A health hazard evaluation (HHE) is performed following the appearance or suggestion of a health problem in the workplace. An HHE usually is conducted by means of a "walk-through" inspection of the workplace and interviews with managers, production supervisors, and employees at the worksite in question. This type of evaluation is seldom conducted by a physician alone; other occupational health professionals — particularly industrial hygienists, safety engineers, and occupational health nurses — typically assume roles of equal or greater responsibility in the HHE team. (Chapter 23 provides an introduction to occupational health hazards and the conduct of an HHE, but special training and experience are required to participate in such an evaluation.)

  Absence control frequently is a source of misunderstanding between the employer and the occupational physician. Management is responsible for identifying individual workers whose performance on the job is declining or failing due to alleged or real sickness; the physician only evaluates the worker's fitness to work and makes appropriate recommendations for actions. The physician should not be held responsible for monitoring absence and should never accept being placed in the position of acting as a "policeman." (These issues are dealt with in detail in Chapters 18 and 22.)

  Employee assistance programs (EAPs) are organized within companies to identify employees with personal problems, refer them for treatment, support and motivate them to complete prescribed therapy, and assist in their rehabilitation. Most EAPs are focused on alcohol and drug abuse and mental illness, but some also address family and adjustment problems, financial mismanagment (particularly credit card overruns), and stress. A typical EAP operates primarily by self-referral; patients then are triaged to local health care or counseling facilities. Except for the initial counseling, EAPs usually do not provide direct treatment. The employer monitors the progress of the worker, and, where treatment requires absence from the job, guarantees return to the same or similar work. (EAPs are discussed in detail in Chapter 26.)

  Health promotion encompasses a variety of activities from the simple to the sophisticated that are designed to benefit workers by preventing health problems and enhancing physical health and well-being. Worksite health promotion programs typically include elements of health education, problem prevention, and physical fitness. (Chapter 27 examines these elements at length.)

The Occupational Environment

Aside from the real opportunity that exists in occupational medicine to prevent injury and disease and to promote good health, the medical treatment of injuries and illnesses is the same in the two systems. However, the overall management of cases may be subject to different influences. For one thing, administration and communication are more obviously part of the day-to-day practice in occupational medicine.

Program Administration

In an occupationally related case, the physician never acts alone; each development is reviewed and discussed among the other players in the system, often generating multiple decisions. Communication among all the parties involved in the form of telephone authorizations, claims, chart reviews, and requests for clarification is often extensive. Maintaining confidentiality is particularly troublesome, as some parties may be entitled to full information about a case, while others are not.

For example, in some organizations, only health care professionals (physicians and nurses) may receive laboratory reports involving biological monitoring or toxicological screening tests on the principle that these tests constitute diagnostic exams for individual workers. In other organizations, industrial hygienists and other hazard control professionals routinely have access to such data on the grounds that the tests are akin to environmental monitoring and may indicate hazardous workplace conditions. Where there is good communication among involved professionals, differences in specific policies should not interfere with the conduct of the occupational health care program. Barriers to communication, on the other hand, can lead to confusion and chaos. (Chapters 4, 5, and 19 discuss the appropriate policies for handling such information in greater detail.)

Many physicians balk at the amount of paperwork involved in workers' compensation cases. Yet there is a logic and a structure to the process, and the forms usually are simple and straightforward, requiring little more than a dictated progress note or a brief hospital discharge summary. Refusal to complete them, delay in filing them, or lack of attention to their content may severely harm the patient, distort health care costs, mislead regulatory activities, and result in health services not being covered by the carrier.

Equally as important in the delivery of occupational health care is the correct handling of health records. Portions of records are subject to review by the patient, by the insurance carrier and employer, and by outside consultants when a claim is appealed. Under some circumstances, records may be subpoenaed. (Records are discussed at length in Chapter 12.)

Program Objectives

Occupational health services do not exist as an end in themselves but as a means to an end, that is, to protect and, ideally, to enhance the health of workers within the special context of the workplace. Occupational health care is a process, not an outcome, and the success and quality of the services it provides ultimately are measured by the absence of problems rather than by a specific end point. In any organization, large or small, public or private, this must be the fundamental principle underlying the occupational health service: that the commitment to sound occupational health practices is ongoing, not limited to a specific problem-solving exercise.

(Health professionals speak of both "an occupational health service" and "occupational health services." The singular term usually indicates a facility, department, or other administrative unit charged with responsibility for occupational health and, usually, safety. This use of the term is analogous to a "service" in a hospital. The plural phrase typically refers to an activity, program, or function in the sense of a service to be provided. The meanings given "occupational health service" in this book parallel current use of the terms in the field and should be clear from the context in which the terms are used.)

The role of the occupational health service is to provide assistance to both the employer and the employee with the aim of protecting the employee from harm in the course of the work. To fulfill this mission, the service must be—and also must be perceived as being—objective and impartial, whether it is organized as part of the management structure or is provided through an external health care facility.

The day-to-day operating responsibility for sound occupational health and safety practices lies with those who carry out and supervise the work: the employee, operating personnel, and managers. The occupational health service exists to serve these various interests equally as consultant, troubleshooter, teacher, auditor, and advocate. To remain effective, it cannot function as a policeman, personnel officer, or scapegoat. Its objectives are to:

- Provide leadership, support, and technical services to the employer and the employee in all areas relating to health and safety in the workplace.
- Develop standards, procedures, reporting systems, and policies necessary to promote sound occupational health and safety practices, and to monitor compliance with them.
- Evaluate, treat, and limit temporary or permanent impairment resulting from injury or illness occurring in the workplace.
- Detect significant health hazards as early as possible and assist the employee and those responsible for the working unit in correcting the hazard before an injury or illness results.
- Assist the employee in managing personal health problems and living a healthy life, with the aim of enhancing quality of life, productivity, and well-being.

Philosophically, the occupational health service helps to create a fair balance between the rights and obligations of both the employee and the employer. It exists first to protect the employee from harm and second to ensure that if the employee is harmed, despite the best efforts of the employer, the care given will be adequate and the compensation for the injury just. At the same time, it must guard against attempts to unfairly hold the employer responsible for situations beyond its control. Like the fulcrum of a seesaw, then, the occupational health service is pressured from two sides simultaneously; in practice, keeping the legitimate interests of labor and management on an even keel requires that the service enjoy a certain degree of independence from the employer in both administrative structure and policy.

When the occupational health service is provided by an outside practitioner on a contract or fee-for-service basis, there is often an inherent conflict between the desire to please the employer, so as to maintain the relationship, and the desire to please employees, so as to attract private patients from among the workforce. If the natural desire to accommodate the expectations and wishes of the two groups leads the practitioner to be more responsive to the needs of both, the results can include such positive outcomes as better service, closer attention to detail, and an incentive to keep up with changing conditions. However, there is a point at which the process of responding legitimately to concerns may become vulnerable to the danger of introducing bias into medical decisions and communications. When the occupational health service is an in-plant facility, the pressures more strongly tend to favor management. It is important for the physician to keep medical judgments objective by remaining open and responsive to both sides while recognizing the potential for conflict.

An enlightened employer sees the long-range benefit—and ethical imperative—of treating employees fairly and providing for their health care. The most enlightened will extend this same logic to promoting the health of their employees. They will ensure that preventable hazards on the job are controlled to the most feasible degree allowed by current technology and appropriate to the magnitude of the hazard to health—beyond any regulatory requirements specifying the legally acceptable minimum.

Those employers who do not subscribe to this philosophy may have a cynical view of occupational health services because of such bad experiences as repeated abuse of the workers' compensation system, union complaints that management views as frivolous, or citation for failure to comply with occupational health and safety regulations that the employer does not accept as valid. One suspects that there is often a process of action-reaction going on, in which constrained management policies are met with hostility on the part of employees. This may be expressed in many ways, including abuse of the workers' compensation system. When this occurs, it is usually up to management to take the first step toward reducing tensions and it almost invariably follows that pent-up frustrations on the part of employees are what have led to an initially disappointing result. Yet, the transition to a mutually supportive relationship between labor and management can be accomplished even in the face of a smokescreen of rhetoric. In such situations, the occupational health service should resist pressure and present an attitude of fairness and mutual respect.

Further Reading

American Medical Association Council on Long Range Planning and Development: The Environment of Medicine. Chicago, American Medical Association, 1985.

American Medical Association Council on Medical Service: Effects of competition in medicine. JAMA 1983; 249:1864–1868.

DeHart R: Guidelines for Establishing an Occupational Medical Program. Chicago, American Occupational Medical Association, 1987.

Enthoven AC: Consumer-choice health plan. N Eng J Med 1978; 298:650–656, 709–720.

Frist TF: A cottage industry no more. The Internist 1983; 23(10):8–9.

Guidotti TL: Limiting MD investment in health field ill-advised. American Medical News (Chicago, American Medical Association) 14 September 1984, p. 49.

Guidotti TL: Occupational medicine at a crossroads. ACP Observer (American College of Physicians) January 1984, p. 5.

Guidotti TL, Kuetzing BH: Competition and despecialization: An analytical study of occupational health services in San Diego, 1974–1984. Amer J Indust Med 1985; 8:155–165.

Guidotti TL: What constitutes an ideal health care system? The Pharos (Alpha Omega Alpha) Summer 1981; 44:20–23.

Lee JA: The New Nurse in Industry. Washington DC, Government Printing Office, National Institute of Occupational Safety and Health, DHEW (NIOSH) Publication No. 78–143, 1979.

Murray R, Schilling RSF: Functions of an occupational health service, in Schilling RSF (ed): Occupational Health Practice. London, Butterworths, 1981, pp. 145–158.

Pear R: High costs determine who controls medicine. New York Times, 18 October 1987, p. E-G.

Relman AS: The future of medical practice. Health Affairs 1983; 2:5–19.

Rest K (ed): How to begin an occupational health program – administrative and ethical issues. Sem Occup Med 1986; 1(1):1–96.

Sedlak J: Occupational health organization, in Parmeggiani L (ed): Encyclopaedia of Occupational Health and Safety, vol. 2. Geneva, International Labor Office, pp. 1504–1511.

Starr P: The Social Transformation of American Medicine. New York, Basic Books/Harper-Colophon, 1982.

The Future of Health and Work: Implications for Health Strategies. Alexandria, Virginia, Institute for Alternative Futures, 1985.

2 THE ROLE OF WORKERS' COMPENSATION

The Industrial Revolution occurred neither suddenly nor at the same time in all parts of the world, but by the mid-nineteenth century it had brought a profound and irreversible change to western society. This was a time for quick investment and rapid expansion of industry, the introduction of new manufacturing processes, mechanization, and long working hours. The introduction of new marvels in transportation, manufacturing, and personal convenience were, however, accompanied by severe disruption and displacement of the human social fabric and by deleterious effects on health. Accident and illness prevention measures at the workplace were virtually non-existent, resulting in industrial injuries that were both frequent and severe. With progress came such unwelcome consequences of the Industrial Age as crushed bodies, torn limbs, blinded eyes, and blighted lungs suffered by the working men and women and even children who were exposed to the new and harsh physical, chemical, and psychological hazards of the factory.

Genesis of Workers' Compensation

At the turn of the century, the sole recourse for the disabled worker was the common law principle that holds an employer responsible for the injury or death of a worker caused by the employer's negligence. In order to benefit from common law, the worker had to bring suit against the employer and prove that the employer had been negligent and had caused the injury. Obtaining this proof was predictably a long, difficult, and expensive process. Few workers could afford to undertake legal action on their low wages and they were also confounded by legal delays. The employers used a variety of legal defenses, including the concepts of contributory negligence by the victims, the assumption of risk by workers accepting a job, and negligence by fellow workers. Judges tended to side with the employer when an industry was vital to the prosperity of a community. The only practical alternative for the disabled worker who had a family to support was to take to begging on the streets.

This state of affairs prompted a few social pioneers to champion the cause of workers, proposing that employees injured at their jobs were entitled to an effective and efficient system of compensation in order to have a chance to survive. This theory took a practical form in 1884, when the first version of the modern workers' compensation system was introduced in Germany.

In the first 10 years of the twentieth century, special employer liability laws were adopted by many counties, but not until 1911 did the first workers' compensation law come into being on the North American continent. Canadian laws followed this initial U.S. venture four years later. A profound change had occurred—now the injured worker was spared the effort of having to prove that the employer had been negligent, as well as the cost and time of a common law trial.

Today, there are over 70 legislated workers' compensation programs in North America. They are found in all 50 states; the District of Columbia; the 10 Canadian provinces; and the territories and areas under federal jurisdiction in both countries. European, British Commonwealth, and the majority of industrialized nations also have workers' compensation systems, some of which are of unusual design.

Principles of Workers' Compensation Law

Workers' compensation was founded as a means of providing a compulsory "no-fault" form of disability insurance for workers injured in the course of employment. Workers are automatically compensated for injuries or illness sustained at work, regardless of fault.

The system is compulsory on two fronts: employers as a group must pay all premiums and compensation as a cost of doing business and workers are obliged to participate and automatically surrender their right to take legal action against their employer for negligent acts.

Workers agreed to forgo their right of access to the courts in return for receiving prompt income and medical benefits for work-related injuries. They also escaped the problems of court delays, legal costs, the necessity to prove negligence, and the uncertainty of outcome. Employers, on the other hand, no longer faced the possibility of being assessed high settlement or restitution costs, since these costs were now pooled and assessed outside of the personal injury litigation system. In addition, the good of the public was served by relieving government and charitable organizations of the cost of supporting uncompensated disabled workers, and by encouraging employers to minimize the occurrence of workplace accidents and injuries.

The fundamental principles that underlie the many workers' compensation systems and programs have evolved over the years since the concept was first introduced in North America. Because so many independent jurisdictions are involved, and because tremendous socioeconomic changes have taken place since 1910, significant variations in virtually all aspects of workers' compensation are found from place to place. It is essential, therefore, that physicians and occupational health administrators have a clear understanding of the workers' compensation law, regulations, and current system of operation in the particular jurisdiction in which they function.

Workers' Compensation Law

In several U.S. states, employers have the right either to accept or to reject the state workers' compensation system. However, in opting out of the system, employers are prohibited from using the defenses of contributory negligence, assumption of risk, and negligence of fellow workers when sued by injured workers. The vast majority of states and all of the Canadian provinces require employers to participate in their workers' compensation systems and to provide the cost of compensation.

Most states require employers to obtain their own workers' compensation insurance. This may be through self-insurance or through commercial insurance firms on a private or employer group basis, depending on what is allowed under the state law. Self-insurance is permitted in most jurisdictions, but is primarily of use to large corporations who have sufficient financial resources and the legal and medical staff to manage it successfully. Such companies have the advantage of being able to deduct the amounts paid out in compensation as business expenses for tax purposes. A few states require companies to be insured in a state-sponsored insurance fund; some, like California, sponsor funds only as insurers of last resort for companies that cannot obtain commercial insurance. In Canada, self-insurance by companies is not permitted and all provinces have their own insurance funds.

In addition to the individual state workers' compensation laws, the U.S. Federal Employees Compensation Act (FECA) exists to govern the compensation for most federal employees. The Federal Employers Liability Act, Veterans Administration, the Black Lung Benefits Act, the Social Security Administration Disability Insurance Program, and the Longshore and Harbor Workers Act provide varying types of compensation for injured workers, although they are not primarily workers' compensation legislation. In Canada, the Government Employee's Compensation Act, administered by Labour Canada, covers federal workers and the Canadian Merchant Seaman's Act covers seafarers.

Workers' compensation is administered by a commission or board and/or the courts in the United States. All workers' compensation in Canada is administered through workers' compensation boards. These organizations are responsible for supervising and ensuring compliance with the compensation act and regulations; investigating worker claims; supervising medical care and rehabilitation of workers; managing all premiums, administrative, and compensation funds; and collecting and analyzing occupational injury and illness data.

Worker Coverage

Although the concept of workers' compensation could apply to all workers, there is no jurisdiction in which all workers receive automatic coverage. Most workers' compensation legislation specifically excludes from coverage certain types of work, generally agricultural employment, domestic help, and casual labor. Other exclusions vary, but workers in these sectors are usually allowed to self-enroll on a voluntary basis. Coverage in the United States includes about 90 percent of all wage and salaried employees.

The Canadian provinces and some U.S. states permit individual employees to be covered, but others exclude employers who have less than a stated minimum number of employees.

All jurisdictions provide workers' compensation coverage for working minors. Some pay special benefits in case of injury to minors and have stiff penalties applied to employers whose young workers suffer work-related injury.

Compensable Injuries and Illnesses

For many years after its introduction, workers' compensation was preoccupied with claims for physical injury. The early factories of the new industrial age were minefields for the unwary, with unguarded gear wheels, shafts, belts, blades, and exposed electrical wiring in great abundance. Burns, fractures, amputations and crush injuries were extremely common and evident to all. On the other hand, occupational illnesses tended to develop slowly over many years with cause and effect being less clear. Only gradually did occupational diseases receive recognition by workers' compensation authorities. Even today, acceptance of some occupational disorders is confined to only a fraction of jurisdictions. The long latency of some diseases, the relative significance of a particular disease to the local economy, and the availability of trained occupational physicians all affect the acceptance of an industrial disease by compensation authorities.

Disorders labelled as "ordinary diseases of life," those which are not peculiar to the workers' own occupation, are not recognized for compensation. Examples of the former are diabetes, sinusitis, and rheumatoid arthritis. However, some diseases that until recently have been considered as ordinary diseases of life (notably coronary artery disease and mental illness, thought to be associated with stress) are now being accepted for compensation in some jurisdictions when workplace circumstances warrant.

Recognition and acceptance of an injury or illness by the workers' compensation authority as being affected or caused by the working environment is the first hurdle that faces the claimant. The next is meeting the time limit for filling the claim for compensation. These time limits vary enormously in U.S. jurisdictions, from a low of 60 days after injury to five years after the last workplace exposure to the hazard. In some cases there is no limit for specified diseases and at least one state will excuse the time limit in certain circumstances. Canadian workers' compensation authorities set a claim time limit that varies from six months after injury or death to five years after the last employment.

Funding of Workers' Compensation

As previously noted, one of the original principles of workers' compensation was that the employers should pay the entire cost of the service. This principle is still followed, albeit with modifications, in today's organizations.

In the United States, workers' compensation premium rates are set on the basis of each industry's injury/illness experience. Experience data are compiled annually by the National Council on Compensation Insurance and each state then sets the specific experience rates for the employers operating within its borders. Canadian rates are set annually by each provincial workers' compensation board by class of risk for each industry. These rates are expected to meet payments for injuries and illness that occur during the year. In both countries the basic annual cost to a company is calculated by multiplying the assessable rate by 1/100th of the company's payroll. Some jurisdictions apply additional rate factors that relate to the industry's or company's accident record in the preceding year, or set number of years, or to the actual compensation costs incurred by injured workers employed by the company. The additional rates are called "experience ratings."

Occasionally, workers who sustain an occupational injury or illness while employed move to another state before initiating a claim. Although most workers' compensation laws are extra-territorial (claims can be made in one jurisdiction for disabilities sustained in another), the administration of such cases depends on the specific circumstances, including the place of employment, the worker's principal residence, and the employer's place of business.

Compensation Benefits

Workers' compensation was originally intended to provide for the injured worker's loss of earnings and medical treatment. Following the two world wars, rehabilitation medicine took on new importance and the techniques of the specialty became increasingly effective. The newly developed fields of social, vocational, and mental rehabilitation were added to the medical aspects of physical rehabilitation. These were included as part of the workers' compensation benefit packages so that today worker benefits take three basic forms: cash for disability, medical care, and rehabilitation.

Cash Benefits
Four types of cash benefits can be awarded; the choice depends upon the particular types of disability suffered by the worker claimant. Whether a disability is partial or total is a matter of the residual function preserved by the individual in relation to the ability to perform marketable work. Furthermore, disability may be temporary or permanent in nature. For example, a simple fracture will almost invariably be a temporary disability; by contrast, an amputation would be permanent. Temporary and permanent disability may each be either partial or total in extent. Severe lung damage, for example, may lead to total disability, with the worker being unable to do work of any kind, while loss of vision in one eye may result in partial disability. Whether an injury is classified as temporary or permanent thus depends on the question of whether complete recovery on a medical or physiological basis is possible.

Under the workers' compensation classification, then, the four types of disability are:
- Temporary total—The disability is total, but recovery is expected.
- Permanent total—The worker will remain unable to undertake gainful employment.
- Temporary partial—The disability does not affect all functions and recovery is expected.
- Permanent partial—There is a permanent loss of one or several functions. Work is

possible, but the workplace may need to be modified or a new line of work undertaken.

This classification parallels that used by occupational physicians in making individual fitness-to-work assessments (Chapter 18). Each serves a similar purpose: to communicate in summary form an individual's ability to perform work. Cash benefits are triggered once the injury or illness has kept the worker off the job for a specified period of time. This post-injury waiting period varies among the states from one to seven days. Most compensation agencies provide a retroactive adjustment to the actual date of injury if the disability continues beyond a certain threshold period.

The amount of cash benefit payable to a worker is usually based on a percentage of the prior normal weekly wage. All states and the Canadian provinces have both a maximum and minimum limit on the weekly benefit. Some states also place a ceiling on the number of weeks or the total amount of cash benefit or both; no Canadian province limits the total amount payable. Time limitations on benefits received in Canada are either the actual duration of a temporary total disability or life, in the case of permanent total disabilities.

Cash benefits for partial disabilities may be made according to a fixed schedule that presumes loss of wages or may be based on a percentage of wage loss or of total disability. Most states augment the cash benefit of the fixed schedule with an extra amount. Fixed schedules are not used in Canada, each case receiving individual assessment using medical impairment ratings as a guideline.

Adjustments may be made to cash benefits when they are paid to dependent survivors or when cost of living changes occur. Almost all states provide an automatic annual adjustment of maxiumum benefits based on the state average weekly wage. Adjustments also may be made if a worker has violated safety regulations, but these are not universal.

Benefits that may accrue to the survivors of a deceased worker include burial allowances and a percentage of the worker's wage. The latter is usually paid to a surviving spouse until remarriage and to children until they reach a specified age.

Medical Care

In North America, medical and hospital benefits for workers' compensation claimants are almost unlimited. All jurisdictions, for example, provide prostheses. In Canada, the resources of the universal medical insurance system administered by each province are available to and are used by workers' compensation claimants, even though the provincial universal health insurance plan and the workers' compensation system are regulated, funded, and administered separately.

Workers have a basic right to refuse any recommended medical care or procedures. However, workers' compensation authorities take the view that a worker who is uncooperative in his or her medical or rehabilitative care risks cancellation of benefits.

Rehabilitation

The rehabilitation aspect of workers' compensation has become an increasingly important part of the compensation benefit package. It is in the interest of both the system and the worker to achieve the greatest possible degree of recovery in the shortest possible time. As a result, in many jurisdictions workers' compensation has become an innovative leader in rehabilitation.

Rehabilitation has been defined as the process of assisting an individual disabled from any cause to achieve a maintainable maximum level of functional independence in relation to self, family, home, and community. Although workers' compensation is concerned with the rehabilitation of workers disabled from occupationally related injury or illness, this definition applies.

If the objective of rehabilitation is to get the disabled worker back to meaningful work as soon as possible, then two requirements must be met. First, the rehabilitation process must begin as early as possible. Second, the process must be sustained until the worker has reached a level of recovery where he or she enjoys functional independence. Accordingly, a link, however tenuous, should be maintained between the newly disabled worker and the place of work, beginning as soon as possible after injury. It may be necessary for the employer to prepare the workplace for the worker's eventual return by installing functional aids to assist and maintain efficiency and safety at work or by finding an alternative position. Such supportive measures must not be planned in isolation, but should be discussed with the disabled worker and the health care providers. In many jurisdictions, funding to assist the disabled is available to employers from workers' compensation or other agencies for worksite modifications.

Traumatic injury imposes a psychological burden on the individual that may be more troublesome and longer lasting than the actual physical damage. Modern medicine has recognized the post-trauma syndrome in which the worker is depressed, anxious, fearful, and suffers severe sleep disturbances. Depending on the individual's view of the injury, this condition may quickly be overcome or may persist for a long time, sometimes for the remainder of life. It may change the worker's personality, so that a previously well adjusted and affable person becomes withdrawn, irritable, suspicious, and disinterested in former pursuits. By all objective measures, the original physical damage may have been repaired and full functional ability restored, but the worker may continue to insist that he or she still is unable to function as before. Even when the individual appears to accept having been restored to full function, he or she may become a hypochondriac and complain of a number of unrelated health problems, none of which ever seem to resolve themselves. Sometimes, the worker's frustrations may concentrate on the rehabilitation agency and its personnel so that he or she becomes persistently dissatisfied with their services.

Such psychological problems inevitably have a deleterious effect on the individual's attitude toward work and toward family and friends. These important providers of psychological support often have difficulty in adjusting to the disabled worker and his or her changed attitudes, but their reaction is important to the worker's recovery.

Clearly, the rehabilitative process in work-related disability is far more complex than simply repairing a fracture or teaching a worker to walk with aid of a cane or artificial limb. The World Health Organization defines the three main areas of rehabilitation as follows:

- Medical Rehabilitation—The process of medical care aimed at developing the functional and psychological activities of the individual and, if necessary, his or her compensatory mechanisms, so as to enable the person to attain independence and lead an active life.
- Social Rehabilitation—That part of the rehabilitation process aimed at integrating or reintegrating a disabled person into society by helping him adjust to the demands of family, community, and occupation, while reducing any economic and social burdens that may impede the total rehabilitation process.

- Vocational Rehabilitation—The provision of those vocational services, including vocational guidance, vocational training, and selective placement, designed to enable a disabled person to secure and retain suitable employment.

Integrating these areas of rehabilitation assumes a global approach. At the state or local level, however, the components of rehabilitation tend to fragment into separate responsibilities of separate agencies. It is therefore not possible to describe the rehabilitative services provided by a typical workers' compensation organization because there is no "typical" pattern. Some (as is the case for most Canadian workers' compensation organizations) have their own rehabilitation centers with a variable mix of medically oriented programs (physiotherapy, prosthetics, remedial and recreational therapy, work assessment, etc.) and vocationally oriented programs (vocational rehabilitation, psychological services, drug and alcohol abuse counselling, occupational therapy, etc.). Other jurisdictions contract out for some or all of these services.

The Compensation Process

The details of the procedure by which a worker's claim becomes a benefit package differ among organizations and across jurisdictions but all procedures follow the same basic steps. The worker or a representative submits a claim. The validity of the claim is then investigated. Should the claim be considered valid, the worker's residual disability is assessed and a decision is made as to the compensation entitlement. Should the claim be declared invalid or if the amount or type of compensation awarded is felt by the worker to be inappropriate, he or she may follow an appeal procedure. The employer also may appeal a decision it feels is without merit.

The Claim

Although a worker may be assisted or guided by others who help, such as a physician, it is the worker's own responsibility to initiate a claim for compensation. In most jurisdictions, the employer is required by law to report any workplace health-related incident that results in a worker or workers being off the job for a specified length of time. This is often a minimum of one to three days. Also, accidents that result in any of a listed category of injuries commonly must be reported. The Occupational Safety and Health Administration also uniformally requires all businesses to report injuries using OSHA Form 200. In a few states, the penalty for failure to report is $100 per day and imprisonment for up to one year.

Standard forms are commonly used in each jurisdiction for the initial claim. (Figure 2.1 reproduces California's mandatory form for physicians.) The form provides the claims office with the basic information on which to base a follow-up and assessment. The form frequently includes information from the employer on the facts of the incident as well as a statement from the treating physician. However, if a form is not available, a worker or the worker's next-of-kin still can initiate a claim by means of a personal letter or by personal appearance at a claims office.

An employer may be legally required to keep a record of all accidents as they occur at the worksite and it is a wise employer who is diligent in doing so. Injured workers or their survivors, for a number of reasons, may delay in submitting a claim and both

Figure 2.1 Doctor's First Report of Occupational Injury or Illness Form (as used in California).

DOCTOR'S FIRST REPORT

OF

WORK INJURY

STATE OF CALIFORNIA

Immediately after first examination, mail original to insurer or self-insured employer Failure to file a doctor's report is a misdemeanor (Labor Code 6413.5). In addition, in the case of diagnosed or suspected pesticide poisoning, you are required to. Send one copy of this report directly to the Division of Labor Statistics and Research, P.O. Box 603, San Francisco CA 94101, send one copy to your local health officer, notify your local health officer by telephone within 24 hours

		Do not write in this space
1	**EMPLOYER** (No. St	
2	Address & City] (Manufacturing shoes, building con-	
3	Business struction, retailing men's clothes, etc.)	
4	**EMPLOYEE** (First name, middle initial, last name)	
5	Address (No. St. & City)	
6	Occupation........Age........Sex	
7	Date injured........Hour........M Date last worked	
8	Injured at (No. St. & City)	
9	Date of your first examination........Hour........M Who engaged your services?	
10	Social Security Number	
11	**ACCIDENT OR EXPOSURE:** Did employee notify employer of this injury?........Employee's statement of cause of injury or illness	
12	**NATURE AND EXTENT OF INJURY OR DISEASE** (Include all objective findings, subjective complaints, and diagnoses. If occupational disease state date of onset, occupational history, and exposures.)	
13	X-rays By whom taken? (State if none) Findings	
14	Treatment	
15	Kind of case (Office, home, or hospital)........If hospitalized, date........Estimated stay	
	Name and address of hospital	
16	Further treatment (Estimated frequency and duration)	
17	Estimated period of disability for Regular work........Modified work	
18	Describe any permanent disability or disfigurement expected (State if none)	
19	If death ensued, give date	
20	**REMARKS** (Note any pre-existing injuries or diseases, need for special examination or laboratory tests, other pertinent information.)	

Name........Degree........[PERSONAL SIGNATURE OF DOCTOR]
(Type or print)

Date of report........Address (No. St. & City)........Tel No

FORM NO 1196-3

the worker and the employer may find it difficult to recall with any degree of accuracy exactly what took place at the time of the accident.

There are, however, time limits within which a worker must file a claim. There are also time limits in which the worker must notify the employer that he or she has suffered an injury or illness. In the United States, the time limit for informing the employer varies from immediately to one year. In some states and in Canada there is no limitation. Workers must file their claim within 60 days after injury in some states, but up to eight years after injury in others. Some states permit workers to file claims up to 25 years after their last exposure to ionizing radiation. In Canada, time limits for filing also vary but to a lesser degree, ranging from six months to five years following injury or death.

Medical treatment and various forms of rehabilitation are often well underway before a claim has been submitted. Provided that the worker has alternative means of financing this initial care, the delay in workers' compensation benefits because of late filing or the agency's continuing investigation of the validity of the claim may not be significant. However, for many injured workers, receiving cash benefits early is vital; for this reason, prompt filing and efficient investigation procedures are necessary.

Once the claims department is satisfied that a legal basis exists for compensation, the treatment and rehabilitation process can be continuously funded according to the prescribed benefit schedule. For a long-term disability, periodic reports on progress will be required from the professionals involved.

Adjudication

Assessing a claim for compensation requires answering two questions: first, was the injury or illness caused or aggravated by workplace events and, second, do the facts fulfill the requirements of workers' compensation law? The first question is, in large part, medical; the second is strictly legal.

Decisions concerning an injury's relationship to the worksite are based on a physician's report that an injury or illness of a certain type has been treated and that recovery requires the worker to be off the job for a certain period of time. This report will be supported by the employer's confirmation that an accident or hazardous exposure affecting the worker occurred at the workplace on the specified date. The agency accepts such simple temporary disability claims without further investigation.

For some claims of temporary disability and for all claims of permanent disability, the procedure is far more complex. The compensation authorities must be satisfied that a claimed permanent disability is indeed permanent. Total lifetime benefits in such cases commonly amount to hundreds of thousands of dollars. Therefore, cases of severe disabling trauma (traumatic amputations, paralysis from falls, serious burns, etc.) are always thoroughly investigated and a great deal of medical advice is required on a continuing basis.

Concurrent with the growing recognition of complex occupational diseases, the adjudication process has involved ever increasing participation by physicians. Many of these diseases, such as the pneumoconioses and heavy metal toxicities, have been recognized for some time as causing compensable disabilities. There are now a vast number of occupational disorders that are newly recognized as occurring from worker exposure to some of the many thousands of hazardous substances and processes involved in the manufacture of modern goods. Detection of these disorders frequently follows years of latency, making attribution to a specific workplace extremely difficult. This problem is compounded in a great many instances by the scarcity of available scientific evidence linking substance exposure with effect. Where this background evidence is weak, the compensation adjudicator naturally has difficulty in accepting the workplace as the cause of the disability and the claimant understandably can become frustrated in his or her claim.

Disability Assessment

Disability is a reduction in the capacity of an individual to meet personal, social, or occupational demands. The reduction or impairment may be total or partial, temporary or permanent. Impairment, in this context, is the loss of use of a body part—actual anatomic loss, as by amputation, or loss of use or derangement of a body part or system or function. The level of impairment suffered by an individual is only one important aspect of determining disability. Also significant in disability evaluation are such nonmedical factors as employability, level of performance required on the job or in a social role, and level of education or training. The physician assesses impairment and advises on causation and fitness to work. The assessment of disability, on the other hand, is a nonmedical determination based on many factors, not merely the level of impairment.

An injured worker who, despite treatment and rehabilitation, remains with a permanent disability is evaluated for the degree of disability. The assessment is based on anatomic, physiologic, or functional impairment and on the consequent loss to earnings capability (i.e., potential wage loss). Full functional disability, which is normally a disability that precludes the ability to undertake any work for which remuneration is paid, is assessed as 100 percent disability. Lesser degrees of disability are given correspondingly lower degrees.

Guides have been published for the clinical assessment of impairment, and each jurisdiction uses one or the other as its own reference. Some of the more commonly accepted ones are:

- The AMA Guides to the Evaluation of Permanent Impairment, 3rd edition, 1988.
- Disability Evaluation and Principles of Treatment of Compensable Injuries, E.D. McBride.
- Evaluating Orthopedic Disability, T.R. Miller, Medical Economics Books, Oradell, N.J., 1979.
- Manual for Orthopedic Surgeons in Evaluating Permanent Physical Impairment, American Academy of Orthopedic Surgeons, Chicago, 1960.
- Injury Ratings: How to Figure Dollar Values in the U.S.A., I.N. Rattner, Crescent, N.Y., 1970.

Reports of disability requested from physicians are easist to interpret when they use standard tests and terminology. The tests are described in the references listed above; Table 2.1 presents some standard terminology describing the intensity and frequency of symptoms or signs, such as pain or shortness of breath.

Sometimes an impairment has existed prior to the injury for which the worker claims compensation. The preexisting trauma not infrequently results in disability greater than the new injury would have produced on its own. In such situations, some states require the employer to pay an amount equivalent to the benefit the worker would have received if the most recent injury had occurred without the presence of any previous impairment. Compensation for the combined injury is then paid out of a so-called "second injury fund." In jurisdictions not having such a system, the employer is usually assessed for the total disability. This latter arrangement has the unfortunate effect of discouraging employers from hiring disabled workers, a restriction that is detrimental to the rehabilitation process as well as to the disabled individual seeking work. However, these workers may be protected by the Rehabilitation Act of 1973 and various state laws. Canadian jurisdictions, at least in theory, do not encounter this problem to the same extent

Table 2.1. Standard Terminology Used to Describe Features of Symptoms and Signs, as Recommended by the American Medical Association

1. Intensity:

    Minimal when the symptoms or signs constitute an annoyance but cause no impairment in the performance of a particular activity.

    Slight when the symptoms or signs can be tolerated but would cause some impairment in the performance of an activity that precipitates the symptoms or signs.

    Moderate when the symptoms and signs would cause marked impairment in the performance of an activity that precipitates the symptoms or signs.

    Marked when the symptoms or signs preclude any activity that precipitates the symptoms or signs.

2. Frequency:

    Intermittent when the symptoms or signs occur less than 25 percent of the time when awake.

    Occasional when the symptoms or signs occur between 25 and 50 percent of the time when awake.

    Frequent when the symptoms and signs occur between 50 and 75 percent of the time when awake.

    Constant when symptoms and signs occur between 75 and 100 percent of the time when awake.

as in the United States. In Canada compensation funds originate from pooled employer premiums and both federal and provincial human rights legislation prohibit employment discrimination on the basis of physical or mental disability.

Appeals

Disputes about compensation are not infrequent and, in fact, are becoming increasingly common. Dissatisfaction occurs for many reasons, but typical problems involve disagreements over the compensation authority's decision on the injury-workplace relationship, the assessed degree of disability, or the size of the cash benefit.

Workers' compensation legislation invariably provides a mechanism for appeals by both workers and employers. In the United States, appeals are made by the plaintiff to a court specified by state law. Compensation appeals in some states may only be made on the basis of compensation law, not on the medical facts of the case. Other states permit appeals on both grounds. The ultimate decision on cases most often is made by a judge or panel of judges. Only a few states permit juries to adjudicate appeals of this nature.

In Canada, most appeals are handled by the provincial workers' compensation board's claim review panel or committee. Legal and medical aspects both are reviewed. The presence of legal assistants at the appeal depends on the provincial regulation, as does the worker's access to his compensation file. Although the appeal hearings may be quite formal, there is understandably concern by workers and labor unions that the organization that assessed the allowable compensation in the first instance not judge the appeal.

The Physician's Role

The physician's role in the compensation process is determined by his or her situation with respect to the workers' compensation organization. If outside the organization, the physician will be involved in the medical treatment and rehabilitation of the injured worker as well as in fulfilling some of the regulatory requirements of the compensation system, including filing required medical reports on the worker's condition. Physicians who are part of the workers' compensation organization are usually involved in some aspect of claimant referral for examination or treatment and medical adjudication of impairment.

Most jurisdictions allow the worker-claimant to choose his or her own physician for medical care or assessment, but this freedom may be limited if the agency has questions or doubts about the accuracy of diagnosis or appropriateness of treatment. It is not uncommon for the insuring agency to have a staff of medical consultants who perform clinical examinations of claimants and provide various aspects of rehabilitative treatment.

Physicians, although not directly responsible for awarding compensation, play a number of critical roles in the process: establishing diagnosis, assessing prognosis for recovery or for permanent or temporary impairment, providing acute treatment, and providing or more often supervising some aspects of rehabilitation. When providing ongoing medical care, the physician in most instances will be required to submit progress reports on a continuing basis. These reports are used by the compensation authority to determine if the level of impairment continues to warrant the level of benefits being paid. The reports are also the basis for closing the file when impairment has become permanent or when the temporary impairment has resolved and the worker is fit to return to work.

Most jurisdictions request the physician's opinion on the extent of impairment. A description of the physical limitations of the worker is normally required. Determination of disability and its degree is left to the adjudicator within the compensation authority. This person bases the figure on the description of limitation provided by the treating physician or an assessing specialist to whom the claimant has been referred. The question of compensability and the amount of compensation must be left to the decision of the workers' compensation authority or to the courts. It is therefore vital that the physician be guided by objective clinical findings as well as by the worker's subjective complaints.

Current Problems and Future Possibilities

Like all human institutions, workers' compensation boards suffer from imperfection and face many problems. Some of the problems are produced by the modern phenomenon of scientific knowledge outstripping the human ability to effect appropriate social change. Others are caused by change within the social and economic structure. Some of these problems have led workers and employers to question the philosophic basis of the workers' compensation system.

In its century or so of existence, the system has been successful in providing varying degrees of compensation to many thousands of injured workers and their next-of-kin.

These workers and families have been spared the inconsistencies, delays, and costs of relying on the regular court system. Employers also have benefited by avoiding the risk of bankruptcy resulting from imposed legal costs for negligence and personal damages and avoiding sky-high insurance rates. Yet, despite these considerable accomplishments, workers' compensation organizations are facing the need for self-examination and possibly radical change.

Worker groups charge that the system is unfair. Assigning compensation costs to employers, on a pooled basis, has not noticeably reduced work-related injuries or illness overall, they say. Treatment and rehabilitation are delayed due to oversubscription of available facilities, and coverage is still not universal and is denied to many employees who are at very high risk of injury, such as agricultural workers. The system has not kept pace with the early recognition of occupational disease, technical advances in disability management, or the conditions of a changing economic climate.

One question increasingly being asked by critics of the system is whether employers should enjoy absolute protection from suits for negligent acts which cause injury or illness to workers. While "tort," or liability law, has evolved and progressed over the decades since workers' compensation law was first drafted, the latter has remained essentially unchanged. Liability law is now much more highly developed and has a vastly wider case law base than it had in the nineteenth century. Workers' compensation cases, generally shielded from tort litigation in trial or appellate courts, have not developed to nearly the same extent.

It is not surprising that workers in some jurisdictions recently have been suing employers in increasing numbers in defiance of the intent of workers' compensation legislation. Some suits have been filed because of a lack of confidence that the workers' compensation system will provide timely, fair, and adequate compensation. Others have been entered as a search for justice, on the grounds that negligent employers deserve punishment. The desire to force the employer to take steps to protect other workers from the same preventable disability is the motivation behind other legal actions. In several states and Canadian provinces, these suits have been allowed to proceed by high court decisions that call into question the conflict between the citizen's right to due legal process and the provisions of workers' compensation law. Access to the courts has been judged the higher good.

Under U.S. case law, children have sued employers of their injured fathers for damages resulting in "loss of companionship and society," and workers their employers for damages due to fraudulent concealment of hazardous exposure. The courts have ruled that the portion of incapacity that may have been caused by any factor unrelated to work is not compensable under workers' compensation.

In 1987, the Supreme Court of Canada overturned a 1986 Newfoundland Supreme Court decision that held that the province's Workers' Compensation Act violated section 15 of the Federal Charter of Rights and Freedoms by prohibiting injured workers from suing employers for negligence. The provincial court had recommended a system similar to one in the United Kingdom in which the right to tort action is retained in addition to normal no-fault compensation benefits. The federal court upheld the legality of the existing workers' compensation system, ending a suspenseful legal challenge to the underpinnings of the system.

Some observers have contended that joining a no-fault compensation system to a tort liability system would be disastrous in North America. For one thing, employers would somehow have to fund both. More importantly, though, litigation already is a common tactic in the United States—and a combined system would open up two avenues for compensation, both of them heavily used by plaintiffs. This would portend a dramatic increase in the costs required to operate a business and a likely increase in the size of the total award received by claimants. On the other hand, of course, injury and illness prevention measures in industry would undoubtedly be taken much more seriously than ever before.

Injury and illness prevention is obviously a vital factor in keeping compensation and premium costs down. Preventive measures are therefore of corresponding benefit to both employer and worker. Yet, prevention has received scant attention by many workers' compensation organizations. A case in point is the data collection procedure, which has routinely compiled information on illnesses and injuries for decades. Until recently, the data were used almost exclusively for the purpose of assigning industry-wide assessment rates—even though their true value lies in their usefulness for planning approaches to prevention. By identifying industries with a high prevalence or incidence of accidental injury or occupational disease, the data allow authorities to concentrate preventive actions where they are likely to do the most good. Such use of workers' compensation data is a relatively recent endeavour for many jurisdictions.

It is true that some workers' compensation agencies offer preventive services to workers and employers, from publicizing safe and healthy work practices to providing safety engineering counselling and occupational hygiene assessments of workplace hazards. These activities are sometimes coupled in the same agency with regulatory authority. However, in most jurisdictions the workers' compensation system remains primarily an insurance service, with occupational health and safety regulatory authority being the responsibility of a completely separate governmental agency.

In times of general economic difficulty, there is inevitable resistance by employers and politicians toward increasing assessment rates for workers' compensation. Unfortunately, poor economic conditions do not necessarily coincide with lowered compensation costs. During economic downturns, many workers file claims that would not otherwise be filed. Employers therefore have tended to demand cutbacks in compensation benefits while, at the same time, organized labor has called for increased employer assessments.

The severe financial pressures plaguing many workers' compensation agencies could be alleviated by a number of tactics. One of the best is directly fostering preventive measures at the workplace. Another approach to controlling financial cost is to encourage employers to keep injuries down by rewarding those with good safety records. So-called "experience rating" schemes modify an employer's assessment on the basis of a company's record of injuries or claims. A low average injury cost record thus results in a lower assessment, a high record leads to an increased assessment. However, this method may be seen by the courts as a violation of the collective liability principle on which the workers' compensation system has been based, and may be viewed as a precedent for departing from the fundamental principles of the system, offering an opening to return to tort actions.

Despite attempts by workers' compensation organizations to provide the most appropriate benefits to each injured worker, they are inevitably constrained by financial limitations. It is generally recognized that in North America, workers with industrial diseases are, on average, financially undercompensated. In addition, many occupational disorders are not recognized by some workers' compensation authorities until the disorder causes overt disability. For example, if a symptomless worker is found on a routine examination to have very early X-ray signs of silicosis and then is medically advised to cease further exposure to rock dust, the worker is unlikely to receive compensation, even for job retraining. A worker without symptoms or functional impairment is not considered to be physically disabled.

Nevertheless, it is clear that some hazardous substances may be absorbed by the body, produce no overt ill effects at low doses, and yet become deadly through gradual accumulation. Lead, mercury, and ionizing radiation are examples of such hazards. The problem in such cases is the vague borderline between the low-dose physiological effects, which warrant cessation of exposure, and the clinically and functionally overt disease, which requires treatment. Treatment may well be the least effective solution at that point. The question is, should compensation in some form, such as vocational retraining, be provided earlier?

There is also the problem of workers' compensation and so-called "lifestyle disorders," such as myocardial ischemia or infarction, hypertension, psychological stress disorders, and pulmonary disease associated with secondhand cigarette smoke exposure. To the extent that a work-related factor is involved, should workers with these disorders receive disability benefits? This was not the intent of the workers' compensation system but public pressure appears to be in favor of some form of disability benefits. Some workers' compensation agencies have been known to award benefits for these lifestyle disorders.

The trend in cash benefits is to compensate on the basis of the actual wage loss for permanent disability rather than to use the physical impairment approach or projected loss of earnings. However, in some jurisdictions a hybrid formula based on actual wage loss and projected wage loss is awarded. Whatever system is used, equitable compensation must be provided, otherwise injured workers will increasingly abandon the present system to pursue equity in the courts.

In recent years, numerous jurisdictional reviews have been held in the United States and Canada in an attempt to improve the workers' compensation system. Some authorities have introduced legislation to protect disabled workers from unjust dismissal; others have begun taking steps toward developing systems that join workers, employers, and rehabilitation specialists in teams to plan the job placement of disabled workers.

A 1972 evaluation by the U.S. National Commission on State Workmen's Compensation Laws concluded with a list of 84 recommendations for improving state compensation laws. Four years later, the Inter-Agency Workers' Compensation Task Force, whose members came from various departments and agencies of the U.S. government, called for reforming existing workers' compensation programs at the state level, with the federal government monitoring progress and providing technical assistance. Both the state commission and the federal task force rejected proposals to replace the individual state workers' compensation programs with a single federal program.

Large gaps in worker coverage still exist in North America, but it is conceivable that workers' compensation may eventually include all workers. Some see workers' compensation as part of a future universal medical care system for all citizens. Others perceive the future compensation organization as vastly improved, but still separate from any public medical care plan. The possibilities for the future are enormous, and much still remains to be done.

Further Reading

Analysis of Workers' Compensation Laws. Washington, U.S. Chamber of Commerce, annual.

Ashford NA, Andrews RA: Workers' compensation, in Rom WN (ed): Environmental and Occupational Medicine. Boston, Little Brown, 1983, pp. 907–912.

Barth PS: Workers' Compensation and Work-Related Illnesses and Injuries. Cambridge, MIT Press, 1982.

Berkowitz M, Barton JF Jr: Permanent Disability Benefits in Workers' Compensation. Kalamazoo MI, W.E. Upjohn, 1987.

Brennan TA: Untangling causation issues in law and medicine: Hazardous substance litigation. Ann Int Med 1987; 107:741–747.

Chelius J (ed): Current Issues in Workers' Compensation. Kalamazoo MI, W.E. Upjohn, 1986.

Darling-Hammond L, Kniesner TJ: The Law and Economics of Workers' Compensation. Santa Monica, CA, The Rand Corporation, Institute for Civil Justice, 1980.

Disability Evaluation under Social Security: A Handbook for Physicians. Washington, U.S. Department of Health and Human Services No. (SSA) 05-10089, February 1986.

International Classification of Impairments, Disabilities, and Handicaps. Geneva, World Health Organization, 1980.

Kanner RE: Impairment and disability evaluation: A review, in Rom WN (ed): Environmental and Occupational Medicine, Boston, Little Brown, 1983, pp. 43–47.

LaDou J (ed): Occupational Health Law: A Guide for Industry. New York, Marcel Dekker, 1981.

Milstein A, Nethercut G, Martin M: Controlling medical costs in workers' compensation. Business and Health, March 1988, pp. 34–37.

Nash IN: Occupational Health and Safety Law. Don Mills, CCH Canadian Ltd, 1983.

Nelson DE: A practical approach to workers' compensation. Amer Fam Phys, 1988; 37:233–238.

Ong JR: Workers' compensation, in Zenz C (ed): Occupational Medicine: Principles and Practical Applications. Chicago, Year Book Medical Publishers, 1975, 83–86.

Petrie P: Workers' compensation at the crossroads. At the Centre (newsletter of the Canadian Centre for Occupational Health and Safety), March 1987; 10(1):1–3.

Richman SI: Why Change? A look at the current system of disability determination and workers compensation for occupational lung disease. Ann Int Med 1982; 97:908–914.

Worral JD, Appel D (eds): Workers' Compensation Benefits: Adequacy, Equity, and Efficiency. Ithaca, Cornell University, ILR Press (New York State School of Industrial and Labor Relations), 1985.

3 OCCUPATIONAL SAFETY AND HEALTH REGULATION

Occupational safety and health and the conduct of occupational medicine in the United States is governed by the sweeping Occupational Safety and Health Act (OSH Act) of 1970. In passing the OSH Act, the U.S. Congress declared that the purpose and policy of the legislation was "to assure so far as possible every working man and woman in the Nation safe and healthful working conditions and to preserve our human resources."

The Act is a landmark in the history of American labor and public health legislation. It was the first major piece of legislation in the the United States that governed occupational safety and health throughout industy. (Previous legislation had dealt with occupational safety and health in equal detail but only with specific industries and with federal contractors.) Even so, the Act was not intended to apply to the numerous employees of public agencies (federal, state, county, and municipal), nor is it enforced, in most instances, in private establishments with fewer than 10 employees. Nevertheless, the public policy and purpose as well as the basic provisions of the Act should apply to all workers through the medium of the occupational physician.

OSH Act Standards & Guidelines

Each employer "shall furnish to each of his employees employment and a place of employment which are free from recognized hazards that are causing or are likely to cause death or serious physical harm to his employees," according to the so-called "general duty clause" of the OSH Act. The Occupational Safety and Health Administration (OSHA), the agency primarily responsible for enforcing the OSH Act, sets the standards, rules, and regulations by which employers are expected to protect their employees in the course of conducting their businesses. However, not all potential hazardous exposures can be anticipated. The "general duty clause" covers all possible hazards, and puts responsibility for eliminating or minimizing hazardous conditions squarely on the shoulders of the employers.

Section 6 of the Act gives OSHA the authority to adopt standards, rules, and regulations governing the protection of health in the workplace. Standards for occupational safety and health adopted by OSHA are to be based on recommendations from the National Institute for Occupational Safety and Health (NIOSH), a separate creation of the OSH Act. There are hundreds of standards, covering much more than chemical exposure. They include, for example: machine guarding, materials handling and standards, noise, radiation, exits, walking and working surfaces, sanitation, fire prevention, welding, staging and shoring, scaffolding, and the operation of machinery. If no specific standard is set for a workplace, there still remains the general duty clause in the OSH Act. When new hazards are introduced into the workplace, temporary emergency standards can be set until permanent ones are established to protect workers.

Most standards for exposure to chemical and physical agents in the workplace were set within the first 22 months of the adoption of the Act. In those hectic first months, OSHA adopted the guidelines and standards that were available at that time. Most of these early standards were adopted by reference to the Walsh-Healy Act, an earlier federal law requiring federal government contractors to comply with occupational health and safety standards, or recommendations by such organizations as the American National Standards Institute. Once adopted by OSHA, these standards could only be changed by a lengthy rule-making process. As a result, many OSHA standards have not been changed since the early 1970s, even though knowledge about many hazards has grown substantially.

In addition to appreciating their history, physicians must also understand the concepts behind OSHA exposure standards in order to interpret them correctly. The most common standard is called the Permissible Exposure Limit (PEL). The PEL is the maximum concentration level of an agent permitted in the workplace; employees may not be exposed to concentrations above that level. Although expressed in legal terms, the concept supposedly is grounded in a toxicological understanding of exposure and the human response to that exposure. Usually, the PEL is stated in terms of an 8-hour time-weighted average (TWA) of exposure. Obviously, in a time-weighted PEL a peak concentration at one point in time can be averaged out by a lower concentration at some other time. For a given substance, there may also be a Short-Term Exposure Limit (STEL), another level above which no worker may be exposed for more than a specified short period of time, such as 15 minutes. Finally, there may be a Ceiling (Ceil) Limit, above which a worker must never be exposed, not even for the briefest time.

Because of the legal nature of the PELs, STELs, and Ceiling Limits under the OSH Act, the layperson may conclude that all exposures in compliance with the standards are "safe" and that all that are out of compliance are "unsafe." This is not necessarily the case. To guide the physician and to help management, an additional authoritative set of standards is often more useful. These are the Threshold Limit Values (TLVs) of the American Conference of Governmental Industrial Hygienists (ACGIH), a professional society that since 1938 has reviewed toxicologic data and developed guidelines for exposure to a variety of hazards. Based on those data, ACGIH has three types of exposure guidelines:

- The TLV-TWA is the time-weighted average concentration for a normal 8-hour workday and 40-hour workweek, to which *nearly all workers* may be repeatedly exposed, day after day, without adverse effect (emphasis added).
- TLV-STEL is the concentration to which workers can be exposed continuously for

a short period of time without suffering from irritation, chronic or irreversible tissue damage, or narcosis of sufficient degrees to increase the likelihood of accidental injury or impaired self-rescue or to materially reduce work efficiency.
- The TLV-C (Ceiling) is the concentration that should not be exceeded during any part of the working exposure.

The ACGIH Threshold Limit Values clearly parallel the OSHA permissible exposure limits. Yet even though all employers covered by the OSH Act must comply with OSHA exposure limits, from a purely health-based approach the ACGIH guidelines may be more useful because they are reviewed every two years and are not subject to a lengthy legal rule-making process.

A third set of exposure guidelines also may be helpful to the physician who practices occupational medicine. The National Institute for Occupational Safety and Health (NIOSH), administratively a part of the U.S. Public Health Service, has research and educational, but not enforcement, functions. One of NIOSH's responsibilities is to review chemical, toxicologic, and control-process data in order to arrive at "criteria for a recommended standard" of exposure and control. These criteria have been published as "criteria documents" by NIOSH. Unlike the ACGIH, whose guidelines are published in a small booklet and whose justifications for guidelines are summarized in only one or two pages for each chemical or physical agent, NIOSH "criteria documents" are often hundreds of pages in length. They take years to produce and are reviewed extensively. Although they are not official standards, they have the advisory authority of having been produced by a federal agency and are designed to be used by OSHA in implementing new standards. With recent cutbacks in budgets, NIOSH has produced fewer criteria documents, and some of them are now over a decade old. However, the thorough documentation behind each recommended standard still makes them very useful.

The physician, then, has a choice of where to look for data to assist management in maintaining a workplace that is safe from harmful exposure levels. Table 3.1 shows the differences between OSHA standards and ACGIH and NIOSH recommendations for a few selected chemicals. This table illustrates three important points: OSHA, ACGIH, and NIOSH may not agree with one another; the basis for a recommended exposure level may differ (NIOSH considers epichlorhydrin to be a carcinogen while ACGIH and OSHA do not); and OSHA standards may not always be the least restrictive (cf. those for inorganic lead), despite their age and the cumbersome legal procedure by which they are amended.

Table 3.1. OSHA Permissible Exposure Limits and ACGIH and NIOSH Recommended Exposure Levels Compared (8-hour Time-Weighted Averages only) for Three Selected Chemicals

	OSHA PEL	ACGIH TLV	NIOSH Recommended Standard
Acrylonitrile	2 ppm (parts per million)	2 ppm	1 ppm
Epichlorhydrin	5 ppm	2 ppm	Carcinogen-lowest feasible limit
Inorganic Lead	0.05 mg/m³ (milligrams per cubic meter)	0.15 mg/m³	0.1mg/m³

A major reversal in OSHA's standard-setting authority occurred in 1980 when the Supreme Court ruled that OSHA had not made a strong enough scientific case to demonstrate that the benefits of regulation should be worth the proposed costs. (Although very visible at the time and widely publicized, the ruling provided little in the way of a legal precedent because it was decided by a bare majority of the court and the opinions offered, even by the justices in the majority, were not uniform in their interpretation.) The Reagan Administration tried to modify the OSH Act by interpretation to permit the use of cost/benefit analysis in setting standards. Initially, this was attempted through a directive from the Office of Management and the Budget. The issue was also brought to the Supreme Court in the case of setting cotton dust standards to prevent "brown lung" disease. The Supreme Court voted 5–3 to uphold current standards and rejected the argument that the government should consider whether the costs to be imposed on industry were justified by the health benefits to be gained.

Nevertheless, in order to be seen as responsive to employers' concerns, OSHA has introduced the so-called "regulatory relief" package, a series of policy changes to reduce the perceived burden of federal regulation of industry. Rather than concentrating on eliminating hazards from the workplace, the policy emphasizes increasing use of such protective gear as respirators and earplugs. In the past OSHA has allowed only temporary reliance on respirators and similar personal protective devices. Occupational health experts argue that protective gear is seldom as effective as engineering controls.

Most standards that have been promulgated by OSHA do not mandate specific medical surveillance practices. Among those that do are the standards for lead, arsenic, cotton dust, and asbestos. The surveillance requirements specify detailed procedures for screening workers and may include: mandatory preplacement testing; mandatory periodic testing at varying, prescribed intervals; post-employment testing; specific tests and procedures; specific methods of performing and interpreting tests and procedures; long-term recordkeeping requirements; and mandated access to records by governmental authorities. Any one of these requirements can have a profound effect on a physician's practice. (For an example, see Chapter 20.)

NIOSH is the primary research arm of the federal government for occupational safety and health. To conduct its research, NIOSH often must rely on access to both medical records and workers in private industry—and while it has no direct role in enforcement, the agency can require that it be given access to confidential medical and exposure records. If conducted according to the proper procedure, it is not considered a breach of physician-patient confidentiality for NIOSH and its contractors conducting agency-approved research to gain access to medical records that are held for employers and employees by third parties, such as contracting physicians and health care institutions.

Physicians must comply when NIOSH approaches them to inspect their records; the agency's regulations regarding subpoena and mandatory access to records have held up in court. When complying with a NIOSH order, physicians and managers should ensure that those requesting access follow the agency's own rules concerning confidentiality and records management (42 Code of Federal Regulations Parts 85 and 85a). In general, NIOSH requires access to private records for purposes consistent with medical ethics: to study the effects of exposure on human beings in order to recommend appropriate public and private responses to the knowledge that is gained. Despite the initial concern a physician might have about breach of confidentiality these activities are not at cross purposes to the basic ethics of medical practice.

Enforcement Activities

The enabling legislation for the federal Occupational Safety and Health Act assumed that most states would eventually take over partial responsibility for occupational health and safety in the private sector under broad federal supervision. Most were slow to do so, however. Only about 25 states have ever had their own occupational safety and health administration. In 1987, funding for the California state OSHA (CalOSHA) was rescinded from the budget and the agency was dissolved by the governor even though its state expenditures totalled only $8 million per year. (Federal OSHA contributed $14 million to the state program.) This action by the governor has been disputed and is before the Supreme Court of California. Even so, federal OSHA has had to step in to provide services. Until that time, CalOSHA had generally been considered the leading state OSHA program.

State regulations, permitted under the OSH Act, must be at least as strict as the federal law and may be even stricter in setting standards and enforcement policies. California's state legislation and standards are much more comprehensive and stringent than federal statutes and standards. However, much depends on the financial resources available. Funding for state OSHAs is shared by the federal and state governments. As budget cuts on the federal level reduce the federal contribution, maintenance of a state agency has become increasingly difficult for state governments.

All employers with at least one employee are required to comply with state OSHA standards, with a few exceptions: federal employees, who are covered by federal OSHA directly or indirectly by interagency agreement; miners, who are covered under the Mine Safety and Health Act; ground workers for airlines, who are nominally covered by the Federal Aviation Administration; and structural pest control workers, who do not seem to be protected under any occupational health law. Many people are under the mistaken impression that small businesses are not covered by the OSH Act. In fact, an employer with fewer than 10 workers on the payroll during any 24 hour period is exempt only from the recordkeeping requirements of the OSH Act; the employer still must comply with all applicable standards.

The OSH Act provides for three categories of violations: imminent danger, serious, and other than serious. Citations for imminent danger are very rare, but when they are made, the shop is closed down immediately until the danger is corrected. Serious violations are those that have substantial probability of causing death or physical harm. Serious violations accounted for just under 13 percent of all violations cited by CalOSHA in 1980.

The size of a fine is determined by the severity of the violation as well as such factors as the size of the employer's business, the apparent good faith of management, and any record of prior violations. If management shows "good faith" in trying to keep the workplace safe, for example, the penalty is reduced by one third. Small businesses enjoy an additional 10 percent reduction. There is no limit on the dollar amount of a fine. In 1987, federal OSHA imposed a fine of $1.6 million on Chrysler Corporation's Newark, Delaware, plant for multiple violations. Such amounts are very unusual, however. (In this case, the fine was widely interpreted as a muscle-flexing effort on the part of OSHA.) After all the factors are taken into consideration, penalties are frequently minimal. In San Diego in 1980, the average fine fell in the range of $30–$60 for minor violations and \$700–\$1,000 for more serious ones. Employers also could petition the CalOSHA Appeals Board, a body appointed by the Governor of California, for relief from a penalty.

A company may be granted a temporary or permanent variance exempting it from a particular standard. The request for variance can be submitted at any time; if it comes after an inspection, it will not affect the citation. Employers also can appeal OSHA actions on violations, fines, prescribed clean up, and deadlines. Employees, on the other hand, can appeal only the scheduling of deadlines.

Standards are enforced through inspections. In general, compliance officers have been much better trained in safety hazards than in health problems. OSHA compliance officers visit workplaces for basically three reasons: for routine inspections made at workplaces where there is a high risk of accidents, such as construction sites; in response to complaints from workers; and in investigations of accidents where there is a fatality or five or more people seriously injured. In 1980, routine inspections comprised only 4 percent of all inspection conducted by CalOSHA; worker complaints were responsible for 34 percent of all inspection, and accidents for 25 percent.

Inspections have three major phases:

- The "opening conference" at which the inspector describes the inspection plan to management and representatives of the employees.
- The "walk around," or the actual inspection tour, during which management and employee representatives are allowed to accompany the OSHA inspector. (Employers now are not required to pay employees for the time spent participating in an OSHA inspection, and this has become a source of considerable controversy.)
- The "closing conference," at which the inspector discusses with management the results of the inspection and means of correcting any hazards, deadlines for action, and the possibility of fines. The employee representative can request attendance at this meeting but management has the privilege of vetoing such representation.

Under Section 11(c) of the OSH Act, an employer is prohibited from firing or discriminating against any employee "because of the exercise by such employee on behalf of himself or others of any right afforded by this act." This section specifically includes the following rights: to file a safety and health complaint; to institute a proceeding under the OSH Act; and to testify at any hearings. Nonetheless, despite the guarantees of Section 11(c), many workers fear that their employer will find grounds to discipline or even to fire them on other grounds or on pretexts should they exercise their rights. Unfortunately, this happens often enough to confirm such fears. Once an employee is singled out as a "troublemaker," management may find it easy enough to accumulate on other grounds real or imagined problems that may lead to the worker's termination.

Employees encountering a job hazard should bring the matter to the attention of the employer. If no action is taken, an employee may then contact the OSHA area office and file a complaint in writing. All complaints are evaluated and priority is assigned by the perceived severity of the hazard. On the basis of this evaluation, OSHA staff decide whether to conduct an inspection. OSHA policy has been to inspect all potential serious violations within three working days. Formal requests for the inspection of hazards not considered serious by OSHA are dealt with either by dismissal or by scheduling of an inspection within 20 working days. If OSHA decides not to conduct an inspection, the union representative or the employee signing the complaint must be informed in writing of the reason the inspection was denied. An informal review may then be requested.

Exceptions to this step-by-step procedure are made for situations of "imminent danger" as defined in Section 13(a) of the OSH Act. This condition exists when there is reasonable certainty that a present danger can be expected to cause death or serious physical harm immediately or before it can be eliminated through normal enforcement procedures. Besides being assessed a fine, an employer found not to be in compliance with OSHA standards may be issued a citation and given an abatement date by which the hazard must be corrected. Since it often costs considerably more to correct a hazard than to pay OSHA fines, abatement dates may be missed or ignored by employers. And although an employer may be assessed a civil penalty of up to $1,000 for each day past the deadline that the danger continues unabated, extensions of the abatement date are common. During this time, employees may continue to be exposed to the hazard.

Many state OSHAs have both consultation and compliance branches. The major difference in the functions of the two branches is that the compliance office is in many respects the employee's advocate, while the consultation service is designed primarily to be the advocate or resource to the employer. Its main purpose is to assist management in correcting a health or safety problem by providing information and education to employers and employee organizations. In practice, OSHA consultation services tend to be confined to simple forms of assistance, such as spot checks, single measurements of hazards, and advice, with limited technical capabilities. Even so, the services provide a point of departure for employers to begin to resolve their problems. Unfortunately, many—perhaps most— smaller employers shy away from using OSHA-sponsored consultation services out of fear that their deficiencies will come to the attention of the enforcement branch. The fear is largely groundless but has substantially inhibited the use of this service. Larger employers usually have access to their own technical experts anyway or can afford expensive consultation services from private firms.

Perspectives on OSHA

Although OSHA has been widely viewed as too weak on enforcement, it clearly has achieved much in fostering a greater and more sophisticated appreciation of the problems of occupational health and safety. Nothing is as important as the message that has come from the introduction of OSHA: change the workplace, not the worker.

The way in which OSHA is viewed depends on the perspective of the viewer. Worker advocates see employees as the victims of occupational disease and disabilities, and charge companies with inflicting suffering through unhealthy working conditions and constraints. Even so, workers are not solidly in support of OSHA as the advocate of their best interest; they do not always see OSHA or other issues narrowly from a "worker" point of view. This may reflect the more conservative politics of the rank and file union member, compared with the attitudes of the past, or may indicate a lack of interest in politics among a substantial alienated subgroup of the working population, many of whom abstain from voting or community involvement.

Employers and managers, on the other hand, show more consistency in holding views against "government regulations." Their advocates typically see management as the victim, and view OSHA, workers, unions, and government in general as inflicting excessive and unnecessary regulation leading to delays, frustration, and increased costs. Intrusion into the production process is not easily accepted by the business manager or owner who expects to control the process.

There remain many paradoxes and inconsistencies in OSHA and the OSH Act. The OSH Act was passed to assure employees of legal protection against occupational injury and disease. However, nowhere in this piece of otherwise enlightened legislation is it explicitly stated that a worker has the right to refuse an assignment that may result in serious injury or death without fear of retribution for the refusal. This right was established only by administrative declaration in a subsequent regulation.

Until the OSH Act was passed, personnel or industrial relations managers rarely had more than the most rudimentary training in safety and health. Few courses or texts in industrial relations or human resources contained more than a mention of occupational safety and health other than in relation to the workers' compensation system. Top management was rarely involved in controlling hazards; hazard control was delegated to maintenance or engineering departments, and supervisors in these departments were directly responsible to line management whose major concern was production, not the improvement of working conditions. The safety director rarely had much influence or support from top management unless a major accident occurred. Many companies regarded accidents strictly from a cost standpoint—they titled their safety and health director the "loss control" supervisor, and labelled workers as "accident prone." This old approach considered safety issues only after an accident or illness had already occurred.

Although the situation is still far from ideal, it has improved considerably. A vigorous effort has been made to clean up the workplace, in large part by directly training workers to recognize hazards, monitor their presence in the workplace, know how to control them and participate in their control, and exercise their rights under the law. As this book goes to press, NIOSH and OSHA are considering actions that may expand the rights of workers to be informed on hazards they encounter in the workplace. (See Chapter 20.) The worker in American industry may become more knowledgeable and aware than ever before.

Occupational Health & Safety Law in Canada

Canada has no national equivalent to OSHA and the OSH Act; Canadian constitutional authority places the responsibility for health legislation with the provinces. As a consequence, there are effectively 13 separate and independent occupational health and safety acts in the country (10 provincial, two territorial, and one for federal employees), each of which is substantially different from the others. Generally speaking, the Canadian provinces exhibit more variation in occupational health regulation and enforcement than in their various workers' compensation plans. (See Chapter 2.)

There is an array of legislative and organizational approaches to regulating and administering occupational health and safety; each approach reflects the political and economic realities of the populations served. In some provinces, occupational health and safety authority for setting standards and for enforcement is vested in a ministry of health. In others, it lies in a ministry of labor, and in still others it rests elsewhere. In several provinces, the regulatory arm is part of the workers' compensation board while in others it is completely independent. Worker representatives have direct input into the development of legislation in some jurisdictions; elsewhere, their input is indirect and informal.

There are also wide differences in the provinces' approaches to standard setting and monitoring. Occupational health and exposure regulations in some provinces (e.g., Ontario) use an approach similar to that of OSHA, detailing the criteria for health and safety procedures an employer must follow. Others (e.g., Alberta) use result-oriented or "performance" standards that allow the employer to develop local methods to prevent exposure or worker illness and injury. Standards regarding the use of a ladder exemplify the difference between these two approaches. The former might require the employer to use an approved type of ladder, made of specific materials with rungs at stated distances apart, supported at a certain angle with a worker holding the base during its use. The latter, by contrast, would require the employer or the industry to develop its own code of practice for use of ladders that would effectively prevent injury to the worker. In the first approach, a citation might be issued if criteria for use of the ladder were not met. In the latter, a citation would be issued only if practices at the worksite could be shown to result in unsafe use of the ladder.

There are advantages and disadvantages to each approach, but both impose a need for monitoring by government. Criteria standards require the government agency to be a policeman; performance standards require the employers to police themselves. Performance standards also are more appropriate for some situations than for others. For example, criteria standards for shoring up the sides of trenches or ditches are indispensable because accidents in such settings are sudden, unpredictable, and too frequently fatal.

Unlike the United States, Canada has no nationally applicable standards for occupational exposure to hazardous substances. Some jurisdictions use the ACGIH TLVs; others use the same time-weighted average system but with altered values. These changed values reflect the provinces' reinterpretation of U.S. and European research and their own conclusions regarding risk. In these cases, a province normally renames the exposure levels, referring to them no longer as "TLVs," but as something else (such as "OELs," or Occupational Exposure Limits) in order not to confuse employers and workers with the terminology for provincial and U.S. values for the same hazardous material.

A great deal more could be written about the Canadian regulatory system, but to do it adequately would require a complete volume. The multiplicity of systems are partly the result of rapid developments in legislation and workers' compensation systems. The changing nature of these systems also makes detailed presentation subject to rapid obsolescence. The physician who practices occupational medicine in Canada must become familiar with applicable provincial legislation and the pertinent governmental agencies operating locally. Physicians serving employers with branch plants or subsidiaries operating in more than one province must be knowledgeable about standards and procedures in each of those jurisdictions.

Further Reading

All about OSHA—the Who, What, Where, When, Why, and How of the Occupational Safety and Health Act of 1970. Washington DC, OSHA Office of Information.

Auchter T: How to get out of an OSHA inspection. Christian Science Monitor, 14 January 1983, p. 5.

Barth PS: The Tragedy of Black Lung: Federal Compensation for Occupational Disease. Kalamazoo MI, W.E. Upjohn Institute for Employment Research, 1987.

Berkowitz M, Burton JF Jr: Permanent Disability Benefits in Workers' Compensation. Kalamazoo MI, W.E. Upjohn Institute for Employment Research, 1987.

Bock G: Blood, sweat, and fears. Time, 28 September 1984, pp. 50–51.

Boden LI, Levinstein C: Regulating safety: OSHA's "new look." Amer J Foren Med Pathol 1982; 3:339–342.

Brandt-Rauf SI, Brandt-Rauf PW: Occupational health ethics: OSHA and the courts. Journal of Health Politics, Policy, and Law 1980; 5:523–534.

Cal OSHA cuts: Political issue. California Political Week, June 1987, p. 3.

Chelius J, (ed): Current Issues in Workers' Compensation. Kalamazoo MI, W.E. Upjohn Institute for Employment Research, 1986.

Crawford J: The dismantling of OSHA. The Nation, 12 September 1981, pp. 205–207.

Gainer WJ: OSHA's assumption of private sector enforcement activities in California. Testimony on behalf of the U.S. General Accounting Office before the U.S. House of Representatives Committee on House Government Operations, Subcommittee on Employment and Housing, 20 June 1988.

Glaberson W: Is OSHA falling down on the job? New York Times, 2 August 1987, pp. 3-1, 3-6.

Guidotti TL: OSHA replaces CalOSHA: What can we expect from federal succession? California Political Week, Special Report, 1988.

Impact of job safety law on employer and workers. U.S. News and World Report, 11 January 1971, p. 88.

Industrial safety: the toll of neglect. Time, 7 February 1969, p. 76.

Job safety bill breaks new ground. U.S. News and World Report, 28 December 1970, p. 57.

Labor Day '69: Some plain talk from George Meany. U.S. News and World Report, 8 September 1969, p. 77.

Mac Sheoin T: The dismantling of U.S. health and safety regulations under the first Reagan Administration: A bibliography. Internat J Health Serv 1985; 15:585–608.

McCaffrey DP: OSHA and the Politics of Health Regulation. New York, Plenum, 1982.

Mendeloff J: The role of OSHA violations in serious workplace accidents. J Occup Med 1984; 26:353–360.

Miller ML, Kennish R: Occupational Health and Safety Administration, in LaDou J (ed): Occupational Health Law: A Guide for Industry. New York, Marcel Dekker, 1981.

Nader R: The violence of omission. The Nation, 10 February 1969, pp. 205–207.

Nash IN: Occupational Health and Safety Law. CCH Canadian Ltd., 1983.

Nixon's call for job-safety rules. U.S. News and World Report, 18 August 1969, p. 63.

OSHA, industry's new friend. New York Times, 5 September 1983, pp. 1–19.

Restraining OSHA: It's just a matter of time. Business Week, 5 May 1980, p. 110.

Scalia A: A note on the benzene case. Regulation (American Enterprise Institute), July/August 1980; 4(4):25–28.

Smith RS: The Occupational Safety and Health Act: Its goals and achievements. Washington DC, American Enterprise Institute, 1976.

Storm-tossed OSHA. New Republic, 17 May 1980, pp. 5–7.

The Safety Bill breaks new ground. U.S. News and World Report, 28 December 1970, p. 57.

The Safety Act's hidden bite. Business Week, 9 January 1971, p. 19.

The overhaul that could give OSHA life under Reagan. Business Week, 19 January 1981, p. 88.

Troubled OSHA faces further loss of power. U.S. News and World Report, 11 February 1980, p. 79.

Unions and Nixon: Disharmony at the start. U.S. News and World Report, 3 March 1969, p. 62.

Weber S: How OSHA enforces the law: A case study. New York, INFORM, 1981.

Weisskopf M: The loud, loud lobby against a chemical carcinogen rating. Washington Post (National Weekly Edition), 17 August 1987, p. 31.

Will reform be the death of OSHA? Nation's Business, April 1980, p. 55.

4 ETHICS IN OCCUPATIONAL MEDICINE

Occupational medicine, although at times a highly technical medical specialty, is also a socially conscious field of health care, dealing with the broader society and issues of ethics, economics, social attitudes, and technology. In a very real sense, occupational medicine acts as a three-way bridge uniting the practice of medicine, the concerns of society as a whole (including the economy), and technological change. It affords an exciting vantage point from which to observe the broader aspects of social change and their influence on health and to address challenging problems that go beyond medical practice.

The field of occupational medicine can boast of both impressive accomplishments in scientific research and outstanding leaders of the profession. Nevertheless, there have been some abuses in the past: occasional incidents of serious negligence or ignorance in which occupational health problems were allowed to continue and benefits due disabled workers were denied without good cause. Occupational medicine has shed some of its past associations and as it becomes increasingly familiar to physicians who have not yet had much contact with it, remaining misconceptions will be dispelled and the unique problems faced by the speciality will become more widely appreciated.

Ethical Issues in Occupational Medicine

Physicians comprise one of the three traditional professions: medicine, law, and the clergy. Each of these professions is distinguished from other occupations in part by the control its members exercise over their own behavior and practice. Physicians have the power to alter people's lives; in some situations their actions even determine life and death. A special, self-imposed code of behavior, above what might be demanded by law, is necessary to guard against a member of a profession taking advantage of this power. The underlying principle in all medical codes is that the interests of the patient always come before those of the physician and are to be protected by the physician against third parties who do not have a recognized, legitimate interest.

Other branches of medicine are characterized by a relatively straightforward two-party relationship between doctor and patient, modified, of course, by third-party payers in some situations. In occupational medicine, third parties are involved as major players in virtually all cases. An ethical code for medical practice, so obviously necessary in the simple, two-party situation, becomes a critical matter in the everyday routine of occupational medicine.

The occupational physician, more than other physicians, deals with individual patients in the presence of third parties who may try to influence the relationship. The occupational physician, bound by the ethical constraints of the doctor/patient relationship, must make rational decisions about a worker's welfare within the context of the employer/employee relationship. Some would argue that the traditional doctor/patient relationship is subtly or even overtly altered in occupational medicine, because the interests of the employer must be served as well. This should not be so, because in order to serve the interests of the employer and provide the fair-minded and objective advice needed, the physician must have credibility and enjoy the trust of the employees. The power of the physician is obvious to workers. If there is any suspicion that this power is being misused, the physician will not be able to serve as an impartial advocate of the worker and as an objective advisor to the employer.

Frequently, an occupational physician or nurse enters into a strictly one-sided commercial relationship with an organization, usually an employer, in order to provide a service purely of interest to the organization. For example, a physician might be retained by an employer to review a disputed claim for workers' compensation or to evaluate the merit of a pending lawsuit. In such situations, the occupational health professional is acting solely as the organization's agent rather than in the service of the patient-worker. There is no doctor/patient relationship in this case. There is nothing unethical with this arrangement, but this agent arrangement must be made known to the worker. There should never be any question over whom the physician is there to serve. This role must be clearly distinguished from the role of the occupational physician in practice as it is outlined here.

Some ethical issues are unique to occupational medicine, such as the appropriate conduct of a health surveillance or monitoring program for exposure-related health outcomes. Others are common to medicine as a whole, such as confidentiality of health records. The major ethical problems in an occupational health service are those that pertain to the role of the physician in balancing the rights of the employee and the employer within the context of the doctor/patient relationship. The clinician has an absolute ethical responsibility to treat the worker with the same care, levels of knowledge and attention, and respect accorded other patients and to provide all patients the highest quality of care that the physician is capable of rendering. When circumstances arise in which these rights and responsibilities create a conflict, something is wrong. The physician must then analyze the situation to determine who is out of line and must stand firm in an unambiguous position, regardless of personal interest and sympathies.

The physician who is seeing a patient on behalf of an employer or insurance carrier has an obligation to report to those parties such information as is directly pertinent to the worker's fitness to work or evaluation of a work-related disorder, and no more. Once an application for employment or a claim for compensation is made, the worker cannot stop the physician from conveying such information without withdrawing the application or claim. The physician also must notify the appropriate government agency of a work-related injury or illness, as a legal responsibility. The worker has an absolute right to know the nature, name, and probable cause of any disorder that is found on examination and the physician has an absolute duty to inform the worker of these findings and of what information will be conveyed to third parties. Under workers' compensation rules, however, the worker may not necessarily be free to select another physician to treat a disorder, beyond the first encounter, with the expectation that unauthorized fees will be paid.

Ethical Implications of Clinical Occupational Health Services

Particular occupational health programs or types of service generate specific ethical issues. These issues are addressed in this book as they arise. All clinical services, however, share certain concerns, and there is general agreement on what constitutes acceptable practice. Among occupational health professionals, informal "standards of practice" for health services hold that:

- The conduct of monitoring and surveillance programs for working populations is not an acceptable substitute for exposure monitoring and control.
- Employers, health professionals, and any other parties involved in monitoring or other health evaluation programs have a moral and ethical obligation—and often a legal duty—to see that the workers under evaluation understand the purpose, degree of validity, and consequences of participation.
- Workers have an absolute right to be informed of their individual results and the implications for their health and well-being and to be assured that this information will remain confidential.
- Employers have no right to information that does not pertain directly to either occupationally related disorders or the capability of a worker to perform the job assigned.
- Unusual or special evaluation techniques, such as a biological monitoring procedure under development and not yet standardized, should be conducted only with the specific consent of the worker, especially if the technique is invasive.
- Commitment to a monitoring or surveillance program implies that the data will be gathered for a purpose and that the findings will be acted upon.

Specific clinical occupational health services have their own ethical considerations as well. The more common services are presented in Table 4.1, along with their characteristic problem areas. These issues are discussed in greater detail where they appear in the text.

Codes of Ethics in Occupational Medicine

The American Occupational Medical Association (now the American College of Occupational Medicine) has developed a detailed code of ethics for the speciality. (See Table 4.2.) While intended for all physicians providing occupational medicine services, the code is particularly appropriate for specialists in occupational medicine since it covers

Table 4.1. Human Rights Issues Associated with Clinical Occupational Health Services

Medical Service	Particular Problem Areas
Fitness-for-work	Consistency of criteria Testing validity and predictive value Access to personal health information Screening for susceptible states
Occupational health monitoring	Collection of personal health data
Occupational health surveillance	"Labelling" of high-risk groups and subsequent anxiety Substitution for control May require removal from workplace on medical grounds
Case finding for occupational disorders	Data can be used by both sides in a disputed case
Case finding for health risks	Inevitably encroaches on privacy, lifestyle "Second chance" before serious consequences arise May require removal from workplace on medical grounds
Occupational health research	Communication of findings subject to "labelling" of high-risk groups and subsequent anxiety

more situations that a specialist is likely to encounter on a regular basis.

The Canadian Medical Association also has established eight basic ethical principles for physicians providing services in occupational medicine, summarized here in Table 4.3. The need for an ethical code arose from considerable confusion over the physician's role as an agent of the employer as well as a health professional in the service of the employee-patient. Because there is a great potential for ambiguity and abuse in such situations, the CMA developed this ethical code as a guide for all physicians providing occupational medicine services, regardless of specialty.

Other major efforts to establish ethical codes that bear on occupational health services are summarized in Table 4.4. The codes proposed under these efforts seem to have certain omissions in common, probably because they tend to use one another as points of departure. The omissions are summarized in Table 4.5, which is not intended as a new code but as a contribution toward a more comprehensive standard.

Ethics in Occupational Medicine Practice

The appropriate handling of confidential occupational health information collected on employees within an organization is central to the ethical behavior of the occupational physician. Organizations can avoid conflict and mistrust between the physician, workers, and employer by drawing up a policy describing how such information will be handled. Such written policies and procedures should be developed, regardless of whether the occupational health service is part of the organization or is an outside

Table 4.2. Code of Ethical Conduct for Physicians Providing Occupational Medical Services (American College of Occupational Medicine)

These principles are intended to aid physicians in maintaining ethical conduct in providing occupational medical service. They are standards to guide physicians in their relationships with the individuals they serve, with employers and workers' representatives, with colleagues in the health profession, and with the public. Physicians should:

1. Accord highest priority to the health and safety of the individual in the workplace;
2. Practice on a scientific basis with objectivity and integrity;
3. Make or endorse only statements which reflect their observations or honest opinion;
4. Actively oppose and strive to correct unethical conduct in relation to occupational health service;
5. Avoid allowing their medical judgment to be influenced by any conflict of interest;
6. Strive conscientiously to become familiar with the medical fitness requirements, the environment and the hazards of the work done by those they serve, and with the health and safety aspects of the products and operations involved;
7. Treat as confidential whatever is learned about individuals served, releasing information only when required by law or by over-riding public health considerations, or to other physicians at the request of the individual in relation to work, but employers are not entitled to diagnoses or details of a specific nature;
8. Strive continually to improve medical knowledge, and should communicate information about health hazards in timely and effective fashion to individuals or groups potentially affected, and make appropriate reports to the scientific community;
9. Communicate understandably to those they serve any significant observations about their health, recommending further study, counsel or treatment when indicated;
10. Seek consultation concerning the individual or the workplace whenever indicated;
11. Cooperate with governmental health personnel and agencies, and foster and maintain sound ethical relationships with other members of the health professions; and
12. Avoid solicitation of the use of their services by making claims, offering testimonials, or implying results which may not be achieved, but they may appropriately advise colleagues and others of services available.

service under contract, and should be made available to all concerned, from the chief executive officer to the newest of recruits.

The policy should explicitly outline procedures that will safeguard the rights of employees, recognize the professional obligations of the occupational health professional, and allow employers to make responsible decisions to achieve productive results. The policy and procedure documents should address the following questions:

• Who are the occupational health service staff?
• What is the content of the occupational health record (i.e., what constitutes occupational health information)?
• Who has ownership of the records?
• Where and for how long are records to be stored?

Table 4.3. Some Applications of the Canadian Medical Association Code of Ethics to Occupational Health Services

Consider first the well-being of the patient.
- Accord highest priority to the health and safety of the individual in the workplace.

Honor your profession and its traditions.
- Strive continually to improve medical knowledge and make appropriate reports to the scientific community.
- Avoid allowing medical judgment to be influenced by any conflict of interest.
- Actively oppose and strive to correct unethical conduct by any person or group.

Recognize your limitations and the special skills of others in the prevention and treatment of disease.
- Seek consultation whenever it is indicated.
- Avoid usurping the position of the family physician, but offer information, assistance, and cooperation in the medical management of the worker.
- Refrain from verifying the genuineness of sickness absence on behalf of the employer.
- Cooperate and consult with others outside the medical profession to prevent illness and promote health to the extent that they are competent and have similar intent and ethics with respect to the health and well-being of the workers.

Protect the patient's secrets.
- Treat as confidential whatever is learned about the worker as a patient; release information only when it is required by law or when it is clearly needed by others to preserve health and life; release information to other physicians according to traditional medical practice.
- Keep the medical records secure; be clear, through written agreement, on who is responsible for the custody of records in your absence and on what happens to them in the event of changes in the health service staff or in the status of the firm; do not permit access to medical records by persons outside the service unless required by law to do so.
- Communicate your judgment to both the employer and the worker when the worker has undergone a medical assessment for fitness to perform a specific job; however, do not give the employer specific details or diagnoses unless the worker has so requested.
- Grant a request by a worker to release medical information to employers or others only if the request has been made without duress; specifies the nature of the information, the purpose for its release, and the person to whom it may be released; and states the time for which it is valid.

Teach and be taught.
- Become familiar with the medical fitness requirements, the environment, the hazards of the work, and the health and safety aspects of the production and operations.
- Advise management and workers or their representatives of hazards to health and of opportunities to improve employee well-being, and assist in necessary actions.

Table 4.4. Recent Efforts in North America to Establish Voluntary Codes of Conduct Pertinent to Occupational Health Services

Agent	Activity	Area of Emphasis
American College of Epidemiology	Proposed guidelines	Occupational epidemiology
American Public Health Association	Occupational Health Section	Occupational medicine
Canadian Medical Association	Code of Ethics for Occupational Medicine	Occupational medicine
American College of Occupational Medicine	Code of Ethics	Occupational medicine
American Medical Association	Statement to U.S. OSHA	Occupational health and exposure records
National Commission on Confidentiality of Health Records	Federation of 26 organizations concerned with medical records	Occupational and exposure records
Canadian Centre for Occupational Health and Safety	Proposed guidelines	Monitoring and surveillance

• Who has access to the records and to whom may information be disclosed?

Occupational Health Services Staff
The occupational health service staff includes physicians, nurses, paramedics, and clerical support staff who are supervised by the physician or nurse. These staff members enjoy a position of trust and neutrality within the organization. They are expected to act in ways that support the obligation of the service as a whole to balance the rights and obligations of the workers with those of the employer without compromising ethical codes.

Content of an Occupational Health Record
The occupational health record varies from place to place, but usually contains: a medical history; work history; preplacement medical record; fitness-to-work assessments and advisements; progress notes; technical records describing exposure situations or accident investigations; employer assistance assessments and referrals; laboratory studies; work hazard exposure records; biological monitoring; toxicological screening results; and consultants' reports. The occupational health record should not be confused with medical records developed for workers participating in voluntary health promotion programs, which have no direct bearing on the employment relationship. Records of medical evaluations for health promotion programs that are not under the direct control of the occupational health service should be kept apart from occupational health records. Employee assistance records, on the other hand, should be incorporated into the occupational health record.

Table 4.5. Overlooked Elements of an Ethical Code in Occupational Medicine

1. A human life is not a negotiable commodity.
2. Both worker and employer are ultimately best served by the whole truth.
3. No short-term benefit to any party outweighs the common harm done by shading the facts.
4. An outsider charged with evaluating a problem has a right to a complete and fair hearing of his or her methods, results, and conclusions and cannot tolerate interference with fact-finding.
5. The history of occupational health has demonstrated repeatedly that when a health hazard has not been proven but is suggested by sound evidence, the worker should be protected.

Ownership and Storage

The occupational health service must establish strict procedures for the maintenance, storage, and disclosure of health information. Adherence to the procedures will foster trust among all parties and allow the occupational health professionals to function in a highly professional and ethical manner. Such procedures serve and protect the legitimate rights of all three parties.

The occupational health record, whether in paper or electronic format, is considered to be owned by the organization or individual who caused and paid for its creation. In workplaces with an in-house occupational health service, the occupational health record is stored in a secure area within the occupational health center. If the record is electronic, access must be restricted to occupational health personnel; ideally there should be a free-standing computer dedicated to records within the occupational health center. If the records are stored on a mainframe or outside the occupational health center, they must be secured by foolproof access codes. All occupational health records should be kept for a minimum of 40 years, or 20 years after retirement, to accommodate a normal working lifetime with the potential for hazardous exposures and the latency factor of occupational disease.

In the case of external occupational health services, the health record should remain under the guardianship of the occupational health service that developed it. If the occupational health service then goes out of business or ceases to exist, the records should be retained by the parent organization (if a hospital or group practice), or transferred to the external occupational health service that has taken over the care of the employees of the particular employer. The records of an individual worker also may be forwarded to the worker's personal physician, if known. If none of these options is practical, the records might be deposited with a government agency with responsibility for occupational safety and health. Records should never be transferred to any employer that lacks an internal occupational health service with a standing policy of confidentiality. Even when the employer has such guarantees, transferring records directly to the employer sometimes may be unwise. Records may contain information that could be damaging to workers in a disputed case, even though such information may be extraneous to the occupational disorder itself, such as information on personal habits or lifestyle. In one such case, an employer used an inaccurate history that was recorded by an outside physician as evidence against a worker's claim for compensation for a work-related injury. In the absence of an internal occupational health service, an employer is never entitled to these records.

Access

Unrestricted access to all parts of the occupational health record is limited to the occupational health professionals and to those personnel who report directly to them.

Employees should have unrestricted access to the parts of their own records pertaining to their personal medical history, work history, fitness-to-work advisements, preplacement medical record, and laboratory reports. In practice, there is rarely a circumstance when an employee would not be permitted complete access to his or her own file. Some parts of the record, however, may require interpretation by the occupational health professional or may contain opinions sought from others whose permission should be obtained before disclosure.

It is generally accepted that the employer owns the record. Managers may misinterpret this principle and feel that they are entitled to access whenever they think they need it. Some employers mistakenly believe they need access to a worker's record to make employment or workplace hazard decisions. The fact is that employers never need detailed medical information—they do, however, require fitness-to-work judgments and interpretations of workplace hazard exposures, such as the nature of an environmental workplace monitoring result or the result of a biological monitoring test.

Rules for Disclosure

From the perspective of an occupational health professional, the rules for disclosure of any part of the occupational health record are clear. Ordinarily, disclosure of any part of the occupational health record will require the written or verbal consent of the worker. Exceptions to this rule include emergency, health-threatening situations or situations in which disclosure is required by law or deemed by the occupational health professional to be in the worker's best interest. When a disclosure is made under these exceptional circumstances, the worker must be informed in a timely way. (It is important to keep in mind that fitness-to-work advisements, while contained within the occupational health record, also form part of the nonmedical records of the company, and thus do not require an employee's permission for disclosure. See Chapter 18.) The principles underlying these rules have been quite clearly stated in the various codes published by the American and Canadian Medical Associations.

Employers have an obligation to protect workers' health and safety and to respect the workers' right to privacy of their personal medical information. "Privilege" is the legal obligation that requires lawyers to refuse to reveal information that has been given to them in confidence by a client. Although physicians and nurses do not enjoy "privilege" under the law as do attorneys, they traditionally have practiced their profession as if they did and the courts have respected their need to guarantee confidentiality. In day-to-day practice, it is assumed by both the patient and the physician that information passed between them in the course of a medical interaction will remain confidential.

An employer does not have the legal right to require a health professional to disclose health information about workers. This situation was addressed by a 1979 Canadian Supreme Court decision in which Mr. Justice Pigeon decided that "an employee's duty of obedience towards the employer does not mean [that] the latter has any power to compel the employee to act in breach of a duty of confidentiality." The employer was trying to force the occupational health professional it employed to reveal health information about a worker of the company and in so doing to violate medical ethics, to the advantage of the employer. The court sided with the occupational health professional's higher obligation to observe the code of confidentiality.

Professional codes of ethical practice, state medical practice acts, and provincial health disciplines acts all support the notion that, excepting emergency or life-threatening situations, all personal medical information should be kept confidential unless its release is authorized by the patient or is required by law. The patient may authorize the release of medical information by written or oral consent. (Form 4.1 provides an example of an authorization for medical release of information.) Occupational health professionals, regardless of their own employment relationships, must adhere to these codes and laws, and employers who maintain an occupational health service or who consult with occupational health professionals must understand and respect the need for such adherence. The occupational health professional can manage the employee-employer relationship and provide effective direction to the employer without using medical terminology or divulging a diagnosis through the fitness-to-work process discussed in Chapter 18.

Occasionally, persons other than occupational health professionals will need to know certain types of health-related information. In the case of personal injury, whoever is

---

Form 4.1. Authorization for Release of Medical Information

I, _____, hereby authorize _____
to release the following medical information about me:

_____
_____
_____
_____

to the following persons(s)/organization(s):

_____
_____
_____

I give my permission for this medical information to be used for the following purposes:

_____
_____
_____
_____

I do not give my permission for any other use or re-disclosure of this information and this authorization is not effective beyond the following date: _____

_____
Signature of person authorizing release

_____   _____
Signature of Witness   Date of signature

(Courtesy of Sharp Rees-Stealy Medical Group, San Diego, CA)

responsible for accident investigation, safety, or first aid will need to know many details about the injury. Occupational hygienists may need to know the results of biological monitoring or toxicological screening. As a general rule, measurements of substances in body fluids can be disclosed if their presence could be due only to an occupational or environmental exposure and are not normally found in the body. However, the occupational hygienist must keep the identity of the individual confidential. If a worker is a participant in a health surveillance or health monitoring program, he or she must be informed of the purpose of the monitoring program and the results of any toxicological screening tests. Abnormal results from such programs should lead to a thorough review of the worker's health, working conditions, and the manner of performing the job. If a level of a potentially toxic substance is so high that the worker must be removed from the job, ethical business practice would require maintaining the employee's income by transferring the worker to another job or making some other arrangement within the organization.

Further Reading

American Occupational Medical Association: Code of Ethics for Physicians Providing Occupational Medical Services. Chicago, 1976.

Ashford NA, Spadafor CJ, Caldari CC: Human monitoring: Scientific legal, and ethical-considerations. Harvard Environ Law Rev 1984; 8:263–363.

Atherley G: Human rights versus occupational medicine. Int J Health Services 1983; 13:265–275.

Bok S: The limits of confidentiality. Hastings Center R, February 1983, pp. 24–31.

Canadian Medical Association: Basic Principles for the Provision of Occupational Health Services. Ottawa, 1988, revised.

Canadian Medical Association: Code of Ethics, 1984. Report of the Commission of Inquiry into the Confidentiality of Health Information. Toronto, Queen's Printer for Ontario, 1984.

Conrad CC: Biomedical ethics: Unique issues for preventive medicine. Washington, American College of Preventive Medicine, 1982.

Cowell JWF: Employee health information: For the record. OHS Canada 1986; 3(6):10.

Cowell JWF: Pre-employment health evaluations: Walking a fine line. OHS Canada 1987; 3(3):14.

Ethics in occupational medicine. Lancet 1980; 2:134.

Guidotti TL: A critique of the guidelines proposed for medical evaluation procedures by the Canadian Centre for Occupational Health and Safety. Occup Health in Ontario, 1988, in press.

Karrh B: The confidentiality of occupational medical data. J Occup Med 1979; 21:157–160.

Lappe M: Ethical issues in testing for differential sensitivity to occupational hazards. J Occup Med 1983; 25:797–808.

Lee JS, Rom WN (eds): Legal and Ethical Dilemmas in Occupational Health. Ann Arbor, Ann Arbor Science, 1982.

Morton W: The responsibility to report occupational health risks. J Occup Med 1977; 19:258–260.

Nethercott JR: Confidentiality and the right to know. Occup Health in Ontario 1984; 5:2–9.

Reiser SJ, Dyck AJ, Curran WJ (eds): Ethics in Medicine. Cambridge, Massachusetts, MIT Press, 1977.

Sammons JH: Access to employee exposure and medical records: A statement of the American Medical Association to the Occupational Safety and Health Administration. JAMA 1978; 240:2175–2176.

Sieghart P: Professional ethics: For whose benefit? J Soc Occup Med 1982: 32:4–14.

Warshaw L: The malpractice problem and the occupational physician. J Occup Med 1977;19:593–597.

SECTION II
OCCUPATIONAL HEALTH CARE DELIVERY

5

THE BUSINESS CONTEXT

All business organizations are influenced by the context in which they operate. The business climate affects the company's financial status, productivity, employee morale, indeed its very existence. Laws and regulations govern how the company will conduct its business. Employee expectations may be high or low, the company may have a particular image it wants to project to the public, to customers, or to clients. Finally, there are the individual characteristics of the business itself, such as its size, type, age, history, location, ownership, and mission.

The Corporate Environment

All large organizations—whether places of business, military establishments, universities, unions, or governments—share a common basic structure (Figure 5.1): the operating line of authority extends from the ultimate leader to the lowest level employee. Along this line all actions take place, with the direct result that goods or services are produced by the organization. The staff line supports the operating line by providing essential services through the financial, legal, human resource, and occupational health and safety functions. This common basic structure does not exist in isolation. To the contrary, it is subject to strong external influences that constitute the context within which business decisions are made (Figure 5.2).

Of all external factors influencing the delivery of occupational health care, the most critical is the company business philosophy (Figure 5.3). Does management, from the most senior levels down to the most junior foreman, show concern for employees and the public's health and safety, obey laws, recognize industry codes of practice, reflect and respect human values? Providing effective occupational health services requires that the business philosophy embrace these values. The occupational health professional may have to help establish and maintain this type of enlightened business philosophy in order to ensure both that the program enjoys a nurturing environment and that it functions as a valuable and essential asset to the business.

Figure 5.1. Basic structure of all organizations.

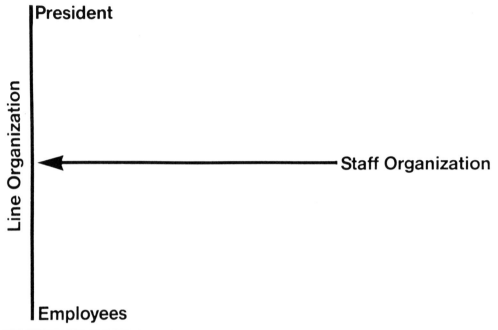

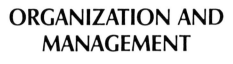

The company occupational health and safety policy, of necessity, must reflect the company's business philosophy, articulate its commitment to employee and public well-being, recognize the relevant laws, define roles, and assign responsibility. (A model occupational and environmental health policy that could apply to any company large enough to have a corporate office, diverse operations, and affiliated businesses is provided at the end of this chapter as Exhibit 5.1) The service plays many roles within the organization and serves many functions. These include:

- Daily routine (operational) functions involving the day-to-day conduct of business and handling of individual cases;
- Short- or medium-term (tactical) functions involving setting consistent standards and short-term benefits; and
- Long-term (strategic) functions to achieve organizational goals involving the reduction of risks and maximizing long-term benefits.

The occupational physician within a corporate setting is responsible for a whole matrix of management and medical concerns, as identified by Walsh and summarized in Table 5.1. These may include concern for environmental health and product liability issues and personal health problems among employees as well as occupational health concerns per se.

Other factors that may influence the actions of the occupational health and safety

Figure 5.2. Context within which business operates.

BUSINESS ORGANIZATION

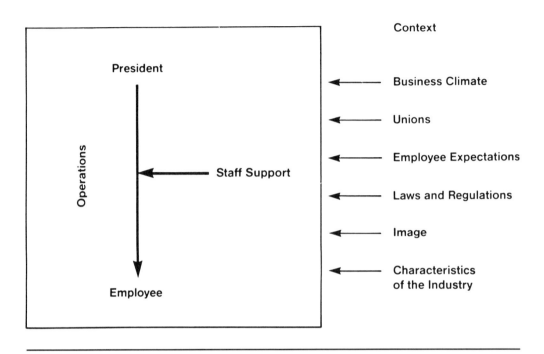

group are the legal and regulatory environment, social and economic forces, and the nature of the relationship between labor and management (Figure 5.3). For example, the company may operate in an environment where aggressive litigation is the rule of the day, or where regulations are stiff and routinely enforced. During periods of prosperity, the occupational health and safety function will not have to scramble for funding, but in lean times may find itself fighting for its very survival, regardless of the impact it may have had on the bottom line. The occupational health and safety department may have to deal with a workforce with special linguistic, educational, and economic problems, or may be swept up into conflicts between labor and management, especially if a union is present and feels that the health and welfare of its membership is not being managed properly by the company. However, a well run occupational health and safety group that understands its role and communicates its mission can have a very positive influence on labor/management relations. The underlying role of the occupational health and safety department in matters of health is to help create a fair balance between employee rights and obligations and those of the company (Figure 5.4).

Figure 5.3. The forces acting on the occupational health and safety department reflect the forces within the context of the company as a whole, with the critical addition of the company's philosophy and policy.

CONTEXTUAL FRAMEWORK – EXTERNAL INFLUENCES

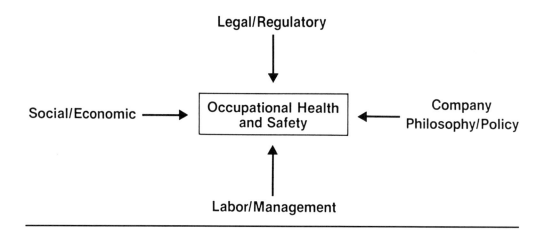

Service Mission and Structure

The occupational health and safety department needs a clearly defined mission statement that is fully supported by the company policy document. A typical mission statement might read as follows:

"The mission of the occupational health and safety department is to provide leadership, support, and service, and to audit the entire organization for compliance with occupational health and safety procedures to ensure:

1. The health and safety of employees are maintained and protected while at work.
2. The health of people living or working near the company's operation is not adversely affected.
3. The company meets or exceeds legislated requirements to protect it from charges and inappropriate liability."

The occupational health and safety unit is a staff rather than operating function. In a large company the organizational positioning of occupational health and safety is quite critical. Especially in circumstances where a company has both corporate and operating occupational health and safety personnel, reporting relationships should be specified and lines of authority defined.

The corporate occupational health and safety group should be headed up by a senior manager reporting as high in the organization as is practical (Figure 5.5). This leader should have strong administrative skills and a technical background, preferably in medicine, hygiene, or safety. The position can be and often is occupied by a physician with

Table 5.1. Matrix of Occupational Health Service Responsibilities in Large Organizations

	Medical Level		
Management Level	Individual (Worker)	Group (Workers)	Community (External)
Operational	Clinical care: case management Fitness-to-Work	Health identification and control	Environmental/product hazard management
Tactical	Health surveillance* Fitness-to-Work	Health surveillance** Comprehensive occupational health service	Regulatory affairs
Strategic	Health promotion*	Health policy, cost containment Health promotion	Risk/liability control

(Modified after Walsh DC: Harvard Business Review, July/August 1984; pp. 84–94.)
* To protect and enhance the health of the individual worker.
** To protect and enhance the general health of workers as groups or populations, recognizing that there will be individual variations.

such a background, but this does not imply that the safety and hygiene functions are subordinate to health. Each group has its own role to play (Figure 5.6) yet should have a close working relationship with the others. In companies with more than 1,000 employees, the occupational health service is likely to be part of the personnel department while safety and hygiene report to an operating manager. But once a company has grown to around 3,000 employees, a single administrative grouping of health, safety, and hygiene may best ensure coordination of services (Figure 5.7).

The corporate group often will be quite small, providing leadership, support, and audit to the occupational health and safety personnel distributed throughout operations. The matrix of relationships so formed depends on professional links as well as formal administrative links (represented by dotted and straight lines, respectively, in Figure 5.8). For example, nurses in the field may receive their health-related direction from medical personnel at the corporate level while they are directly supervised by an operating manager in the field.

Regardless of the medical standing of the corporate vice president for occupational health and safety, a corporate medical director is needed to provide direct professional leadership to the occupational health programs. This position is particularly important in companies where occupational health nurses handle most of the routine services. Part-time occupational health physicians seldom are able to provide the close support needed by the nurses. The corporate medical director should report to a vice president of occupational health and safety or someone else at the policy-making level, and should have sufficient power within the organization to influence or set policy and establish standards of practice. Some large companies have neither a senior manager nor a company medical director responsible for occupational health and safety; some use outside medical consultants primarily or exclusively. Neither of these models works well—such arrangements keep the medical consultant as an outsider, unable to wield the authority to set policy or to make changes. In such settings, authority is diffuse and

Figure 5.4. The occupational health and safety department must strike the balance between the rights and obligations of the employee and the company.

Help Create a Fair Balance

Employee Rights and Obligations   Company Rights and Obligations

coordination difficult. These arrangements usually reflect a fundamental lack of commitment to occupational health and safety on the part of senior management.

A successful occupational health and safety service can be achieved only in an organizational environment that is based on a sound business philosophy that requires the company to care about people and to obey laws. Lacking this underlying value system, occupational health and safety policy and programs cannot achieve their potential.

Implications of Labor Relations

The state of relations between an organization and its employees has an important effect on the occupational health service. Most obviously, the presence of a labor union in the workplace will affect day-to-day operations of the service. For example, the union representing employees may negotiate for improved working conditions and occupational health services as part of the collective bargaining process. Unfortunately, occupational health services that are the direct product of collective bargaining are vulnerable to abrupt changes in policy and financial cutbacks, and may be used as a pawn or distraction in contract negotiations. Preserving the occupational health service as neutral ground in such circumstances requires effort and commitment from both sides...and this commitment can only come from a mutual understanding of the occupational health service and its actual role in the workplace, regardless of the designs of either party.

If both the union and management agree that the organization is ultimately responsible on both a moral and legal basis for protecting its workers, then a mutually agreeable approach can be negotiated. However, management acknowledgement of its responsibilities must be met by union acceptance that the employer is able and willing to fulfill its responsibilities. If an environment of trust and cooperation can be established, health and safety will enjoy a uniquely neutral place in the labor/management relationship and the well-being of workers will be ensured. Unfortunately, many agreements falter and health and safety issues become swept into and confused with other often controversial labor/management matters.

Today, society demands that workers not be maimed, killed, or diseased because of the work they do. To ensure this, labor, health, and human rights laws have been enacted. Many employers clearly do manage in a responsible manner, applying advanced

Figure 5.5. The corporate occupational health and safety department should report as high in the organization as possible.

DEPARTMENTAL STRUCTURE – REPORTING

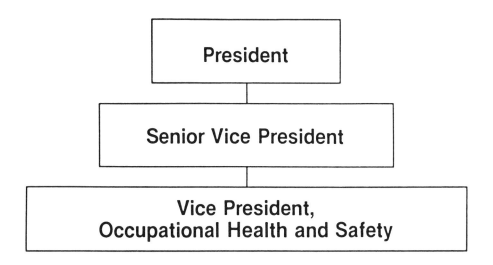

technical knowledge and providing professionally trained individuals to occupational health and safety programs. Yet many workers in many organizations still are not properly protected. Thus, unions should and will remain vigilant. Management's role is to establish and to apply the policies and programs necessary to protect employees; the union's role is to ensure that these policies and programs are fair, appropriate, and accessible. Unions and management both should be equally concerned with safe work practices, safe work environments, health surveillance examinations, fitness-to-work procedures, confidentiality of health records, freedom of choice, and alcohol and drug abuse rehabilitation programs. In the area of health and safety their interests should coincide. Conflict arises when management believes the union is making unreasonable demands or the union thinks that health and safety issues are being skirted or addressed in an unfair, incompetent, or unethical manner.

Union Contract Provisions
The collective bargaining agreement negotiated between an employer and its union (or unions) sets the tone of their relationship by listing many rules of behavior for the workforce. Sometimes the terms of the agreement contain only broad standards; more often they include very specific policies and procedures.

Issues concerning the well-being of workers, individually and as a group, traditionally have formed an important and often controversial part of collective agreements. And in recent years, agreements have broken important new ground in occupational health and safety. Most insist upon some form of worker participation in programs that

Figure 5.6. The occupational health and safety department may develop units for each of its major functions, each on an equal basis with the others.

ORGANIZATION AND MANAGEMENT OF OCCUPATIONAL HEALTH AND SAFETY

REPORTING STRUCTURE

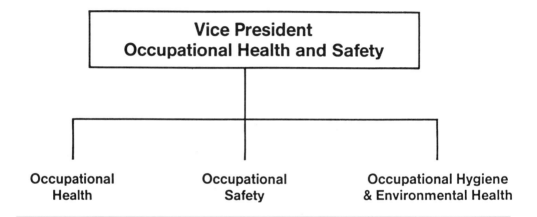

deal with worker health and safety; some unions have even negotiated the exclusive right to provide occupational health services to the workforce and sponsor their own facilities or plan.

A common form of direct worker involvement is the joint health and safety committee. In some jurisdictions such committees are even mandated by state or provincial law. In others, legislation merely suggests that they be formed. The powers of these committees vary greatly—the group may exercise total control over health and safety matters or may serve merely as a forum for discussion or as advisors to management.

The provisions contained in the bargaining agreement in no way remove the employer's right to run the organization, yet they very definitely bind management and the workforce to a contractual arrangement that ordinarily will be upheld by the courts. These rules, which are in force for the life of the contract, typically include an arbitration mechanism for settling disputes.

The union may intervene in individual worker compensation or benefits claim and fitness-to-work assessments in addition to advocating changes in the workplace and acting as a conduit for complaints regarding working conditions. The union representative may assist the employee in filing a claim, arguing an appeal, or researching the background to a complex problem. Absent contractual provisions or specific authorization from the worker, the union representative is no more entitled to personal medical information (other than fitness-to-work judgments) than is an employer representative.

Figure 5.7. Once a company has grown to 3,000 employees, a single administrative grouping is needed to coordinate the three occupational health and safety functions.

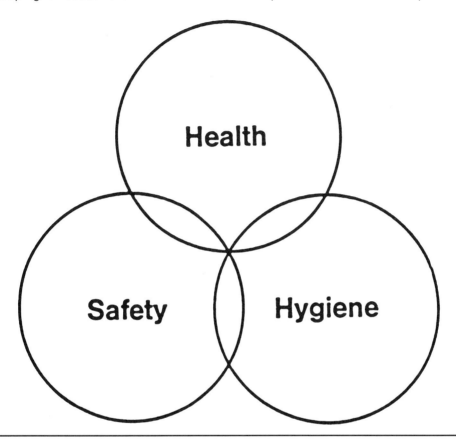

The employee, of course, is free to authorize release of medical information to whomever he or she wishes and almost always will do so if the union is taking up the case. If the contract stipulates that specific information is to be or can be released, the union has valid authority to receive the data. In all cases, however, consideration of ethics must guide the physician. (See Chapter 4.)

Non-union Worksites

The occupational health service in or serving an organization without union representation has a different set of problems and opportunities. As a creation of the employer uninfluenced by a union, the service often commands greater support from management, but sometimes is subjected to considerable and unrelenting pressure to see things management's way. Communication with employees is often more difficult because there may be no organized representation and no vehicle for conveying information other than through supervisors, who may have their own agendas. Information tends to become distorted as it passes through such channels. In this situation, full use must be made of all means to communicate directly with employees: joint worksite health

Figure 5.8. The matrix of professional relationships and reporting relationships in an occupational health and safety department.

Organization and Management of Occupational Health and Safety

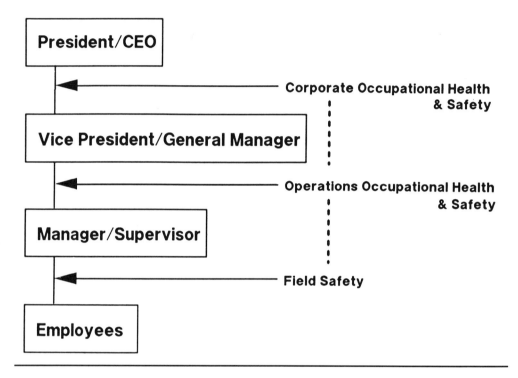

and safety committees (required by law in some jurisdictions), employee councils, quality circles, recreation associations, and newsletters.

Unions tend to promote improved but not ideal working conditions in most industries, in part because the process of collective bargaining makes it hard to focus attention on this one issue when wages, hours, and benefits all are on the table. By contrast, non-union plants often tend to extremes—the absence of union representation may lead to unacceptable conditions in one plant yet may induce the management of another to provide excellent benefits and working conditions as a means of ensuring employee satisfaction and warding off possible organizing attempts.

In all situations, the responsibility for protecting worker health rests squarely with management. Management must fulfill this obligation diligently and in a non-patronizing manner regardless of whether a union is looking over its shoulder.

Prudent non-unionized employers encourage worker involvement in health and safety strategies, frequently through voluntary joint health and safety committees. Such participatory mechanisms tend to be most successful where management already has established a relationship of trust with the workforce. Although it is the employer who ultimately writes the rule book, creative ways must be found to involve the workforce in formulating and implementing health and safety rules. Employee welfare is one sector of the corporate world that benefits considerably from an attitude of creative cooperation. Organizations that tend to mismanage employee health issues usually tend to mismanage other critical areas in their business as well, and in the long run are more likely to fail and disappear. The enlightened ones prosper because they recognize the need to be consistent with social change.

Services to Small Business

Small business is an important sector of the U.S. economy, comprising 96 to 99 percent of U.S. corporations, according to the U.S. Small Business Administration (SBA). This number represents roughly 6.25 million establishments, many of them very small retail, service, and farming entities. Obviously, small business is very big business in the aggregate. Equally as important is its role as the nursery for innovation and technological advancement—its vitality is most evident in the highest levels of technology. Nevertheless, while small business leads much of the economy and is valuable beyond the volume of its revenues, it faces severe problems in profitability and finance.

As a subset of North American business and industry, small business is very heterogeneous. There is no generally accepted operative definition of what constitutes a "small" business. The current working definition used by the Small Business Administration is based on a sliding scale that takes into account a company's sales, ownership, assets, numbers of employees, and other factors. This definition is exceedingly complex, relies in large part on prior rulings, rests on SBA adjudication, is not consistently used by U.S. federal and state programs, and is virtually impossible to apply for statistical purposes outside the agency. (A proposed simplified definition published for preliminary comment by the SBA in 1980 was retracted because of problems associated with categorizing multiindustry firms and reclassifying some 250,000 organizations so as to make them ineligible for SBA assistance.) In the absence of a precise definition, the term "small business" is taken here to mean a small operation within the context of a particular industry, be it a machine shop, a dry cleaning establishment, or a computer manufacturer.

Large corporations have several advantages over most small firms in complying with good occupational safety and health practices. These include a much larger pool of technical talent to identify and correct hazards; established in-house medical programs; favorable cash-flow and capital margins that allow resources to be put into occupational health and safety; and the capacity to assign responsibility for full-time management of safety and health programs to specific employees. The small firm almost invariably is working on a much narrower margin and by definition has at its command far fewer resources in capital, personnel, and facilities.

Furthermore, small businesses are unable to capitalize on economies of scale. One estimate suggests that for companies with fewer than 50 employees the cost of regulatory compliance (occupational, environmental, and socioeconomic) is seven to ten times as great per employee as for firms with 50 to 250 employees. A slightly lower differential probably applies to companies with fewer than 500 employees as compared to those with more than 500. Organizations with 20 to 250 employees have an injury rate higher than that of either smaller or larger corporations. Small business, then, has a particularly acute need for occupational health services delivered at reasonable cost.

A recent survey conducted in the state of Colorado and reported by Buchan confirms that industries with fewer than 100 employees rarely employ full-time occupational health professionals. These industries depend instead either on a part-time physician or nurse or on community-based services. By contrast, the majority of large industries employ at least an industrial hygienist. The smaller industries polled in the survey were much less likely than large industries to offer basic services, such as preplacement examinations, periodic health evaluations, and industrial hygiene surveys. Interestingly, a third of industries surveyed were of the opinion that present levels of occupational health services provided for them were not adequate to meet their and their employees' needs. However, there was no consensus expressed on how to better address these needs.

Unfortunately, the dispersed nature of small business makes the task of serving its needs in a coordinated fashion difficult at best, given practical limits on cost and local accessibility. The logistics permit only a dispersed network of facilities; yet the very decentralization of the network makes it all the harder to provide services at a consistent standard. It is difficult to exert quality assurance without control and smaller service units are more likely to be responsive to what the client wants, rather than what the client needs. On the other hand, a smaller, local service unit is likely to establish a closer relationship with the employer client and to become more aware of the client's constraints and perceived problems. The resulting situation is both good and bad: it enhances responsiveness to the employer client but may also create a cozy, uncritical, dependent relationship that excludes the worker. Smaller service units also may themselves even qualify as small businesses, and may suffer from many of the same resource constraints as their clients. It is common, for example, for small facilities of the "industrial medicine clinic" model to open without staff qualified in occupational medicine and to limit their activities to treating routine injuries and performing periodic or preplacement evaluations, without realizing the larger potential of their services.

Although the logistical problems of providing consistent occupational health services to small business are formidable, the potential rewards more than justify the effort. As noted above, most of society's economic activity and employment arise from small enterprises. This is true not only for the United States and Canada but for every economy around the world, regardless of the economic system. Developing services for small-scale industry is therefore an important strategy to improve occupational health standards in general. The effect of even small improvements consistently applied will be multiplied by the larger numbers of workers involved. From the standpoint of marketing, small business ultimately represents a much larger market for occupational health services than large corporations. The latter are more likely to have internal resources to resolve their health problems and may already have their own plant occupational health services or corporate occupational health department. Small business must cope as best it can and usually must turn to resources in the community in order to obtain assistance in solving its problems.

The direct benefits of prevention-oriented occupational health services for small enterprises are also proportionately greater than for large concerns. Few small businesses can absorb the consequences of absence or disability of a trained employee or manager without the loss being reflected in business performance. The direct costs associated with workers' compensation assessments, retraining and recruitment, and administrative overhead for dealing with absences would seem to provide an incentive for small business to use sound occupational health services, particularly those oriented toward prevention. Additionally, employees of small enterprises usually develop a more personal relationship with their managers than workers in corporations; indeed, in very small enterprises the workforce may be made up mostly or entirely of family members. One would think, then, that small enterprises would demand preventive services up to the limit they could afford. In practice, however, this is rarely the case.

The managers of small enterprises have many competing priorities and often perceive occupational health and safety as a regulatory burden imposed on them rather than as an integral part of operating a business. Many managers in small business have no clear idea of the hazards of their workplace or recognize only one or a few highly visible hazards. This should not be surprising because their interest and expertise are in business, not health. Invisible threats, such as cancer-causing chemicals, tend to be lost among urgent day-to-day matters of business. A handful of these managers, especially owner-managers, also take the attitude that acceptance of some risk is a necessary part of success in their business and that if they have taken risks themselves, their employees should be prepared to do so as well. Many, especially in industries requiring skilled work, see their employees as autonomous and knowledgeable tradespeople who know their job well and need no additional supervision. In many cases, the employee is a craftsman or has a skilled trade and knows more about the process than the manager. Managerial interference might even cause friction in such settings.

The great majority of managers of small business, however, are simply not knowledgeable about the cost-effective prevention of injury and illness in the workplace. The successful provision of sound occupational health services to small businesses therefore requires two levels of activity: (1) helping solve problems through effective consultation and (2) educating managers as to the value and appropriate utilization of services. It is not reasonable to expect all managers of small businesses to solve their own occupational health problems. They must have help based nearby in their own community.

Managers and owners of small businesses tend to be conservative in their approach to occupational health services, limiting use to the care of injured or ill employees and to screening activities required by law. Most perceive preventive or health promotion services with some skepticism, but the depth of this attitude depends in large part on the nature of the industry and attitudes in the community. Small firms involved in professional services or up-scale retail or service functions have shown interest in participating in community-based health promotion activities, as long as the financial burden is not excessive. Employee assistance programs designed to serve many small firms have been successful, usually when the firms served are dependent on a few key people. Even so, treatment and rehabilitative services are accepted more readily than preventive-oriented services. Occupational hygiene—evaluating and designing controls for hazards in the workplace—is not a familiar concept to many small business managers, who assume that such services will incur an excessive cost. All occupational health services available to small businesses should include provisions to educate and guide managers in achieving greater cost-effectiveness through selective utilization of available services.

To the owner or plant manager, occupational health coverage is a consumptive rather than an investment cost. There is no guarantee that a heavy investment in prevention or hazard control or health promotion will forestall the occurrence of a future injury or illness; the cost is tangible but the benefit is not. Furthermore, employees come and go and a heavy investment one year may be lost with personnel turnover the next, particularly since the benefits usually are apparent only in the long term. In larger companies costs associated with disability and failing performance may be reduced by company medical programs, but to a small company the costs of maintaining health services are out of proportion to the visible benefits. It can be demonstrated that intensive safety control applied to companies with high injury rates does appear to reduce downtime, lower insurance premiums and workers' compensation levies, and improve morale. Even so, it is doubtful that small businesses that perceive themselves as low in risk to begin with can be motivated to institute expensive in-house programs except when these are used as benefits to attract exceptionally talented employees.

Costs for occupational health services, therefore, must be kept as low as practicable for small business. One approach to reducing the costs of providing occupational health services to small business has been used in Durham, England, where a sliding fee scale takes plant size into account. Under this system, larger employers partly subsidize the cost of services to smaller employers in the same industrial park. This program has been successful, at least in part, because the impetus for establishing the facility came from the local employers themselves.

The severe shortage of professionals skilled in occupational health and safety also affects the supply of services to small business. One way to overcome this problem might be to increase training in occupational safety and health in medical school and expand postgraduate continuing medical education in occupational medicine. This academic measure is unlikely to resolve the problem, however, because few small businesses are in a position to retain physicians for corporation-sponsored health services and because medical services alone are not enough to resolve most occupational health problems. Equally as important are industrial hygiene services and management changes. More viable solutions are to:

- Provide clinic-based occupational safety and health services to serve many employers;
- Expand the use of non-physician health professionals, particularly nurse practitioners and industrial hygienists; and
- Simplify routine procedures so that, for example, lay personnel using a checklist could inexpensively conduct a health hazard surveillance and a physician untrained in occupational medicine could perform a standardized medical examination appropriate to a particular hazard.

Exhibit 5.1. Corporate Occupational and Environmental Health and Safety Policy

Purpose
To confirm the company's commitment to protect the health and safety of its employees and of persons living or working near company operations, and to assign responsibility for the actions and decisions required to maintain this commitment.

Policy Statements
1. Protect the health and safety of employees by establishing programs and services designed to promote and maintain the health and safety of employees both while at work and while away from work.
2. Protect the health and safety of persons living or working in areas near company operations by establishing procedures and programs that minimize the impact of these operations on the environment.
3. Establish and maintain practices and services that meet or exceed legislated standards by implementing company occupational health and safety standards that reinforce or, where appropriate, exceed current legislated standards.
4. Provide leadership, support, and review on occupational health and safety matters to help affiliated businesses meet their obligations.
5. Require that all contractors comply with company occupational health and safety policy by inserting specific health and safety clauses within their contracts and by performing periodic inspections of the contractors' operations.
6. All employee health information is considered by the Company to be given in confidence and shall be retained in confidence within the confines of occupational health units in locked storage areas.
7. All relevant codes of ethical practice, legislation, and common law governing the behavior of health professionals will be respected.

Responsibility and Authority
Management of all company operations and subsidiary and affiliated companies are responsible for their operations' compliance with this policy, and are required to ensure:
1. Compliance with all laws relating to employee health and safety, including occupational health and safety, public health and safety, workers' compensation, and human rights acts.
2. Compliance with company occupational and environmental health and safety standards.
3. Compliance with programs designed to promote employee and public health and safety.
4. Immediate notification of the next level of management of any health and safety matter requiring the attention of the corporate occupational health and safety department or an appropriate government agency.
5. Employees are responsible for providing reliable information so that their interests and thoset of the company can be best served.

Occupational Health and Safety is Responsible for:
1. Providing leadership, support, audit and services to operating components of the company and its subsidiary and affiliate companies in all areas relating to employee and public health and safety.
2. Developing, in coordination with operating components, company occupational health and safety standards, practices, services and reporting methods necessary to comply with company and legislated standards.
3. Monitoring and auditing the operating components' compliance with legislated and company health and safety standards.

(Continued)

Exhibit 5.1. Continued.

4. Developing programs and services designed to promote the health and safety of the employee and the public.
5. Developing and maintaining health records consistent with all relevant codes, laws, and ethical guidelines.
6. Preparing quarterly and annual reports for senior management on company performance relating to occupational health and safety. These should include recommendations for action at the corporate level.

Reservation of Authority
All employees engaged in those specialties relating to the occupational health and safety department are professionally responsible to the vice president, occupational health and safety, who is provided with the authority to affect their appointment, promotion, compensation, or termination.
    All procedures, guidelines and communications relating to occupational health and safety will be based on this policy.

Exceptions
No exceptions.

Further Reading

A Comprehensive Guide for Establishing an Occupational Health Service. Atlanta, American Association of Occupational Health Nurses, 1987.

American Medical Association Council on Occupational Health: The role of medicine within a business organization. JAMA 1969; 210:1446–1450.

Boden LI, et al: The impact of health and safety committees. J Occup Med 1984; 26:829–834.

Buchan RM: Delivery health services to small industry in Colorado. Occup Health Safety. September 1979; 48(6):42–45.

Charleswater Associates, Inc: The Impact on Small Business Concerns of Government Regulations that Force Technological Change: Final Report. Washington DC, Government Printing Office, Small Business Administration Contract No. SBA 2098-PRA-75, September 1975.

Cowell JWF: Organization and management of occupational health and safety programs. Proceedings, Medichem 1986: Fourteenth International Congress on Occupational Health in the Chemical Industry. Ludwigshafen (Germany), 1986.

Cowell JWF: How to set up an occupational health service. OHS Canada 1986; 3(6):32–38,58.

Cowell JWF: Organization and management of occupational health and safety programs. Occupational Health in Ontario 1985; 6(2):75–86.

Fallows J: American Industry—What ails it, how to save it. The Atlantic. September 1980, n.v. (246):35–50.

Hittig EH: Is safety really worth it? Inc. October 1980; 2:65–66.

How defining "small" became big deal for SBA. Inc. July 1980; 2(7):20.

Howe W, Gibson W, Wiggett IJ: Organizing a group occupational health service in County Durham. J Soc Occup Med 1983; 33:88–92.

King MH: Management, labour and the occupational medicine physician. Can Med Assn J 1984; 131:17–19.

Kusnetz S, Hutchison MK (eds): A Guide to the Work-Relatedness of Disease. Rockville MD, National Institute for Occupational Safety and Health, 1979, DHEW (NIOSH) publication No. 79–116, pp. 1–20.

MacKinnon B: Work-related injuries and illnesses: small employers, 1977–1985. Edmonton, Alberta Community and Occupational Health, 1987.

National Institute for Occupational Safety and Health: Development of Clinic-based Occupational Safety and Health Programs for Small Business: Proceedings of a conference held 1–3 May 1977, Cincinnati OH, Washington DC, U.S. Government Printing Office, 1977.

Northern Telecom: Health and Safety in the Workplace—A Model Program. Don Mills, Ontario, CCH Canadian, 1988.

Ryan EJ: Occupational health services to small business current approaches. In Occupational Safety and Health Symposia (Proceedings of the 38th American Medical Association Annual Congress on Occupational Health, Tucson, 14–16 September 1978). Cincinnati OH, National Institute for Occupational Safety and Health, 1979, pp. 111–115.

SBA proposes "simpler" size standards for aid. Inc. May 1980; 2(5):24,26.

Small Business Health and Safety Guide for Chemical Waste Disposal. Cincinnati, American Conference of Government Industrial Hygienists, 1985.

Stewart M: What we must do to speed growth for small business. Inc. September 1980; 2(9):18–23.

Strasser AL: Occupational medicine in small industry. Occup Health Safety 1980; 49:19–21.

Supplemental Data System: Occupational Injuries and Illnesses, California. Washington DC, U.S. Dept. of Labor, Bureau of Labor Statistics, 1978. National Technical Information Service accession number PB-288 432.

Walsh DC: Is there a doctor in-house? Harvard Business Review 1984 (July–August); (4)84–94.

Walsh DC: The vanguard and the rearguard: Occupational medicine revisits its future. J Occup Med 1988; 30:124–134.

Walsh DC: Corporate Physicians: Between Medicine and Management. New Haven, Yale University Press, 1987.

White House Commission on Small Business: Excerpts from the Report to the President. Inc. July 1980; 2(7):22.

6

CONTRACT SERVICES

The Arena of Occupational Health Practice

In some parts of the world, including Sweden and the Canadian province of Quebec, occupational health services for small business (and some large industries at low risk) are provided by the public sector through community-based facilities. Often these are community health clinics that also provide personal health care. However, in Sweden, especially, a separate and effective network of occupational health centers exists to provide both preventive and acute care. In most other countries the private sector assumes major responsibility for occupational health care; even in Finland, which has an extensive network of municipal health centers offering occupational health services, employers still obtain most services from private facilities.

The private sector does have a few advantages over the public sector in providing occupational health care. As summarized in Table 6.1, the private sector is able to move fast, to raise its own capital, and to adapt quickly to changing circumstances. While the public sector clearly is better able to ensure a consistent standard of service and compliance with publicly determined policies and priorities, even the most efficiently managed public network of facilities must follow policies and priorities that reduce its local adaptability and speed of response. Rather than being reinvented, the private sector needs only to be redirected towards other avenues, such as providing continuing education to the sole practitioner or the few practitioners in a small town or encouraging the establishment of new facilities, either free-standing or attached to existing hospitals or medical groups.

The private sector provides most occupational health services to small business in the United States. Indeed, there are so few models of publicly sponsored services providing direct care in the United States that the public sector can be ignored for all practical purposes in this chapter. (In Canada, however, publicly sponsored and supported services are an important component of the system in many provinces.)

On a small scale, outpatient clinical services for small business have been provided

Table 6.1. General Characteristics of Private and Public Models of Health Care

	Private Sector Approach	Public Sector Approach
Model of operation	Entrepreneurial	Bureaucracy
Incentive	Economic	Political
Capital investment	Private capital	Public funding
Speed of development	Depends on incentives— may be very rapid	Deliberately paced
Adaptability	Rapid	Slow
Coverage	Uneven	Even
Quality assurance	Highly variable	Minimal standards

for decades by private practitioners and, more recently, by group practices. These services, however, have been largely inconspicuous since they constitute only a small part of the activities of such practices. In-plant services, which are sometimes shared among several employers, are described in detail in Chapter 5.

Many models for providing occupational health care to multiple employers exist within the private sector. The most common are:

• Occupational medicine in primary care practice;
• Individual or partnership consultation practice in occupational medicine;
• Multispecialty group practice;
• Hospital-based clinics; and
• "Industrial medicine" clinics.

Less common are such varieties as union-sponsored occupational health services (which are concentrated in New York although there are three examples in Canada). Union-sponsored clinics tend to play highly specialized roles within the system and are clearly oriented toward the needs of individual workers rather than toward employers. In addition, a few health maintenance organizations have established occupational medicine clinics, such as the one operated by Kaiser-Permanente in San Diego.

Occupational Medicine in Primary Care Practice

The typical primary care physician considering occupational medicine as a special interest, for a clinic, or as a part-time commitment, already is capable of handling some of the necessary medical and surgical functions—but the same physician may not be as well prepared for other activities of particular importance in this area of medicine. Table 6.2 compares skill content areas or knowledge needed for community-based practice in occupational medicine against those applicable to primary care, such as family practice or general internal medicine.

The diagnostic and other cognitive skills of clinical practice must be combined with specific training in workplace hazards and toxicology to solve occupational health problems. For example, physicians in clinical occupational medicine practice often screen large groups of persons who are in good health, frequently by using legally mandated

Table 6.2. Skills and Knowledge Needed in Occupational Medicine
Compared to Primary Care

Primary Care	Occupational Medicine
Diagnosis	Identification of Work-Related Disorders Evaluation of Causation Interpretation of the Occupational History
Functional Patient Evaluation	Evaluation of Impairment Fitness-to-Work Evaluation
Health Services*	Occupational Health Care Organization Program Management and Evaluation

Clinical Epidemiology*	Epidemiologic Basis for Health Promotion and
	   Disease Prevention
	Epidemiologic Basis for Health Surveillance and
	   Monitoring
	Risk Assessment

Commitment to Prevention	Primary Prevention of Workplace Exposure Hazard Recognition
Clinical Management	Fitness-to-Work Evaluation Evaluation of Impairment Office Surgery and Orthopedics*
Medical Fund of Knowledge	Knowledge of Workplace Hazards Specialized Knowledge in Toxicology, Epidemiology, Ergonomics, Occupational Hazards

* Of variable importance, depending on practice and setting.

or employer-required protocols that may be obsolete or illogical or that feature such sophisticated, and problemmatical, elements as drug testing and biological monitoring. The logic and methods of clinical epidemiology are invaluable for proper design and interpretation of screening programs. Similarly, the practice of occupational medicine in all settings, not only in corporate medical departments, requires administrative skills beyond those of office management. Communicating successfully with all parties involved (including workers' compensation boards, employers, workers, unions, regulatory agencies, and insurance carriers) requires insight into the occupational health care system.

Properly practiced, occupational medicine is oriented primarily toward prevention. Both clinical intervention and fitness-to-work assessments are part of a broader picture that encompasses health surveillance and monitoring and the introduction of programs and changes in the workplace that protect and, ideally, enhance the health of workers as groups. In this respect, occupational medicine practice, particularly at the higher levels, tends to be less clinical and more administrative in nature. Prevention, particularly on a group level, requires different skills and expertise than treatment-oriented management. The clinician who aims at providing more than just routine occupational care must obtain these skills and specialized knowledge.

The physician considering part-time service in a local plant must gain as complete an understanding as possible of working conditions and hazards in the workplace. A first step on this road to knowledge is a long and detailed tour of the facility that focuses on unusual or troublesome work stations. Visits to maintenance, custodial, and representative administrative areas also are essential and should not be omitted or cut short. Of particular interest are occupations requiring special preplacement tests or periodic screening programs—the physician should observe these jobs carefully and identify their particular physical requirements or hazards.

Physicians who are considering whether to start a clinic or incorporate an increased load of occupational health care services into an existing practice also should conduct some preliminary research:

- First, evaluate the position and capabilities of the practice, including its location and the preparation and interests of the physician associated with it. A clinic or full-time practice in occupational medicine is not likely to succeed unless it is located in an industrial area, is prepared to handle minor trauma, and is efficient at processing workers' compensation claims.
- Second, review the profile of industry in the area. Larger, capital-intensive corporations generally will be more selective in referring cases and may require some assurance of the practitioner's expertise. Small industries, especially in manufacturing or construction, generally look for low costs, trauma care, and minimal waiting time. Certain technologies, such as high-technology electronics, present exotic or uncommon hazards requiring specific and sometimes extensive preparation to manage them appropriately.

Consultation Practice in Occupational Medicine

Developing a referral practice in occupational diseases also requires some research: where will cases come from, who will see them first, and why should they be referred to one particular consultant over another? More and more, consultation practice in occupational medicine today depends on meaningful credentials and several assured sources of referrals. Occupational medicine is practiced in a fishbowl. Opinions and findings are under review by workers' compensation boards, employers, insurance carriers, unions, and, frequently, the courts. Each is either a potential source of or a potential obstacle to referrals. Generally, parties do not object to a competent opinion (although they may disagree in individual cases), but each is very sensitive to inadequate documentation, incomplete records, and delayed reports—and reacts silently by steering referrals elsewhere. Moreover, complex cases (precisely those that are most likely to be referred) often go to court or to arbitration. When the possibility of litigation looms, the suitability of a physician as a possible witness often influences the selection of a professional to evaluate a case. The physician's formal credentials in occupational medicine become important in such situations. The testimony of an expert witness with board certification in the field or at least a fellowship in one of the important organizations (such as the American College of Occupational Medicine) or membership in an important selective organizations (such as the American College of Preventive Medicine) will usually outweigh the credibility of testimony by a witness lacking specific credentials.

Occupational medicine consultation clinics have intrinsic problems that must be addressed in any viable plan. One reality is that they are economically tenuous. Occupational medicine consultation clinics, unlike primary care clinics for occupationally related injuries, are seldom profitable in the private sector. At best they are self-sustaining as a result of revenue generated from a case mix that includes a large percentage of patients requiring low-cost low-intensity screening and preventive services. The typical individual case referred to a consultant for clinical evaluation is extremely time-consuming, and fees recovered from the workers' compensation board or the insurance carrier often cover only a fraction of the overhead and personnel cost. For example, physicians in one university-based clinic spend on the average from 1½ hours to 4 hours on a single patient referred by a general practitioner: ½ hour to 1 hour for interviewing; ½ hour to 2 hours for reviewing medical records and searching the literature; and ½ to 1 hour for preparing the consultation report. For these services, insurance pays approximately three-quarters of what a specialist would bill for medical services provided in 1 hour. Thus, billings cannot support such a clinic.

Although their services are greatly needed, economics dictate that occupational medicine consultation clinics are not a remunerative form of practice. Solutions to this problem lie in developing a mix of cases as described; in basing services at such institutions as universities where physicians are on salary and overhead is subsidized; and, possibly, by associating the clinic with a medical facility that also deals with occupational injuries at the primary care level.

Occupational physicians starting out are wise to target a specific industry, employer, or group in order to become known as an expert in the health problems of a common occupation. Many clinicians have entered occupational medicine practice by taking a particular interest in firefighters, bus drivers, or, increasingly, performing artists. The physician new to occupational medicine also would do well to assume responsibility for the employee health service of a medium-sized hospital. Hospitals are good training grounds for many of the realities of occupational medicine. For example, they require periodic health surveillance of patient-contact personnel; involve numerous occasions of worker exposure to chemical, biological, and physical hazards; and, because they are usually unionized, often are involved in collective bargaining or labor disputes involving benefits. Despite their size, hospitals tend to be very conservative employers and have only rudimentary occupational health services. Directing a hospital employee health service is a good way to observe the good and the bad in occupational medicine practice. It also provides a "captive" patient base for later expansion of services.

Consultation Reports

Writing consultation reports is a special skill that consulting physicians must learn in order to be effective. A good consultation letter should be concise, informative, helpful to the referring physician or agency, and as specific as possible in recommending measures that will benefit the patient.

Two actual letters of consultation are reproduced here. The first (Exhibit 6.1) was prepared by an experienced occupational physician who was involved with a very complicated case. It summarizes the case in enough detail to stand alone as a record, clarifies the issues of primary concern, stipulates what steps were taken with regard to the confidentiality of health information, educates the referring physician without assuming a condescending tone, outlines the recommended management of the case, and ends cordially. Compare this report with the second letter (Exhibit 6.2), which was written by a well qualified specialist at a prestigious medical school. Despite the second clinician's excellent credentials, this consultation report is not as effective as the first.

Exhibit 6.1. Model for Effective Consultation Report
(This consultation report is recommended as an effective model.)

RE: Mr. A.
Dear Dr. B:

Thank you for referring Mr. A to us for evaluation. I have also received the subsequent communication from Dr. C, occupational health physician for the D Corporation. I have discussed with Mr. A the propriety of sharing information with Dr. C and have obtained his written permission to disclose pertinent information. He has no objection and the corporate policy of the D corporation precludes communication of confidential information from the Occupational Health Department to management. Thus, by copy of this letter I am reporting to Dr. C as well in communicating our findings.

Mr. A's history is well known to you but I shall summarize it for the record. He is a 32 year-old male chemical plant worker who since November 1985 has had a series of unexplained abnormalities on blood tests taken as part of his routine periodic health surveillance. The cause of his mild liver function abnormalities is not clear but may be associated with exposure on the job or endogenous causes, of which there are two possibilities. Mr. A has had a persistant abnormality of his serum cholesterol, raising the possibility of an hyperlipoproteinemia. He is also an obligate heterozygote for one of the mucopolysaccharidoses, which affects his son.

His past medical history is unremarkable except that his family history is very strong for coronary artery disease and stroke in all close relatives. He does not smoke and has not drunk alcohol for at least eight years. He is on a diabetic diet but is not taking medication except diclofenac for back pain, as needed. (This drug is known to elevate transaminases and can cause jaundice and hepatitis.) He has no known allergies. He has no history of hepatitis or mononucleosis and has received no transfusions.

Physical examination showed a normal liver span and no palpable spleen. He showed no xanthomata, although he did have hyperpigmentation over his shins.

Examination of his pattern of abnormality shows little discernible pattern with the LDH and the alkaline phosphatase elevated. The transaminases are variably elevated, only once being synchronous, on 18 July 1985. In each case the elevations have been minor, except for the elevated SGPT on that date. By comparison, however, the serum cholesterol has been consistently elevated and the triglycerides have been consistently and markedly elevated. A lipoprotein electropheresis was performed on the request of Dr. C, of the D Corporation, on 27 November 1986. This shows an elevated pre-beta and beta bands interpreted as being either a primary or secondary type IIB pattern.

This presents us with a very interesting diagnostic dilemma.

I have reviewed what little literature exists on the liver function of individuals with this disorder and have consulted with our local University Hereditary Diseases Program in an effort to search out what is known. Liver function abnormality in children affected with the disorder apparently occurs quite late as a result of the storage disease and is nonspecific in its presentation. Although we can find no specific report of heterozygotes being tested for liver function abnormalities, its absence in the early stages of homozygotes strongly argues against its presence in their parents, in the absence of another cause. Logically, there is no reason why the heterozygote condition should interfere with normal liver function. Thus, I think that we can safely dismiss this as a cause of his condition.

Occupational exposures are of concern. His most significant exposure is benzene but there are several other chemicals in the two units in which he works that could be hepatotoxic. In each case, however, for these chemicals to cause liver function abnormalities he would have had to have been exposed at very high

(Continued)

Figure 6.1. Continued

concentrations. Such concentrations do not appear to be at all likely in his workplace. The extremely variable pattern of the abnormality also argues against a
chemical hepatitis since one would expect the transaminases to be more consistently elevated. Thus, I believe that we can conclude that occupational exposure is
unlikely to be the cause.

Mr. A does, clearly, have a type IIB hyperlipoproteinemia and given the family
history, it is almost certainly primary. He clearly is significantly affected clinically
and is at some risk if his elevated serum cholesterol level is not brought under control. It is my conclusion that his unusual pattern of liver function abnormalities
probably is the result of a low-grade fatty liver associated with his hyperlipoproteinemia. This would explain its variable presentation, the lack of associated
clinical abnormalities, the occasional elevation of the alkaline phosphatase (which
would be quite unusual in chemical hepatitis) and its association with the lipid
abnormalities.

Given the history and the relatively benign clinical course of his condition, I
would be reluctant to recommend a liver biopsy. You may, however, be more confident in the diagnosis if a liver scan is performed to rule out a space-occupying
lesion or if a serum 5′-nucleotidase is elevated, confirming the hepatitic origin of
the elevated alkaline phosphatase in the absence of an elevation in the bilirubin,
since this pattern is characteristic of fatty liver. I would suggest following Mr. A very
closely because of his hyperlipoproteinemia but I would consider the liver function
abnormalities a very minor part of the problem likely to correct itself when the lipid
abnormality is brought under control.

Thank you very much for referring this most interesting case. I must say I
enjoyed sorting it out and appreciate the opportunity. Please let me know how he
gets along and please do not hesitate to give me a call if I can be of further
assistance.

Sincerely,
"Doctor E"

Note that in the second consultation letter the clinical description is vague and is
not convincingly associated with the exposures on the job identified by the consulting
physician. This is in part because the consultant appears to have had no idea of what
exposures might have been entailed in the patient's actual job. The note is awkward
in style and there are mistakes (e.g., "symptoms of 3 kinds" when in fact four are given).
The wording (e.g., "These have been present to some degree for over 1 year and thus
are not intermittent...") is vague and rambling and suggests that the particulars of the
case have not been carefully thought through. The findings on physical examination
do not relate to the patient's complaint (e.g., fluid retention is described in the complaint but no mention is made of the presence or absence of edema on examination).
Cystic acne is, of course, very unlikely to be associated with the kinds of chemical
exposure encountered in a department store or following exposure to lacquer, but the
consultant seems to have made no attempt to find this out. Instead, the consultant offers
a very general opinion that could lead to the patient's losing her job. The letter does
not even address the patient's own concerns about monitoring her improvement but
instead reports test results (e.g., pulmonary function tests) that seemingly have nothing to do with her complaints. Finally, the letter is condescending to the referring physician by suggesting that the case be referred to another physician in order to provide
"a continuum of medical attention."

Exhibit 6.2. Example of Ineffective Consultation Report
(The following example is *not recommended* as a response to a serious referral.
It is presented just as it was received.)

Dear Dr. X:
    I examined Ms. Y after reviewing the reports you kindly sent me. Her symptoms
are of 3 kinds.
    1) Eyes—watery, burning, pink to red conjunctivae, swollen lids. Exacerbated after
       visit to department store, around lacquer, handling new clothing. May occur
       during suspected exposure to a chemical of some kind or 2 hours later.
       Other provoking factor—photocopying devices, manufacturing area of her
       present job.
    2) Gagging sensation in throat, soreness in throat. This symptom may be asso-
       ciated with (1) above, and seems to increase with increased concentration of
       chemical.
    3) Rash on face, chest—deep, hard, painful nodules, embarrassing. These have
       been present to some degree for over 1 year and thus are not intermittent, as
       (1) and (2) above.
    4) Accumulation of fluid everywhere, especially the mucus membranes if the reac-
       tions are severe.
    This set of symptomatology is dated from the visits to the Z factory between
March and May, 1982, that were previously documented.
    Environment at home—no unusual exposures or contacts. Has 2 Siamese cats
for many years. Now living alone.
    Mrs. Y wants to know if her reactions can be cumulative and cause permanent
illness. She does not want to undergo standard diagnostic allergy tests, but would
prefer a blood test that could be checked regularly to determine if she is
improving.
    Physical exam: BP 112/80   T = 36.8°C   FEV1 = 2.6 L   FVC = 3.1 L   PEFR = 430 L/M
    EENT, lungs and heart were within normal limits. A cystic acneiform eruption
was present on the cheeks and upper torso.
    Impression: Variable non-specific symptoms attributed to various chemical
exposures dating to a series of work-related factory exposures in March-May 1982.
    Advice:
    1) There is no reason to believe that she should not improve provided that excess
       chemical contacts are avoided.
    2) A personal physician, perhaps an internist, should be obtained in order to give
       Mrs. Y a continuum of medical attention.
    3) She may wish to consult a dermatologist about her skin condition.

Sincerely,
"Doctor F"

The second letter demonstrates how not to write a medical consultation letter. It
incorporates almost every serious mistake a consultant can make, and therefore is well
worth studying as an example of what should be avoided.

Consultation Forms
Just as the consultant has a responsibility to be responsive to the questions being raised,
the referring physician or agency has a responsibility to state clearly what is being asked.
The sample consultation form presented as Form 6.1 contains most of the basic information a consultant in occupational medicine initially needs to know and provides a
convenient format for requesting a consultation when required.

Form 6.1. Request for Consultation

Patient's Name: _____ Insurance #: _____

Address: _____ No Insurance #:   ☐ Check

_____ Phone: _____

Referring Physician: _____ AHCIP Referral #: _____

Address: _____ Physician's Phone: _____

_____ Specialty: _____

Patient's Current Occupation: _____

Occupational Status: ☐ Employed   ☐ Disabled   ☐ Unemployed   ☐ Retired

Chief Complaint: _____

What Questions Do You Wish Us to Address?: (Please use reverse of this sheet if needed.)

_____

_____

_____

_____

_____

Other Physicians Who Have Evaluated Patient For This Problem: _____

_____

_____

Do You Wish Us to Telephone Our Findings Immediately?: ☐ Yes

Date of Request: _____ Doctor's Signature: _____

Multispecialty Group Practices

Multispecialty group practices are organizations in which specialists in compatible areas of medical practice pool expenses and resources. The group may be a single large clinic or a network that includes satellite clinics. Group practices were considered a radical departure for medical practice when they began 60 or 70 years ago, but their numbers are increasing in the United States as practitioners weigh the benefits and costs of solo practice against those of group practice. Group practices have grown explosively, in both numbers and size, and have been in the forefront of the trend toward health maintenance organizations. Developing group practices often participate in health maintenance organizations and similar prepaid plans and base part of their development on the strategy that these "captured" pools of patients are likely to use the group's services on an ongoing basis. Group practices in the United States often enter occupational health services for identical reasons: to "lock-in" large employee populations who will be more likely in the future to use group facilities for personal and family health care. Group managers who adopt this strategy presuppose that these workers are more likely to need personal and family health services rather than occupationally related care, but this practice may lead to serious conflicts of interest and may tend to subordinate occupational health care to other objectives.

Historically, multispecialty group practices have done well in providing occupational health services, in large part because the availability of physicians and ancillary health professionals in major specialties under one roof eliminates the need for referrals outside the group to other clinicians who may not be subject to the controls on cost and utilization that the group has imposed on itself. The group possesses the depth needed to handle most problems within the standards of medical practice, and the wide scope of medical expertise usually available within the group often is complemented by the latest diagnostic equipment, extensive laboratory and x-ray facilities, and a pharmacy. The group may even own or control a hospital or use a nearby hospital for after-hours examination of injured employees. Serious problems requiring hospitalization usually are handled by group physicians with admitting privileges to hospitals, but increasingly groups are opening their own urgent care centers as well. These provide the type of care previously available only in emergency rooms—with the advantage that the group physicians can provide continuity of supervision and enjoy access to medical records.

Multispecialty group practices most often are founded to provide personal health care; often they do not perceive occupational medicine as a high priority until competition becomes intense. Then they rush into developing occupational care without appropriate preparation. The nascent service may find itself subordinated to personal health services whenever decisions are made regarding allocating resources, recruiting staff, marketing, and opening satellites. One way of avoiding this situation is to keep the administrative structure of the occupational health service as autonomous as possible within the group, even at the expense of some duplication. One of the major criticisms by employers of group medical facilities is that injured employees may have to wait longer to be treated because they are competing with non-industrial patients, including children, for available physician time. Administrators who are insensitive to an employer's concern over lost time may see no need to expedite the paperwork of registration and to reduce waiting periods. Furthermore, groups suffering financial problems or poor cash flow also may be tempted to shift overhead expenses onto the apparently lucrative occupational services contracts. In so doing, they raise costs to employers and destroy the attractiveness of the group-based option. (A model demonstration program in occupational medicine is being developed by the Denver-based Center for Research in Ambulatory Health Care Administration for its principal client, the Group Practice Management Association. This activity may provide new or improved approaches to setting up group practices and preliminary data for evaluating them in the future.)

In Canada, multispecialty group practices are less common than in the United States because the health care system does not encourage them. However, where they do exist they tend to be trend setters and often provide at least a limited range of occupational medicine services.

Hospital-Based Occupational Health Clinics

Hospital-based occupational health services are increasingly popular in large metropolitan areas in the United States. Hospitals are setting up services in order to cultivate a patient base likely to enroll in their health maintenance organizations and use the hospital and its outpatient clinics for their personal health care. Some hospitals do a very credible job providing specific occupational health services; others develop their programs more as a marketing device, often merely as extensions of their emergency rooms, with little real commitment of resources or quality assurance.

A 1986 survey conducted by the American Hospital Association (AHA) found that 8 percent of responding institutions had some form of external occupational health service and another 12 percent were planning to introduce such services. Not one hospital in San Diego offered such services in 1974; by 1984, 6 hospitals had occupational health services. Most hospital programs are rudimentary, either an extension of emergency room care or an isolated community outreach program. A few, however, are well developed and comprehensive in their provision of services. For example, Pacific Presbyterian Medical Center in San Francisco has provided an extensive service for a number of years. More recently, community hospitals have entered the field in large numbers. The MedWork Program of Decatur Memorial Hospital in Illinois is an example of an extensive service emphasizing community service and outreach.

The AHA survey also found that most hospitals promote their services through selective business contacts rather than by media advertising. Several hospitals are using occupational health services to build up "wellness" or health promotion programs. Virtually all use the services to increase the use of other hospital departments, such as radiology, clinical specialties, and laboratories. More hospitals are charging on a fee-for-service basis rather than packaging services within a contract. Somewhat under half of the hospitals use both, as determined by the client employer's preferences and circumstances.

The AHA survey report concluded that hospitals reap many benefits from becoming involved in occupational health. Among them are:

- New sources of revenue;
- Heightened awareness of the hospital as a strong community resource for preventive health care;
- Diversification of services;
- Fostering of a strong constituency among such influential groups as business leaders;
- Greater visibility through exposure in the news media;
- Increased utilization of other hospital services;
- Increased referrals for hospital medical staff members;
- Improved hospital employee recruitment opportunities through the addition of attractive employee health and wellness programs; and
- Enhanced opportunity to serve the community's health needs. (Many of these same benefits also accrue to individual physicians and group practices providing occupational health services.)

University teaching hospitals may have additional reasons to become involved, particularly for educational or research purposes, but they, like community hospitals, also are responding to economic realities. Many academically oriented medical centers have offered such services in the past as part of training programs in occupational medicine. These include San Francisco General Hospital (affiliated with the University of California at San Francisco), Harvard, Johns Hopkins, Mount Sinai School of Medicine in New York, and the University of Toronto.

Industrial Medicine Clinics

Industrial medicine clinics are free-standing facilities that are not associated with hospitals or multispecialty group practices. Their patients generally are drawn from local employers with whom they often have contracts for services. They serve many employers, usually in a well defined geographical area, such as a town or an industrial park. They are usually independent operations with a small professional staff, limited facilities, and streamlined procedures designed to facilitate the management of acute injuries and the rehabilitation of temporary disabilities. They emphasize episodic care of acute injuries or illnesses and periodic health evaluations as mandated by law or by company policy; revenues are generated primarily from workers' compensation fees for the former and third-party payments from the employer for the latter. In a few cases, industrial medical clinics have grown quite large and diverse, but usually their growth comes from either budding or merging—by establishing satellites or spin-off clinics and by creating larger health care systems composed of several clinics.

The industrial medicine clinic is characterized by certain basic features: a central facility serving multiple client employers; expansion of medical staff with primary care providers; an emphasis on medical care with less involvement in prevention; close attention to market trends; and a relatively small nursing and support staff. In general, the independent industrial medicine clinics rely on a medical staff and an administrative staff. Line responsibility for administrative functions is vested in a full-time administrator, who establishes systems for financial management and billing, supplies, and personnel. Medical functions are coordinated and supervised by a chief of staff who oversees a full-time medical staff that may consist, in a large clinic, of occupational physicians, general surgeons, primary care practitioners, nurse practitioners, and a part-time affiliated or, less frequently, resident corps of specialists.

A small number of clinics provide industrial hygiene services on a fee-for-service basis. Such services usually do not fit in well with the medical orientation of the clinic, however, and are seldom well utilized. Likewise, mobile clinic vans and contract in-house nurse practitioner services are sometimes available. The relatively low-risk industries that form the principal client base of these clinics usually do not warrant such elaborate and expensive activities.

The specific services provided by industrial medicine clinics often include physiotherapy as well as medical evaluation and treatment. Physiotherapy tends to be intensive for two reasons: the goal is to return the worker to the job as quickly as recovery can be attained and frequent visits to a physiotherapist are useful in monitoring progress. When the worker is sufficiently improved, the physiotherapist can alert the physician at once, without the delay between doctor's appointments that would otherwise result. Because fees for physiotherapy are much less than for medical services, this is more cost-effective and efficient for the insurer, whose primary concern is to return the claimant to work as soon as possible in a condition that will not lead to reinjury or further decline in health.

Employers are naturally anxious to minimize the time an employee spends out of the workplace. Access to radiology and laboratory facilities must be expedited and waiting time minimized. Record handling is best performed by an administrative staff fully conversant with Occupational Safety and Health Administration disclosure guidelines.

Special record formats and questionnaire instruments and the appropriate training of ancillary supporting staff, such as clinic nurses and aides, can relieve the physician of routine low-yield activity.

The concept of an industrial medicine clinic is not new. The Detroit Industrial Clinic, P.C., of Southfield, Michigan, was established in 1920; the Occupational Medical Clinic, Ltd., of Phoenix, Arizona, in 1961. But only in recent years have these clinics become prominent in the United States as providers of occupational health services. Changes in the workers' compensation system and in the health care system in general have made clinics attractive models for entrepreneurs interested in providing direct health care services in settings with low overhead. However, excessive emphasis on profits has led some critics to charge that industrial medical clinics have little regard for the quality of care provided and little commitment to preventive services, which typically are more expensive and less appealing to employers seeking to contain short-term costs.

The very term "industrial medical clinic" is problematical. Clinics generally are identified as such by the operators themselves, despite the disfavor within the specialty of occupational medicine over the phrase "industrial medicine." Very likely, retention of the term "industrial" is a defensive position, since seldom does the staff include specialists in occupational medicine. Also, "industrial" may be construed as showing an affinity for the employer whereas "occupational" may suggest some consideration of workers' point of view. In most cases, however, either the name is a holdover from past practice or the founders themselves did not consider the implications of the term.

The proliferation of industrial medicine clinics in the United States has had dramatic effects on the delivery of occupational health services. Such clinics have allowed small businesses easy access to services and have consolidated into a viable format services previously rendered by individual private practitioners. The operation and staffing of these clinics are of concern, however. These clinics are intensely competitive and frequently bid against one another for contracts to provide care to the employees of corporations and public agencies. The resultant isolation and veil of secrecy have impeded professional dialogue and sharing of case information. Even more disturbing is the frequent lack of involvement by occupational medicine specialists in these clinics — their absence suggests that prevention and knowledgeable consultation are subordinated to episodic acute care.

There are a few exemplary industrial clinics and some individual physicians doing credible clinical work at otherwise undistinguished clinics. Yet concerns with professional qualification and the entrepreneurial style of many of these facilities have raised doubts about the quality of care they provide. In the absence of evaluable data on treatment and outcome, these doubts cannot be readily rebutted. The closed and secretive nature of many, particularly proprietary, clinics makes objective evaluation exceedingly difficult. No broadly recognized accreditation body exists for this sector of health care — industrial medical clinics may be the largest sector of American medical practice to exist outside of a formal or informal network of communication, representation, and peer contact that promote quality assurance.

The rise of the industrial medicine clinic over the past two decades has been almost entirely overlooked in the medical literature. Whatever their limitations, industrial medicine clinics have clearly proven themselves to be an economically successful format thus far. Yet although the clinic is the dominant occupational health care provider in many American communities, it is coming under pressure from such competitors as urgent care centers. Urgent care centers are growing at an even more rapid rate and offer a convenient alternative for the provision of episodic acute care and routine general services. Such centers have a broader base of patients and are usually supported by the financial and marketing resources of much larger organizations. In at least one case in California, a corporate body that owns urgent care centers has successfully competed for a contract to provide in-plant occupational health services. Even if occupational health services represent only a small fraction of the total volume of services provided by urgent care centers, their share of the market for such services may become considerable in a very short time. The absence of even a nominal claim to special expertise in occupational health care on the part of most urgent care centers is, therefore, disturbing.

Further Reading

American Hospital Association: Profile of Hospital Occupational Health Services. Chicago, American Hospital Association, 1986.

Begin C, Demers L: Quebec's multi-instititional health arrangements. Health Management Forum (Toronto), Winter 1986, pp. 31–42.

Conrad DE, Parker-Conrad JE: Hospital-based occupational health programs. AAOHN (American Association of Occupational Health Nurses) Journal 1987; 35:251–253.

Cullen MR: Occupational medicine: A new focus for general internal medicine. Arch Intern Med 1985; 145:511–5.

Freshnock LJ, Jensen LE: The changing structure of medical group practice in the United States, 1969 to 1980. JAMA 1981; 245:2173–2176.

Guidotti TL: The private sector and occupational health. Health Management Forum (Toronto) Summer 1987; 8(2):26–34.

Guidotti TL: Desirable characteristics of the teaching occupational medicine clinic. J Occup Med 1984; 26:105–109.

Guidotti TL: Interaction between a medical group and a school of public health: A case study of a productive affiliation. Amer J Prev Med 1985; 1:30–35.

Guidotti TL: The general internist and occupational medicine. J Gen Intern Med 1986; 1:201–202.

Huston P: Group practice: Poised to flourish — at last. Medical Economics 1983; 212–229.

Moxley JH III, Roeder PC: New opportunities for out-of-hospital health services. New Engl J Med 1984; 310:193–197.

Rosenstock L, Heyer NH: Emergence of occupational medical services outside the workplace. Amer J Indust Med 1982; 3:217–223.

7 PREPARING FOR AN OCCUPATIONAL MEDICINE PRACTICE

Occupational medicine is that specialty that identifies, treats, and, in particular, seeks to prevent disorders related to work, and that promotes positive measures to improve the health and fitness of workers and the working population. This medical specialty has existed for almost three centuries; curiously, however, occupational medicine remains unfamiliar to many physicians. It is one of the oldest boarded specialties in the United States, but since its inception has had a low visibility and, despite explosive development over the last 10 years, remains a small specialty. Although it is one of the most dynamic and rapidly advancing areas of medicine, most of its challenges and accomplishments are scarcely known to outsiders.

The past history of occupational medicine has been rocky. The specialty regularly cycles from respectability to apathy, often within a decade or two. It has had to live down past abuses and image problems, and a general perception of stagnation in the 1960s. The present cycle of expansion began in 1970, stimulated by an increased government role, the response of industry to rising costs, and certain scientific advances in toxicology and epidemiology. In past years, the emphasis in occupational medicine has shifted strongly in the direction of prevention and health promotion.

The expansion of occupational medicine practice has created some unique problems. The growth of small "industrial medicine clinics" that provide services to smaller businesses that lack resources to hire full-time occupational health personnel has been rapid and poorly monitored. Quality control has therefore emerged as a major issue. Meanwhile, the conscientious occupational physician must continually integrate new advances in toxicology, epidemiology, immunology, oncology, and clinical medicine, and must constantly explain his or her actions and thinking in basic lay terms.

The organized specialty of occupational medicine is now at a crossroads because the supply of trained and interested physicians falls far short of demand. An expanding demand for occupational health services has led other medical specialists and primary care practitioners, including internists, to become more involved in the specialty.

Relatively few physicians in North America (about 1,000 in the United States and somewhat over 100 in Canada) have specialty credentials in occupational medicine. These paltry numbers make clear that for some time to come physicians will continue to move into the field from other specialties or from primary care practice. Presently, most occupational physicians enter occupational medicine practice from other specialty practices, particularly family medicine, internal medicine, and general surgery. In many ways, occupational medicine is a primary care specialty for employed adults. Academically, its board examination and training programs are handled as a subspecialty of preventive medicine.

Increasingly, primary care physicians are advised to become involved in occupational medicine, and many physicians have begun to practice in an occupational health service. Although these physicians may not consider themselves occupational medicine specialists, they are practicing occupational medicine.

Especially in institutional settings, physicians who are new to the organization, phasing in retirement, or seeking new roles have been assigned to head occupational health services, regardless of their background. The best of them can be very good indeed, but seldom are they prepared for the challenges they will face in providing occupational health services. Indeed, they often do not have the insight to see where improvements might be made or to understand why their practice of occupational medicine is less than optimal. As in any aspect of medicine, a commitment to the provision of good health care is a prerequisite for a satisfying and satisfactory practice. A professional commitment to this field will yield handsome benefits but only if properly oriented to the complex technical and social aspects of the field.

Occupational Medicine as a Specialty

Physicians who have approached occupational medicine in a spirit of inquiry and discipline have found many opportunities for research and for a satisfying and demanding practice, particularly in academic and group practice settings. The key to success in this effort, however, is a willingness to learn the specific technical content of occupational medicine and to recognize the existing structure and institutions of the field. Those who are prepared to do so and who are committed to the field will find it challenging and rewarding.

In practice, most occupation-related disorders are injuries on the job. These disorders, and the performance of periodic health examinations, are usually what is meant by the now-obsolete term "industrial medicine." Occupational medicine embraces these functions and the management of occupation-related diseases, and places new emphasis on the prevention of health hazards in the workplace and on strategies for health promotion. The types of medical cases typically encountered by the occupational physician include dermatological problems, eye conditions, respiratory disorders, poisonings due to hazardous chemicals, cancer related to work exposure, and neuropathies. In addition, employee assistance programs and health promotion programs may be supervised by the occupational physician.

The physician working in occupational health services must face certain challenges:

- Fixed fee schedules in workers' compensation cases. In some jurisdictions, fees are low compared to personal health care services.
- Competition in fee schedules for discretionary services. Services not covered by workers' compensation are usually priced low in order to attract client employers.

- Difficulties in marketing prevention-oriented services. Employers are not always sold on the value of prevention.
- Labor-management interaction. The position of the occupational physician, standing between the worker and management, complicates some issues.
- Large administrative burden and frequent involvement in litigation. Many physicians do not wish to become involved in cases that may require extensive medico-legal involvement.
- Frequent ethical dilemmas. (This subject is discussed in detail in Chapter 4.)
- Infrequent recognition and reward for outstanding quality of care.
- Lack of recognition and institutional support for excellence in sponsoring institutions, particularly hospitals and medical groups.
- Disproportionate weight played by marketing, rather than medical, factors in success.

Although compensation for services can be low in some states and rates are often set in competition, a well managed occupational health service can be very profitable. The greatest drawback to the field, however, is the lack of understanding, appreciation, and interest among other physicians and administrators.

The world of occupational medicine is different from most other specialties. Rarely does an occupational physician admit a patient to the hospital, for example. The practice of occupational medicine can be very disconcerting to physicians who are oriented to traditional primary care; teamwork, administrative ability, and versatility in handling different types of complaints play a greater role here. Just as a surgeon relies on the operating room team, the occupational physician soon finds that he or she depends heavily on other groups of skilled health professionals, such as occupational health nurses, safety engineers, and industrial hygienists, each with its own training, certification, and licensing arrangements.

The complexities of medical practice are further exacerbated for the occupational physician, who must deal continually with strong economic, political, and social pressures, including workers' compensation, disability claims, law suits, government regulations, labor-management relations, budgeting, and other issues far removed from usual office practice.

Preliminaries to Practice

There are several compelling justifications for physicians in primary care specialities, such as general internal medicine and family medicine, to become involved in occupational medicine. These include a responsibility to give attention to an important determinant of their patients' health; the need to reverse past neglect and indifference; the substantial opportunities for creative research; the compatibility of occupational medicine with primary care practice; and the need to expand and improve the quality of occupational health care in community settings. It seems clear that all physicians, not just occupational medicine specialists, who choose to enter into this type of practice stand to benefit from the relative openness of occupational medicine as compared to other areas of medical practice. However, concomitant with this opportunity is a responsibility to apply to occupational medicine the same professional dedication and standards that traditionally have been applied to the skills drawn from other specialty fields, such as office gynecology, when they fall within primary care practice.

A physician seeking to enter occupational medicine from another type of practice should:

- Become informed about the field.
- Define personal and practice objectives.
- Review the profile and needs of local industry.
- Become knowledgeable regarding local occupational health problems.
- Plan the proposed service.
- Identify staff, facilities, and resources.

Ideally, these steps should be taken in the order given. Unfortunately the sequence is all too often precisely the reverse. A hospital, group, or clinic may decide to open an occupational medicine facility using whatever resources are at hand, next conduct a market survey to determine how to sell the service, and only then put a physician in charge who may or may not have a clear idea of the objectives of the service and of the field as a whole. Such an approach clearly is not recommended.

The proper strategy is to plan the service methodically, with informed leadership from the outset. Institutions that want to enter the field should be agreeable to allowing the physician to prepare for practice in a new field and should be ready to release the physician from other duties while this preparation is underway.

Becoming Informed

Initially, some assistance can be obtained from consultants who are knowledgeable about occupational health services; eventually it will be necessary to have a local "expert" direct the enterprise. There are many ways to gain the specific expertise necessary for a successful and satisfying practice that incorporates occupational health care. Some medical schools, such as the University of Cincinnati and the University of California at San Francisco, have condensed "mini-residencies" in occupational medicine. (These are not true residencies and are not necessarily accepted by certification bodies, but require a full-time commitment for several weeks.) The American College of Occupational Medicine sponsors a Basic Curriculum in Occupational Medicine, an intensive three-part course. The Medical College of Wisconsin has developed the Academic Program in Occupational Medicine, a comprehensive, self-paced extension curriculum that relies on tutorials, interactive computer systems, and proctored examinations that provide the equivalent of a year-long academic program for practicing physicians and even awards an accredited master's degree in public health. Many medical schools and the major specialty organizations sponsor continuing education programs, any one of which is usually strong on either scientific or administrative aspects of occupational medicine practice (but rarely both). Continuing education for nursing staff involved in the clinic or office is also well worthwhile and should be budgeted for. Visits to the better clinics are very valuable; and discussions are likely to be more candid if one goes out of town. Whenever the opportunity arises, the physician should arrange for plant tours and visits to industrial sites in order to follow changing conditions in the workplace and to observe different industries. Staying current requires reading at least one major textbook in the field and following the journal literature (principally the *Journal of Occupational Medicine* and the *American Journal of Industrial Medicine*).

At some point, the physician who intends to enter medicine full-time will have to consider whether to become board certified. In the United States, the American Board of Preventive Medicine (ABPM) certifies specialists in occupational medicine after a formal residency. There is no pathway to certification in the United States that does not require a physician to interrupt practice and return to a residency. In Canada, the Royal College of Physicians and Surgeons, like the ABPM, examines and certifies specialists who complete a formal residency. In addition, however, the Canadian Board of Occupational Medicine examines and certifies specialists in the field after preparation by nontraditional routes, such as part-time courses, self-study, and supervised experience. Table 7.1 provides the addresses of these certifying agencies.

Defining Personal and Practice Objectives

Physicians or managers of health care facilities may choose to enter occupational medicine practice for any number of reasons:

- To develop an additional source of revenue or patients for general care;
- To meet a need for services in community;
- To develop clinical research opportunities;
- To establish a base for education and training; or
- To satisfy personal interests.

Although the physician's professional objectives are critical to the ultimate success of the service, they are seldom well defined. If the primary objective of the occupational health service is to serve as a source of financial revenue, it will be structured differently and have different expectations for performance than if it is set up to meet a community need or to support education. Services set up for profitable operation will need to specify objectives in order to target certain industries and to plan for anticipated growth. If the objective of the clinic is to generate referrals, it will be staffed differently than if it is to be self-contained.

Considerable confusion may arise when objectives are not spelled out. For example, in one typical case involving a large group practice the new occupational health service was heavily criticized by others within the group. It was criticized by the specialists for failing to meet their expectations for referrals; by the family practitioners for creating complications in the satellite clinics because of the need to separate occupational from personal health services; by the administration for wasting time on providing preventive services that were not well compensated; and by the support staff for disrupting the comfortable routine. But when the occupational health service brought in 1,500 new patients, accounting for more than 10 percent of the revenues for the group, the organizers were vindicated.

Understanding Local Needs and Problems

The organizers of an occupational health service must ascertain the types and frequency of the disorders they are most likely to encounter, as well as the risks peculiar to the industries they aim to serve. Hearing conservation and noise control programs merit particular attention, because excessive exposure to noise is a problem common to many industries and workplaces and noise-induced hearing loss is an entirely preventable occupational disorder. Noise-induced hearing loss is one occupational disorder that virtually all services must be prepared to recognize and prevent. Other occupational illnesses vary with the specific hazards of the industry and cannot be generalized

Table 7.1. Examining and Certifying Bodies in the Specialty of Occupational Medicine

United States
American Board of Preventive Medicine
c/o Wright State University
School of Medicine
P.O. Box 927
Dayton, OH 45401
(513) 278-6915

Canada
Royal College of Physicians and Surgeons of Canada
74 Stanley St.
Ottawa, Ontario K1M 1P4
(613) 746-8177

Canadian Board of Occupational Medicine
c/o Medical Services
290 Yonge Street
Toronto, Ontario M5B 1C8

easily. An occupational health service must know in advance what to expect and must be prepared to deal with what comes.

The occupational health service also must be knowledgeable about the nonmedical characteristics of local industry in order to be responsive to community needs. Such knowledge comes from learning about the relationships among major employers in the area; the organization and ownership of local industries; and the special features of the workforce with respect to ethnicity, level of education, socioeconomic class, and unusual patterns of disease prevalence. Good sources of information are local chambers of commerce, local newspapers, the reference sections of local libraries, schools of business, and by interviews with corporate leaders.

One may think one knows a great deal about the economic base of the community, but there are often surprises. The presence of one or two major factories in a community may obscure the extent to which the local economy is dependent on other enterprises—automotive repair and servicing, fast food operations, agriculture, tourism (including hotels and motels), and medical care (a major industry in its own right). Each of these businesses generates a sufficient rate of injuries and illnesses to require occupational health services.

Planning the Service and Identifying Resources
The staff is perhaps the most critical element in starting up a new occupational health service. Planning for the service must include identifying essential roles and staff positions and then filling them with the most qualified and suitable people who can be recruited. Too often, positions are defined around the perceived strengths or limitations of the staff who happen to be available at the time, regardless of whether these people have any interest or background in the field. Often they enter their new positions without even a formal job description and go on to merely recreate their old roles and habits. There is nothing wrong with reassigning employees who have shown their

worth, but the occupational health service must never be a dumping ground for redundant personnel.

Similarly, occupational health facilities are often started up with bits and pieces and spare equipment. If the organization is not prepared to give the service the same support due any clinical activity, it should question its reasons for entering the field.

There should be a sense of mission about the occupational health service. It should play an important role within both the life of the community and its home institution. The physician in charge should be seen as a pioneer, not an outsider. Too often, the job is given to an otherwise qualified and well meaning physician or surgeon who is poorly prepared in this field or about to retire. The occupational health service is not well served by such actions and will never reach its potential unless its leadership is strong, committed, forward-looking, and commands respect.

Further Reading

American College of Physicians Department of Health and Public Policy: Role of the internist in occupational medicine: A position paper of the American College of Physicians. Philadelphia, American College of Physicians, 14 September 1984.

Cullen MR: Occupational medicine. A new focus for general internal medicine. Arch Intern Med 1985; 145:511–515.

Graduate Medical Educational National Advisory Committee: GMNAC Summary Report. Hyattsville, Maryland: Health Resources Administration, U.S. Department of Health and Human Services, 1980.

Guidotti TL: Occupational medicine at a crossroads. ACP Observer American College of Physicians, January, 1984; 4:5.

Guidotti TL: The general internist and occupational medicine. Gen Intern Med 1986; 1:201–202.

Preventive Health Care Committee of the Society for Research and Education in Primary Care Internal Medicine: Preventive medicine in general internal medicine residency training. Ann Intern Med 1985; 102:859–861.

Rosenstock L: Occupational medicine: Too long neglected. Ann Intern Med 1981: 95:774–776.

8

MARKETING SERVICES

Increasingly, sound marketing has become the key to the survival—not just the prosperity—of multiemployer occupational health services. Until the mid-1970s, marketing was considered a dirty word by physicians and hospital administrators. Medical care was viewed as a professional service performed in a setting of mutual respect between the patient and the medical care provider. Twenty years ago, physicians more or less dictated to their patients what services they would consume and insurance companies paid the bill without complaint. The physician would prescribe a treatment or specify a diagnostic test without much regard for the opinions of the patient. Issues of comfort or adaptation to life were considered secondary matters not part of the professional responsibility of the primary health care practitioner. The idea that physicians or medical facilities might be in competition for the same patient was seldom voiced openly.

This attitude has changed dramatically in most metropolitan and many rural areas of the United States. In the current competitive environment, marketing is viewed as necessary, both to preserve financial viability and to respond to patients' needs in a timely manner. The latter role of marketing is just as important as the former, salesmanship aspect. Health care facilities and individual physicians not only must convince the public that their provision of medical care is superior or more desirable, but also must accommodate the needs and preferences of patients and their families. They must do so to retain their share of the "market" of patients seeking medical services. What is required in this effort is a good deal more than just redecorating the waiting room and subscribing to a wider range of magazines. Retaining market share may entail introducing classes, group discussions, and patient education programs; providing services that aid in daily living; relocating to quarters that are more convenient for patients; and making changes in billing and other business procedures.

Needs Assessment

Marketing must be considered as a means of not only promoting a product or service but also determining what the consumers of that product or service require. Ultimately, marketing requires adapting to the needs of the consumer. Applied to health care, marketing implies listening to the consumers of medical care and shaping services to the convenience or benefit of the user.

The distinction between consumer and user is an important one: the "consumer" who selects and purchases a health service may not be the same as the "user," as when an employer arranges for services to be provided to workers. (Unless they are ill or injured, workers may not even be "patients" in the usual sense but more akin to "subjects," as when they are participating in a screening or surveillance program.) Employers who enter into contracts with medical facilities in order to obtain basic medical care select the provider on criteria that are quite different from the criteria applied by a patient seeking a personal physician. The quality of medical services, unless very poor, is difficult for the layperson to evaluate except on superficial grounds. Employers therefore are more likely to select a provider of occupational medical care on the basis of cost and convenience of location and hours. In most cases, they will not attempt the difficult task of comparing the equipment in medical facilities or the qualifications of the staff. Primary services required in occupational health programs, such as the acute care of work-related injuries or the provision of routine screening evaluations, do not even require elaborate or sophisticated facilities and specialized expertise. So employers first and foremost look for the provision of prompt basic acute care and inexpensive periodic or preplacement evaluations. The identification of occupational diseases, the appropriate application of rehabilitation services, and the provision of prevention-oriented services are secondary considerations in the minds of most managers.

A prime requisite in satisfying both the needs of the employer and the expectations of workers is time: minimal waiting time for workers and short turn-around in reporting findings and processing paperwork. Superb diagnostic skills among the physicians at the clinic may seldom be used and rarely appreciated, but considerations of timeliness and good patient flow often determine the success or failure of a clinic.

A marketing representative can help collect feedback on the use of occupational health strategies. When a clinic is just getting started, however, door-to-door data collection is an expensive and inefficient strategy. A simple survey of area employers is a less expensive alternative and puts literature in the hands of the appropriate company managers at an early stage for marketing purposes. A survey also suggests that an occupational health facility is concerned about the needs of local industry and is making a genuine effort to be responsive.

Surveys have their limitations. They can be very useful in determining the needs of a community or in evaluating the changing needs and the perceptions of current clients. They are not scientific studies, however, and rarely achieve high return rates from busy and distracted managers. Return rates of 15 to 20 percent are usual for these surveys. Nevertheless, just by distributing the survey questionnaires, an occupational health service will have conveyed a positive, businesslike impression to the managers receiving them.

The survey questionnaire provided as Appendix 4 has been tested several times in the field and has achieved an unusually high rate of return (between 20 and 30 percent). While not acceptable for purposes of scientific accuracy and validity, this return rate is substantially better than most direct-mail marketing surveys. The Survey on Occupational Health Services is intended to determine the perceived need for various occupational health services emphasizing medical care (Part I) and the employer's use of facilities and occupational health personnel (Part II), as well as provide the respondents with an opportunity to express their own feelings and to communicate their own sense of priorities (Parts III and IV). The survey can be designed to provide anonymity to the respondent or can be used openly.

A for-profit clinic, or a satellite providing occupational health services, should be established only as a commercial venture, never as a means of penetrating a new community for the purpose of expanding the patient base for personal health care. Occupational health services should not be used as a "inducement" to consolidate the position of a facility in the community. To do so subordinates the commitment to provide occupational health services and ultimately undermines the quality of services and the attitude of the staff.

The economic viability of a new facility can be enhanced in advance by agreements with employers — either informal letters of agreement or formal contracts. Most employers prefer the former, a non-binding agreement that allows them to use the services of the new satellite on a trial basis and according to a specified fee schedule.

An occupational health service must respect the physician-patient relationship and maintain the ethical standards common to all health care facilities, including the duties to retain medical records and provide respectful services. However, the management of occupational injuries and illnesses represents a different commitment to health care than is expected in a family practice setting, one that does not imply a standard of continuing care. Just as the occupational health clinic cannot ask employer clients and workers for an emotional bond of loyalty, it should display little sentimentality over decisions affecting the continuity of care to clients and their workers. Satellites that are not economically successful should be closed within a reasonable time period and their resources used elsewhere.

The exception to this general rule comes when a community is expanding rapidly. In this case, it may be desirable to establish a base of operations early on in order to preempt competition. Since a larger organization has resources that a smaller competitor would lack, a hospital or large medical group practice can ride out as an operating expense a longer period of underutilization than could be absorbed by a smaller clinic. Of course, this stategy is fundamentally dependent on sound marketing and the selection of a good location. Wrong decisions may prove disastrous when a commitment has been made to a location that turns out to be ill advised.

Principles of Marketing

Five concepts underlie the marketing of occupational health services and render it different from the marketing of personal health services:

- Locate the facility where the workers work, not where their families live.

- Respond to local needs and prepare the facility to give good service to local employers and their workers.
- Develop a mix of large and small employer clients.
- Keep occupational and personal health services strictly separate.
- Communicate with employer clients as regularly as possible.

Location

Many physicians, attempting to provide both personal and occupational health care within the same facility, locate in areas where the growth in residential population is likely to be greatest. Residential population in a neighborhood means little in the provision of occupational health services, because workers often live some distance away from their jobs, seldom in the same neighborhood. Clinics or other facilities that are placed in a residential community to serve an expanding patient base for general medical services often are in a poor position to provide occupational health care to workers in industrial districts.

Building up an occupational health service requires taking the facility and programs to the worker. The employer will not send workers long distances for care if alternatives are closer. Most routine occupational health services do not require extensive specialty care and are perceived as basic medical practice, within the capability of any qualified physician. Right or wrong, "adequate" is considered good enough by managers contemplating using a certain clinic; an excellent reputation often counts for little if the injured worker is not regarded as requiring specialized care. This attitude also holds true for periodic health evaluations (except for executives), preemployment evaluations, and other forms of fitness-to-work evaluations. Most managers assume that a physical examination is all that is required and believe that any competent physician can perform one.

Locations best suited for occupational health services are areas of high industrial growth. In particular, lower technology industries, such as assembly line manufacturing or automotive repair, tend to produce more work-related injuries and illnesses than capital-intensive high technology or automated industries. Table 8.1 illustrates the difference in injury rates for various industries in California. Labor-intensive industries, particularly those employing large numbers of untrained or partly trained workers with a high turnover (such as fast food operations or automotive repair shops) tend to produce more acute injuries. Generally speaking, lower technology manufacturing industries are more likely to generate large numbers of occupational injuries, while higher technology industries often present exotic problems in toxicology. Virtually all industries, including financial or information services with mostly desk jobs, generate large numbers of back complaints. Office operations and financial or information services are comfortable with a larger proportion of preventive and educational programs and may create a greater demand for health promotion activities.

Industries tend to congregate. Large employers will often be surrounded by many smaller ones, providing support services and goods. In many cities, the downtown area has become the center for finance, management, government, communications, and information. Retailing and manufacturing-related industries have moved to the periphery. Older health facilities serving the downtown area must determine whether the mix of services they have provided in the past is now appropriate. They also must consider where their local industrial base is going in the area.

Table 8.1. Injury Rates by Industry, California, 1980[1]

Industry[2]	Total No. of Injuries	Disabling Injuries per 1,000 Workers
Mining	3,706	85.2
Construction	33,607	75.6
Transportation and Public Utilities	24,187	48.7
Manufacturing	97,381	48.5
Finance, Insurance, and Real Estate[3]	6,571	10.5
Agriculture	18,298	46.9[4]

1. Source: California Work Injuries and Illnesses 1980. Sacramento, Division of Labor Statistics and Research, August 1982.
2. These industries represent 30% of the workforce, but are responsible for 43% of lost time injuries.
3. Given for comparison.
4. Because most agricultural workers are not covered under workers' compensation and may include casual workers, this is probably an underestimate.

A case in point is a clinic established by a large group practice in a commercial development on the periphery of a large suburb in a major metropolitan area. The location was selected as convenient for both industry in an adjoining city and young families in a residential area of that same suburb. On a map, it appeared to be close to a concentration of homes and to a very large industrial district. However, the building housing the clinic was accessible only by car—it was separated by a hill from a local housing development and by enormous parking lots from a shopping center. Mothers with children, the disabled, the elderly, and those dependent on public transportation all found the location highly inconvenient. The major employer in the area never sent injured workers to the clinic because several physicians were within a shorter distance by car. The drive across town took 15 minutes in normal traffic, even though this employer was on the same street. Professional marketing services costing thousands of dollars were engaged to promote the use of the clinic but had little effect. After three years, the satellite closed; during those three years, several small industrial medicine clinics established themselves much closer to the major employer, which was the primary market for occupational health services.

Responsiveness

Occupational health services must be responsive to local needs. For example, as downtown industry is replaced by a clean, white-collar office and service workforce, the demand for health services will change radically. Expanding an existing clinic in the downtown area may be less advisable than, for example, developing a satellite in a rapidly growing suburb. A downtown location may continue to make sense if prevention-oriented and health promotion programs are added to the range of services already available. While the type of industry in the area will be the key factor in generating demand for services, some problems, such as back pain, are found in virtually every industry and office.

More entrepreneurial health services frequently are tempted to market a service before making the investment necessary to provide it. By doing so, they can determine whether the demand justifies introducing the new service. This tendency must be avoided because it destroys the credibility of the clinic in the long term. Services that are being marketed must be in place before they are heavily promoted. The facility must not risk earning a reputation for unreliability among local employers.

Diversification

Whenever possible, the employer clients served should represent a mix of industry size and type. Although it is certainly desirable to have a few large clients to ensure a large volume of services, there is a real danger in depending on a few big contracts that could disappear overnight. This is particularly true if those employers are in the same industry and are subject to the same economic trends. Successful occupational health services usually develop a mix of large and small businesses, in a variety of industries. Small business, of course, is "big" business in the aggregate and is just as important as big business itself in supporting a stable and profitable occupational health service.

Separation

Occupational health services must be separated from personal health services. The types of services needed in an occupational setting are very different from those needed in residential communities, where childhood illnesses and accidents and the health problems of the aging are the order of the day. Occupational and personal health services tend to mix poorly in the same facility and attempts to blend the two are often sources of dissatisfaction on the part of patients, workers, employers, and even staff. Mixing patients suffering occupational disorders with patients awaiting general medical and pediatric care causes unavoidable delays annoying to employers, long waiting lines abhorred by both workers and employers, and a discourteous attitude on the part of the staff resented by workers. Even when she is given priority, a harried mother with screaming children may not appreciate learning that the physician is busy with a routine fitness-to-work evaluation, even though the worker has been waiting for hours. Furthermore, creating a two-class system of medical care within the office promotes an attitude on the part of the staff that the patient is "just an industrial." This attitude can affect the length of time workers are kept waiting, the promptness with which their paperwork is handled, and even the courtesy with which they are treated.

There is no equitable way to get around this problem. Patients who are waiting to be seen, especially with children, unfortunately feel slighted when workers, often with minor or inapparent health problems, pass through the waiting room and bypass the lineup. Giving priority to workers simply does not work in a clinic situation. Employers, on the other hand, expect rapid reporting, fast service, and adequate quality of care. Time off the job because of injuries or routine evaluations costs the employer money that the smaller business particularly can ill afford to lose. Uncertainty over how long the employee will be away from work compounds the loss, by causing confusion, inefficiency, and difficulty meeting production schedules. It is best to insist on a strict separation whenever possible between occupational health services and general medical services, preferably by separating the two into different facilities altogether. Even for a small private practice, waiting rooms should not be shared if occupational health services are more than a small fraction of the total number of cases.

Communication

Communication with employer clients is of utmost importance. If employers are dissatisfied with the service provided them, they often will simply send injured workers elsewhere. The manager handling occupational health services has a responsibility to act in the best interest of the employer and feels that he or she owes the health facility no explanation. It is therefore very important to cultivate clear lines of communication with the representatives of employer clients, as well as with workers using the facilities, to ensure that their needs are being met in a satisfactory manner.

One way to promote such communication is by circulating a newsletter to staff responsible for workers' compensation and occupational health matters in each employer's organization. This makes the health care facility less anonymous and promotes a more personalized relationship that is more difficult to break without explanation. These newsletters give tips on health that can be reproduced in company newsletters, news of the health care facility and its personnel, and items of interest to local industry regarding occupational health, all the while reinforcing a positive image of the clinic. Newsletters should be written and produced as professionally as possible.

An even better way to communicate is direct face-to-face contact between marketing representatives and managers. Physicians should not be used for this purpose; many physicians are not good at public relations and their time is much too expensive to use in on-site visits beyond the initial assessment of the needs of a new client. Physicians also are often perceived as threatening and imposing to non-physicians and will usually be treated more formally and with less candor than a non-physician. A good marketing representative, on the other hand, can visit at regular intervals and will get a more candid view of problems or complaints. The best marketing representatives for occupational health facilities are relatively conservative in appearance, convey a professional manner, have some health-related experience, and are willing to work closely with the professional staff of the facility. Because they are trained in both health and marketing, albeit in another context, former pharmaceutical representatives are often excellent candidates for clinic marketing representatives.

Properly trained and instructed, a marketing representative can serve as the eyes and ears as well as the human face of the health care facility. Even so, caution must be exercised to keep the overenthusiastic types in line. Turning marketing responsibilities over to a contractor or independent representative without supervision can be a very dangerous—and expensive—proposition. Marketing representatives must not oversell the capabilities of the clinic and must not be too quick to agree to employers' requests for specific services, since some of them may be ill-advised or even unethical. For example, one clinic discovered that its marketing representative had negotiated a contract with an employer client that committed it, on paper, to perform routine back X-rays on new employees for screening purposes. The marketing representative did not know that this procedure is no longer considered acceptable practice in occupational medicine. The representative had spent considerable effort persuading local industry that there was need for this unnecessary and questionable service and had put the clinic in an extremely embarrassing position.

Figure 8.1. A "market cube" presents the following three dimensions of occupational health services: range of service, users of service, and level of service. Each subdivision of the cube represents a particular level of a particular service provided to a given category of user.

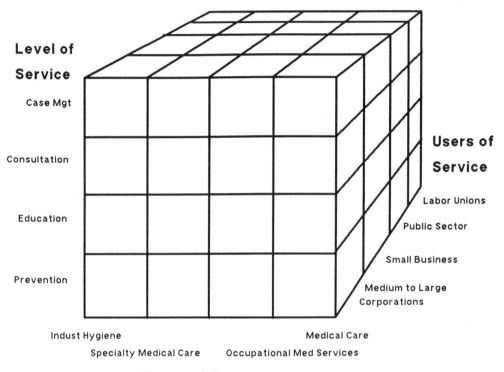

Level of Service

Case Mgt

Consultation

Education

Prevention

Users of Service

Labor Unions

Public Sector

Small Business

Medium to Large Corporations

Indust Hygiene

Specialty Medical Care   Occupational Med Services

Medical Care

Range of Service

Services Offered

A sound marketing strategy requires a knowledge of the range and levels of services that can be provided and the potential users of each of these services.

Figure 8.1 is a diagram known as a "marketing cube" that allows a three-dimensional representation of the possible combinations of levels of service, range of services, and users or "consumers" of these services. Bringing these three dimensions into one illustration helps to visualize the possibilities and opportunities for growth.

The range of services, presented in the horizontal dimension, is the easiest to conceptualize:

- *Medical care,* as used here, includes routine health services usually performed on-site in a large employer's facilities, including first aid and acute care.
- *Industrial hygiene services* are provided not by physicians but by industrial hygienists trained for the purpose. (See Chapter 1.) These assessments, measurements, and

engineering functions must be provided on-site, usually supported by a laboratory elsewhere.

- *Specialty medical care* is rendered on a referral basis for special problems.
- *Occupational medicine services* include specialty care provided by occupational physicians, particularly fitness-to-work evaluations, health surveillance, and health monitoring.

Occupational health clinics providing services for multiple employers usually emphasize basic medical care and occupational medicine services. Large group practices are also in a strong position to provide specialty medical care. However, relatively few facilities provide industrial hygiene services together with medical care. If they are not available in-house, employers hire consultants to provide them with the industrial hygiene services they need. This split between medical and engineering services may not be logical or efficient from the standpoint of resolving the employer's problem, but it reflects the different professional roles of the physician and the engineer. In cases where industrial hygiene services have been offered by medical clinics, they often have been undervalued or subordinated to the medical services, despite the critical role of industrial hygienists in controlling hazards. One means of dealing with this problem is for the clinic to enter into a joint venture or special relationship with an industrial hygiene consulting firm.

The level of services, on the vertical axis, represents a continuum:

- *Direct case management* includes the familiar components of diagnosis, treatment, rehabilitation, and follow-up. The management of specific problems that arise in the workplace, such as hazards that have been identified or clusters of health problems suggesting that a hazard must be searched for, requires direct intervention to correct the situation.
- *Consultation* is a less direct intervention, and requires particular insight and expertise into not only the problem but also the needs, motivations, and resources of those asking for assistance.
- *Education* includes not only formal training sessions but also opportunities to increase the awareness and sophistication of clients so that they will value more highly the services they use.
- *Prevention* is the foundation of sound occupational health practices.

The users of the services, shown along the base of the cube in Figure 8.1, may include larger businesses, small businesses, public agencies, and, possibly, labor unions. Individual workers do not constitute a market for occupational health services in the same way that they and their families form a market for personal health care. The "consumers" of health care are those who use the system and make the choices. In the occupational health care system, it is usually the employer who makes the initial choice and who purchases (directly or through workers' compensation) health services on behalf of the worker. Even when an individual worker changes physicians, or seeks requests from a personal physician for an occupational health problem, the workers' compensation system constrains the choices available to him or her by allowing only a limited number of charges and by refusing to pay for unauthorized referrals. The essential target in marketing occupational health services therefore must be the employer. As a practical matter, the workers' needs must always be met but the employer's needs also must be reasonably satisfied or the relationship between provider and client may be brief.

Figure 8.2. Most clinics and practitioners limit themselves to providing acute medical care and clinical management of cases for employees of a mixture of larger companies, small business, and public agencies, including city or state departments.

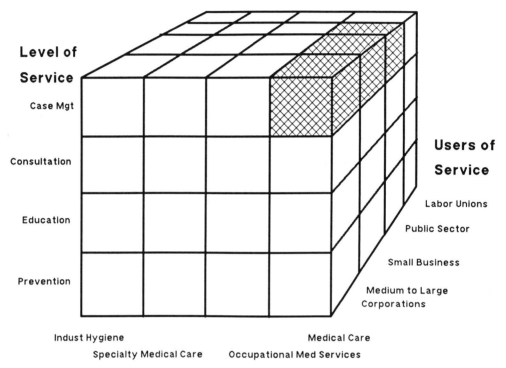

Labor unions often have their own insurance plans and sometimes have their own medical consultants or services. They are potential sources of referrals, usually for disputed or difficult cases. Workers who are members of a union tend to rely on their union more than their personal physicians for advice on medical referrals for occupational problems. Although unions sometimes contract for educational and preventive services for their members, they usually prefer to work with academic or non-profit organizations.

Most medical services are limited to a narrow corner of the cube, as is illustrated in Figure 8.2. Facilities with larger staffs and specialty expertise enjoy expanded opportunities, as shown in Figure 8.3. The addition of industrial hygiene expertise, either to the health facility or by collaboration with a consultant, can open up additional opportunities not otherwise accessible, as illustrated in Figure 8.4, and developing programs oriented toward education and prevention fill up the cube even more, as is shown in Figure 8.5. While no occupational health service is ever likely to develop all potential marketing possibilities, an appreciation of what can be done may lead to new directions that are profitable and worthwhile.

Figure 8.3. Occupational health services that have access to greater resources, such as hospital-based units or those associated with group medical practices, are in a position to provide specialty care and more in-depth consultation on technical aspects of occupational medicine.

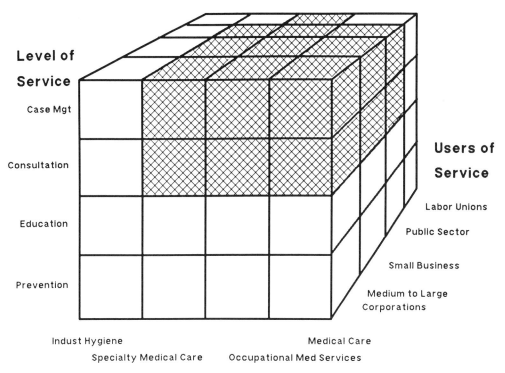

Medical services deal with the treatment of individual cases or preventive services to groups of workers. Opportunities may arise as a result of routine medical practice for health professionals to provide consultative and educational services. Physicians may not be well utilized, on a cost-effective basis, by providing only educational programs. However, highly professional programs, designed with input from physicians can be provided at reasonable cost by health educators or nurses and are very popular among some types of employers and groups of workers. Industrial hygiene services are usually provided on the case management or consultation level, but the market for such services includes periodic assessments for purposes of prevention and to ensure compliance with government regulations.

Executive Health Services

Executive health services, often a perquisite of employment for corporate officials, can be a cost-effective means of protecting valuable human resources. They are intended

Figure 8.4. The addition of industrial hygiene expertise expands the technical capabilities in health hazard evaluation and controlling, and allows a more comprehensive range of services to be provided to clients.

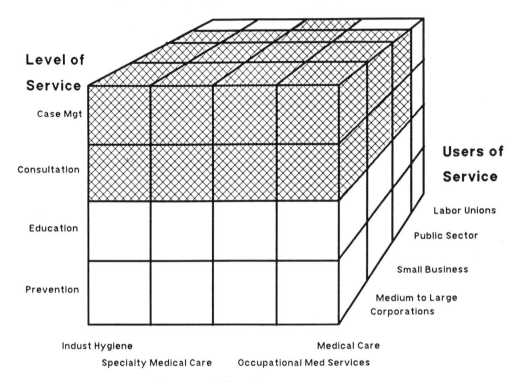

to identify and correct health problems at a very early stage in key management personnel, who often are subject to stress and onerous travel and who, as a group, tend to neglect their health needs. When compared to screening programs for more general public health purposes, executive health services are very attractive programs for well situated medical group practices and hospitals to increase their profitability by catering to an affluent clientele. Patients receiving executive services may in the future choose the institution for additional health care needs and even, in cases of extensive wealth, as beneficiaries of their philanthropy.

Because major companies are dependent on the decisions made by their senior managers, they provide benefit packages to attract and retain the most skilled executives. Certain health care institutions have recognized this fact and have created resort settings, where major executives can have health evaluations on an annual or other periodic basis, combined with recreation and fitness programs. Outstanding examples of these programs include those at the Greenbrier in White Sulphur Springs, West Virginia, and Loma Linda's Rancho Loma Linda near Dulzura, California. Except in such high-prestige settings as the Mayo Clinic and the Cleveland Clinic, executive health

Figure 8.5. The addition of programs in health education and health promotion completes the range of services that can be provided to clients.

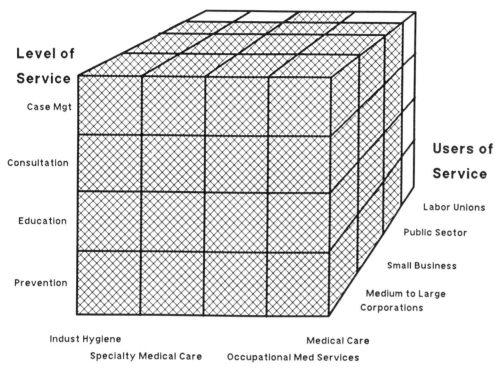

Level of
Service

Case Mgt

Consultation

Education

Prevention

Users of
Service

Labor Unions

Public Sector

Small Business

Medium to Large
Corporations

Indust Hygiene   Medical Care
    Specialty Medical Care   Occupational Med Services

Range of Service

evaluations lacking a resort atmosphere usually fail. Unless the clinic has a world-class reputation and is seen as such, executives would rather combine the health evaluation experience with a vacation in some desirable location.

A congenial resort setting should be selected as the location for an executive health service. A wing or a floor of an up-scale hotel could be equipped to serve as the diagnostic clinic. Highly individualized services related to fitness, health education, habit control, and nutrition could be offered, along with ample opportunity for the executive to enjoy sports and relaxation. (See Chapter 27 on health promotion.) Health problems that are detected in the course of screening tests could be further evaluated in a medical center or by the executive's own physician, as needed.

There are a number of pitfalls that institutions should consider before deciding to develop their own executive health services. When these services are formed within existing clinics and medical groups, internal stresses may affect other aspects of health care. It is not unusual for other patients and staff to resent the special treatment afforded to the executives. Staff sometimes undermine efforts to cultivate the executive service by allowing delays to occur, and by refusing to give executives priority over other patients. The creation of a "two-tier" approach to delivering medical services also leaves the institution open to criticism for appearing to be discriminating in favor of the affluent and against the needy. Workers directed by their employers to occupational health services in the same organization that serves their supervisors may suspect that their cases will be prejudiced or treated less sympathetically because the institution has engaged in an apparently "cozy" relationship with their bosses. These problems can be overcome by insisting on as complete a separation as possible between the executive health service and the rest of the clinic. Ideally, this should be in a separate facility, where a resort or a recreational atmosphere that would be inappropriate for most occupational health services may add to the appeal to busy executives.

These programs do present an excellent opportunity to encourage sound health practices among people who are leaders in their communities. The executive participants are likely to be more receptive to concepts of health promotion than they might be at home. Programs on stress reduction, smoking cessation, prevention of alcohol and drug abuse, health education, motivation, and exercise are usually combined along with screening for early signs of common diseases. Lifestyle-oriented programs present a healthier alternative to the hard-driving executive workaholic stereotype. These programs, combined with a vacation opportunity for the executive and spouse, are very attractive in today's health-conscious society. Health promotion programs can be offered at extra cost or as part of a package within the executive health service.

Executive health programs should be based on sound principles of preventive medicine. Too frequently, the services actually provided are obsolete screening protocols emphasizing extensive clinical testing that may not be justified by the natural history of the disorders being screened for and the predictive value of the tests applied. Tests incorporated in a program should be reasonably cost-effective as well as reliable and safe.

Marketing Brochure

A sample brochure appropriate for marketing purposes is presented as Exhibit 8.1. This brochure originally was developed for use by an occupational health facility that serves many employers. Literature of this type can raise the visibility of occupational health services in an often fiercely competitive market, particularly when combined with regular visits by a marketing representative. The brochure is reproduced with permission from the Sharp Rees-Stealy Medical Group, San Diego, CA.

Exhibit 8.1. Employer's Guide to Occupational Medicine Services

ALLOW US TO INTRODUCE OURSELVES!

We are specialists in occupational medicine. We provide a complete range of services, offering everthing the employer needs, from treatment of industrial accidents and preplacement and periodic examinations to sophisticated consultations in toxicology. We can even design company-wide programs to prevent health problems among employees.

Occupational medicine is our commitment and our specialty, not our hobby.

We have a better idea. In providing occupational medicine services, we are committed to:

- EXCELLENCE. . .Not mere adequacy.
- EFFICIENCY. . .No fooling around.
- FLEXIBILITY. . .The services you need, not the services we can sell you.
- CONVENIENCE. . .Services when you need them, not just when we make them available.
- PREVENTION. . .Not waiting until the situation is out of control.

We have on our staff trained specialists in the key fields of medicine needed to provide high quality occupational medicine services for your employees.

HOW CAN WE MEET YOUR EMPLOYEES' NEEDS?

Care for the injured employee is the most basic service of occupational medicine. We provide to your employees comprehensive care for prompt treatment, timely follow-up, rehabilitation, and a speedier return to health and productivity. We are ready to assist in each and every one of the following areas:

- Acute care of the injured employee.
- Evaluation and treatment of occupational illnesses.
- Rehabilitation and evaluation for return to work.
- Consultation for workers' compensation appeals cases.
- Disability evaluation.
- Specialty referral for complex cases.

QUALITY CARE FOR YOUR EMPLOYEES

Maintaining the health of employees is just as important as treating acute injuries. An employee who is later found to have been unfit for his or her job assignment can be an expensive proposition in terms of liability, bad feelings, and lost productivity.

Providing preplacement and periodic examinations is a responsibility not to be taken lightly. Routine examinations should never become like an assembly line, where the doctor just goes through the motions. We rotate physicians performing routine examinations and limit the number that they conduct at any one time, to ensure that they do not get tired, bored, or lose their mental sharpness.

We believe that preplacement and periodic examinations are opportunities to help employees maintain their good health and to sustain them in a healthier, more vigorous, and more productive state in the work place. We focus on identifying both the employee's strong points and limitations and matching them against the job description provided to us by the employer for preplacement evaluations. We also look for early signs of correctable health problems in order to warn or educate the patient about his or her personal health and to minimize the loss to the employer in reduced productivity and health costs. The Occupational Safety and Health Act requires surveillance programs for employees exposed to specific occupational hazards; our specially designed programs conform to OSHA standards, meet the needs of employees and employers, and are scientifically and medically sound.

(Continued)

Exhibit 8.1. Continued

Periodic evaluations we provide on a routine basis include the following:
- Preplacement examinations.
- Periodic personal health evaluations.
- Lifetime health monitoring programs for managers.
- Surveillance programs for employees exposed to asbestos, noise, lead, pesticide, and other occupational exposures as required by OSHA and for employee exposure not regulated by OSHA.

WHERE CAN THE EMPLOYER TURN FOR HELP IN SOLVING PROBLEMS?

We help area employers solve their occupational health problems. Expertise that is not immediately available through our staff can be secured for clients through our network of affiliations and contacts. We visit the employer's plants, so that our medical staff will see the kind of work that employees perform and gain a clear picture of the possible job-related hazards. In the event that a problem arises, our staff is ready to meet on short notice with management and, if requested, employees, help formulate a solution to the problem, and educate all those concerned about the health implications of the problem. In particular, employers setting up a new plant or expanding an old one are invited to call us for a no-charge consultation on the occupational health needs that may be involved in the development of the plant.

We offer the following kinds of problem-solving services:
- Plant visits and on-site consultation.
- Technical consultation and problem-solving by occupational health experts.
- Health hazard evaluations (in-depth studies of a particular problem).
- Plant walk-throughs and identification of occupational hazards.
- New and expanding plant services.

AN OUNCE OF PREVENTION. . .

Prevention of occupational health problems is the best care of all. For a relatively modest investment up front, an employer can promote the health of workers through programs designed to educate, entertain, and involve employees while breaking their bad life-style habits. The best health promotion programs are those that capture the imagination of the employees and encourage their participation and commitment. These are precisely the kinds of programs that raise employee morale and lead to a more closely knit workforce. We can arrange for the preparation and supervision of a program tailored for the employees in any area of a firm. We are able to provide programs for all sizes of operations, ranging from the smallest to major corporations. We will be happy to analyze the situation in your organization to determine if such a program would be appropriate.

The variety of programs that can be developed include:
- Smoking cessation.
- Fitness and exercise.
- Stress reduction.
- Back injury prevention.
- Nutrition.
- Cardiovascular risk reduction.
- Hypertension control and monitoring.
- Mental health.
- Other programs tailored to the needs of your organization and workers.

THE TROUBLED EMPLOYEE

The troubled employee is a difficult problem for any organization, large or small. Employee Assistance Programs can salvage employees who have much

(Continued)

Exhibit 8.1. Continued

experience and very real skills to contribute to the organization. A well timed but firm intervention can be the key event in the employee's life. We do not ourselves provide Employee Assistance Programs. These programs are highly specialized and require extensive expertise in nonmedical as well as medical areas. Nonetheless, we can help your organization evaluate the options from a medical point of view and select appropriate employee assistance services— treatment of alcohol or drug abuse; mental health counseling; psychiatric care; family or financial and credit counseling; and support for individuals undergoing unusual life stresses. We also can play a gatekeeper role in the diagnosis of substance abuse and the referral of employees for treatment.

CONSULTATION SERVICES

We recognize that not all companies are best served by contracting for services at a central location. The proper structure and development of programs at the work site may be necessary to meet the specific needs of a plant or facility. We are prepared as a consulting service to assist any client in developing its own programs, based on an analysis of what is cost-effective in the situation.

Some of the services that we can provide in this area include the following:
- Designing in-plant employee health services.
- Designing occupational health records systems.
- Designing occupational health information systems.
- Providing continuing education for plant medical and nursing personnel.
- Developing absenteeism monitoring programs.
- Conducting epidemiologic investigations of occupational illnesses.
- Performing needs assessment on the employee population.
- Developing specific prevention-oriented programs.
- Trouble-shooting problem areas and designing program evaluations.

RAPID REPORTING AND PROCESSING KEEPS YOU INFORMED AND WITHIN THE LAW

Providing excellent medical care is not enough in occupational medicine. Federal, state, and local regulations must be complied with and reporting deadlines must be promptly met. Our reporting system ensures that within hours of seeing your employee our staff will be making a preliminary report by telephone or on a short form. This will be followed by a final written report summarizing the findings that pertain to occupational performance and estimating the likely time off work and the level of impairment. Supplemental reports and fitness-to-work evaluations are handled in the same expeditious manner.

Clerical and billing services are provided by personnel specifically trained in the administrative management of workers' compensation cases and supervised by knowledgeable administrators.

Our doors are always open to discussions of the needs of your organization and procedures to meet those needs.

Further Reading

The Health Care Marketer's Handbook. Health Care Marketer, 4550 Montgomery Ave., Suite 700N, Bethesda, Maryland 20814. (Serial publication.)

Mages PM: Marketing medical services. Group Practice J, March/April 1982, pp. 14–20.

SECTION III
OFFICE ADMINISTRATION

9   STAFFING AND PERSONNEL NEEDS

There is no simple formula for staffing an occupational health service. Generally, however, for industries lacking exceptional physical or chemical hazards, the following guidelines are appropriate:

- Where the employee population numbers fewer than 200, easy access to informed medical care is adequate.
- For 300 employees, a full-time occupational health nurse is usually needed; each additional 750 employees requires another such nurse.
- A workforce of about 500 employees justifies hiring a full-time industrial hygienist.
- A workforce of about 1,000 employees requires the services of an occupational physician, on at least a part-time basis. With more than 2,000 employees, the physician should have full-time status.

These crude guidelines, of course, do not take into consideration the hazardous nature of some industries or the requirements imposed by regulations. An occupational health nurse may be quite sufficient for several hundred employees in an office building but an occupational hygienist may be essential for a small company in a high-risk industry. There is no simple formula for staffing an occupational health service but for medium-risk industries the recommendations above will not be far out of line.

Factors Affecting Staffing Levels

As with all medical facilities, the staffing of an occupational health service depends on several factors that reflect the mission of the organization and the health patterns within the industry and the community. Some of these factors are:

- Number of patient encounters expected per year.
- Type of injuries or illnesses to be expected.
- Degree of organizational autonomy enjoyed by the service.
- Administrative responsibilities of the service.
- Budgetary constraints of the organization.

• Anticipated peak utilization of the service and variations during the year.

The last two factors should carry the least weight in considerations of health service staffing. Any organization that lacks the resources to support or to contract for an adequate occupational health service, relative to its needs, is in serious trouble—such programs are not disproportionately costly and they protect the organization from liability. On the other hand, peak needs should never be the basis for full-time staffing projections, as they burden the operation with redundant staff for most of the year. A more cost-effective approach is to anticipate the peak load on the occupational health service and to employ part-time personnel to assist during these times. For example, if all periodic screening tests, such as audiometric testing, are performed in a single month, temporary or part-time staff can perform these duties while the full-time staff deals with preplacement screening on an ongoing basis throughout the year. (An alternative, of course, is to spread such examinations out through the year.) Seasonal industries usually schedule screening tests during their lightest months to minimize disruptions to production.

The most common types of patient encounters handled by an occupational health service usually do not require the presence of a physician. A well trained occupational health nurse is able to handle virtually all routine services and to triage cases requiring a physician's attention. Most routine occupational health programs (such as preplacement evaluations), although repetitive, require strict adherence to a set of criteria and procedures. Nurses perceive such duties as a professional challenge and often perform them exceptionally well, taking pride in their abilities. Physicians often do not perform as well when conducting the same routine tasks. Furthermore, it is to the advantage of the organization to protect the physician's time by permitting nurses or trained technicians to provide routine services whenever appropriate. The occupational physician then can concentrate on more complex matters—managing problem cases, developing programs affecting large groups of workers, and handling policy issues. An efficient occupational health service usually functions on a day-to-day basis through the efforts of an experienced head nurse who enjoys the confidence of a physician prepared to delegate routine duties.

Staffing Patterns in Industry

The majority of occupational health services function solely or primarily with nurses. A registered nurse with special training in administrative aspects of occupational health may be the only staff necessary in offices or other low-risk settings. For more complex situations, however, a certified occupational health nurse (COHN) is preferable and the additional cost is not excessive. (See Chapter 1 for a discussion of COHN qualifications.) A COHN is more versatile, and can handle most common occupational health problems with occasional physician back-up. However, these specially trained nurses are in relatively short supply. (At the end of this chapter is a sample position description for an occupational health nurse.)

Physicians staffing industrial occupational health services may be classified as either plant or corporate physicians. Plant physicians may be full-time, but often are part-time, supplementing their community-based practice with service to a local employer. To be useful to the employees and the employer, the plant physician must master the skills associated with occupational medical practice and become knowledgeable about problems common to or characteristic of the industry, ideally through continuing education. (Refer to Chapter 7 for discussion of preparation for practice in this field.) Depending on the types of hazards encountered in the industry, the employer may want to identify specialists willing to provide services in dermatology, lung disorders, orthopedics, or general surgery on an as-needed basis. Within their specialties, these physicians also can be engaged to review procedures and to set down guidelines for the management of routine problems. The employer and the physician should have a contractual agreement so that both understand the nature of the medical services to be provided.

Corporate physicians are usually full-time medical directors of large companies; less frequently, they are occupational medical consultants providing services as needed. Corporate physicians are involved in formulating policy, procedures, and standards that affect groups of employees. Plant physicians generally have a more limited and more focused range of activities and spend more time providing direct care to ill or injured employees or handling the administrative aspects of individual cases. The corporate physician represents the organization to regulatory agencies, to workers' compensation boards, and to the public and media. As the senior officer for health affairs in the organization, the medical director must have the credibility and credentials to speak with authority.

For a company, a corporate physician is a substantial investment in a valuable human resource. Considerable training in occupational medicine, preferably including specialization complete with formal certification as a specialist in the field, is needed if this investment is to be worthwhile. (Refer to Chapter 5 for more extensive discussion of the organization and staffing of company-based occupational health services.)

Staffing in Clinics and Medical Groups

The pattern of physician staffing is somewhat different in clinics and medical groups that provide occupational health services. In this type of setting, a trained occupational physician may direct a service in which care is provided by non-specialists or even, at times, locum tenens (doctors on short-term assignments). Such a system works reasonably well because the group structure is based on interaction among the physicians and other providers of care.

Properly trained occupational physicians are in too short a supply to comprise the entire clinical staff in most situations; nevertheless, a core group of physicians who have occupational training is essential. The core medical staff may be augmented with temporary or part-time help by family practitioners, internists, general surgeons, and even by locum tenens. An occupational medical clinic may require the regular services of a dermatologist but may only need occasional access to a pulmonary physician, cardiologist, neurologist, or to any of several other medical and surgical specialists. Table 9.1 presents recommended physician staffing patterns for occupational health facilities, depending on volume and type of services offered. Quality assurance for occupational medicine practice is maintained by frequent consultation, continuing education, records review, and spot-checking for quality control of case management. (Refer to Chapters

Table 9.1. Physician Staffing Suggested for a Large Clinic Serving Many Employers

1. Staff in residence or in close proximity:
   Occupational physician (direction and supervision)
   Primary care (family or general practitioner or general
     internist)
   Surgeon (general surgery and burns)
   Dermatologist

2. Staff on call for consultation:
   Ophthalmologist
   Pulmonary specialist
   Clinical toxicologist (access to laboratory important)
   Cardiologist
   Psychiatrist
   Radiologist (should have particular interest in chest
     films and interpreting lung disorders)
   Orthopedist
   Rehabilitation (physical medicine) specialist

13 and 14 for more extensive discussions of quality assurance and evaluation.) In this situation, continuing and in-service training is particularly important.

The capabilities of the basic unit of physician and nurse may be extended by other health care professionals providing special services, such as audiometric technicians, with their routine screening tests for hearing conservation. Depending on the programs offered by the service, others that may be needed include substance abuse counsellors in employee assistance programs (EAPs); physician assistants or nurse practitioners in large services with heavy acute care needs; physiotherapists in settings where musculoskeletal injuries are a problem; and fitness leaders in health promotion programs. (Many of these professions are discussed in Chapter 1.)

Other specialized occupational health and safety professionals not involved in direct patient care provide functions that complement the occupational health service. Safety engineers are trained in the management of physical hazards, such as fire and accident prevention. They are usually experienced in the operations of a plant and often receive their education in a series of short courses to become mid-level managers responsible for safety. Industrial hygienists, on the other hand, are usually university graduates or certificate-holders who are educated in special academic programs emphasizing toxic hazards, engineering principles, and management skills. There is a considerable overlap between the two in practice, and both professionals are trained to be highly versatile. In contrast, radiation protection or control officers (health physicists) have specialized training in their field and are usually limited to that function. The best way to judge the qualifications of each professional is by the relevance of their prior experience to the needs of the organization they are joining, and by the quality of their work as reflected in reports and programs for which they have been responsible. Other special occupational health professionals, such as toxicologists and epidemiologists, are also required on the staffs of some large organizations with special needs. In most of industry, however, these professionals are usually brought in as consultants to deal with specific problems, as is the case with experts in other areas, such as acoustical engineering.

Staffing Strategies

An occupational health service should be a team effort. The service should be organized as simply as possible to coordinate medical and administrative activities. All lines of administrative authority and responsibility should converge on one person, the director. Communication must cut across departmental lines but the service must possess sufficient autonomy to function efficiently in order to meet its own objectives, consistent with the long-range goals of the organization.

As occupational health services expand, two problems arise with respect to quality: maintaining cost-effective staffing levels and managing the stress placed on the entire system by a growing caseload. While the latter problems can only be approached by anticipating demands and strengthening the weak points of the system, there are several ways to minimize the burden of personnel costs until a facility is entirely self-supporting. One approach is to use mid-level health practitioners to perform duties that might otherwise be handled by physicians. Another is to use locum tenens to fill staffing vacancies instead of hiring new physicians on a permanent basis.

Mid-level health practitioners, such as physicians' assistants and nurse practitioners, are highly effective in occupational medicine settings and are very cost-effective. Since the financial goal of an independent occupational medicine clinic is profitability rather than expansion of the medical staff, productivity should be the standard for selecting personnel positions. A well paid nurse practitioner may be a productive alternative to an additional partner in a group practice – and at a substantially lower cost. Since many occupational medical problems are relatively straightforward and the different problems easily identified, quality of care is not an issue as long as the medical supervision is adequate.

Locum tenens can substantially expand the pool of medical personnel available to meet peak needs, permitting the clinic to offer extended hours and making possible on-site screening activities in plants without disrupting usual staff coverage. A locum tenens arrangement does not commit the clinic to an ongoing position and can be both filled and terminated on short notice.

It is important to hire support personnel who are particularly bright and skilled and to pay them competitively. Much of the administrative complexity of occupational medicine comes from dealing with various regulations, client expectations, and requirements to report to government agencies and insurance carriers. These are all easily learned by the intelligent layperson, who then can shield the medical and administrative staff from considerable distraction by handling such matters at a lower level. On the other hand, an inept support staff can cause no end of trouble. In the private practice of occupational medicine, administrative or paperwork problems result in lost referrals, cancelled contracts, and a bad reputation among insurance carriers.

Finally, the routine administration of an occupational health facility is usually best centralized under one person who has the time and the responsibility to learn the nuances of the system. Rarely is it satisfactory for occupational health services to be managed as part of the "span of control" of a manager entrusted with other responsibilities. A designated coordinator or an administrator who knows how the system operates is of great assistance to the occupational health professionals working within the facility. A conscientious coordinator can easily save enough dollars through efficient management to justify the cost of the new position.

Because the key position in most organizations is the nurse, a sample position description for an occupational health nurse follows as Exhibit 9.1.

Exhibit 9.1. Sample Position Description: Occupational Health Nurse.

A. Qualifications
  1. Eligibility for registration with the state or provincial association of registered nurses;
  2. Training and/or experience in occupational health, including occupational health nursing, industrial safety, industrial hygiene, toxicology, adult education, relevant legislation; and
  3. Certification, preferably as an occupational health nurse (COHN).

B. Supervision
  The occupational health nurse practitioner functions as a health professional under the administrative direction of _____.

C. Duties
  1. Health Services
    a) Assessment of the effects of workplace conditions and the workplace environment on the physical, mental, and social well-being of the individual workers and groups of workers. This includes but is not limited to:
    • participation in the diagnosis, treatment, or recommendation of treatment, in conjunction with and under the direct supervision of a medical practitioner;
    • investigation of occupational environment of those employees presenting with an illness attributable to workplace hazards (this may be undertaken with the industrial hygienist);
    • participation in health hazard evaluations and workplace tours ("walk throughs"); and
    • participation in fitness-to-work determinations, health surveillance, and monitoring programs in conjunction with and under the direct supervision of workers.
    b) Action to improve workplace conditions and the physical, mental, and social well-being of workers. This includes but is not limited to:
    • in consultation with medical practitioners, recommendation of therapeutic alternatives appropriate to an early return to work;
    • research and the preparation of reports and briefs; and
    • activities required on behalf of the employer or worker, as appropriate, in pending workers' compensation claims.
  2. Oversight
Provides supervision and instruction for nursing or other health professions during placement within the organization.
  3. Technical Resource
Provides expertise to committees and units within the organization regarding occupational and environmental health matters.
  4. Education
    a) Provides and participates in educational programs in occupational health and safety within the organization; and
    b) Participates in activities to maintain and enhance competence in the practice of occupational health.
  5. Research
Participates in epidemiological and other research that may be conducted.

Further Reading

American Board of Preventive Medicine: Certification in the specialty of occupational medicine. J Occup Med 1982; 24:546.

Arthur D. Little, Inc: Costs and Benefits of Occupational Health Nursing. Washington, Government Printing Office, National Institute for Occupational Safety and Health Publication DHHS (NIOSH) 1980, pp. 80–140.

Brown ML: Occupational Health Nursing: Principles and Practices. New York, Springer, 1981.

Gallagher PM: Occupational health nursing: Autonomy and interdependence. Occup Health Safety 1981; 50:43–47.

Knight AL, Zenz C: Organization and staffing, Zenz C (ed): Occupational Medicine: Principle and Practical Application. Chicago, Yearbook Medical Publishing, 1975, pp. 77–82.

Permanent Commission and International Association on Occupational Health: The Nurse's Contribution to the Health of the Worker. London, 1969.

Seaver ME: Teamwork: Industrial hygienists and occupational health nurses. Occup Health Safety 1982; 51:30–32.

10   FACILITIES AND EQUIPMENT

Occupational health services function best when they occupy facilities that are designed with their purpose in mind and equipped appropriately; they function less well when making do with reassigned space and second-hand equipment. In-plant occupational medical facilities illustrate this rule; since the needs of such facilities are generally more comprehensive, they provide a more complex example for purposes of planning. While the needs of community-based clinics are more variable (depending on the setting, the nature of local industry, and their institutional relationships), many of the points discussed in this chapter apply equally well to clinics of this type, whether independent or associated with a hospital group.

Facility Design

The site and design of the clinical facility ideally should be determined by reference to a successful model with a similar service pattern. While there is no one design that meets the needs of all organizations, facilities do share general principles of space allocation, access, configuration, interior fixtures, and equipment.

Previous reference works have suggested as a rule of thumb a minimum of 200 square feet for a facility, augmented by roughly one square foot for each employee over 200 up to about 1,000 square feet total. However, many others consider this space formula too small for efficiency of operation, particularly since it does not take into account the needs of proactive health services, such as health promotion or employee assistance. For a modern facility, a more reasonable rule of thumb would up the requirements by about 50 percent: a minimum of 1,500 square feet (30 square meters) should be provided, with an additional 1.5 square feet (0.25 square meter) per employee above 200 employees.

Access is critically important to the facility. The occupational health clinic should be easily reached by motor vehicles and by ambulance attendants using a stretcher. It should be barrier-free for the handicapped and close to where employees work.

Cramped quarters in a central location are preferable to a new and spacious facility on the periphery of a worksite. In industries where the job site is large, or where the workforce is spread out or remote, the clinic should be near the traffic flow into and out of the area. In office buildings or in satellite dispensaries, the clinic may be located on an upper floor only if access to an elevator can be assured through key-controlled override systems and a parking place for an ambulance can be guaranteed in an emergency. Otherwise, it is better for the clinic to be positioned on the ground floor in order to provide easy access.

The floor plan of the clinic is an important determinant of its efficiency. In general, there should be a central receiving and triage area, where injured or well employees can be seated comfortably. The entrance between the waiting area and the clinic area should be barrier-free and wide enough to accommodate three people standing abreast – or two people supporting a fainting person or handling a stretcher. At a minimum, two examination rooms should be provided, each with separate entrances that open onto a corridor screened from view of the waiting area. At least one examination room should be equipped to handle minor surgery and the stabilization of trauma cases, which may be encountered more frequently in heavy manufacturing or other industries with a high injury rate. This room should have easy access to an ambulance parking area and should be large enough to allow several persons to surround the examining table. The other examination room can be equipped less elaborately to serve as a consultation room. Each examination room should have a curtain and a stool that can be used by patients when they undress.

The clinic area must be equipped with a toilet and shower; an additional toilet must be provided for the staff. If radiation decontamination is anticipated, the clinic may need a separate shower with its own entrance and an anteroom equipped with supplies for the purpose. A rear exit also is desirable as an alternative to staff coming and going through a crowded waiting room and for transferring injured workers to ambulances, without the necessity of carrying them through the waiting room. Administrative areas, offices for professional staff, areas used for interviews, or space for small group health education programs should be easily accessible and soundproof for confidentiality. Recordkeeping areas and file cabinets must be secure and inaccessible to casual visitors. These basic areas should be within steps of one another.

Two examples of floor plans for occupational health services are provided in Figures 10.1 and 10.2. The former represents a plan for a busy clinic with two health providers practicing; the latter is a plan for a center emphasing prevention, workers' compensation evaluation, and counselling of injured or disabled workers. Both plans were compromises to accommodate the existing space.

The best floor plan for a particular facility will depend on the space available, anticipated patient volume, staffing, and services to be provided. Traffic flow is particularly critical; the facility planner should identify and separate wherever possible paths taken by different types of patients, areas in the corridor where paths cross, and the locations where the patients are likely to stand waiting. Privacy is essential; the interior of examination rooms should never be visible from the waiting area.

Besides these considerations, there also should be sufficient space for additional activities appropriate to the needs of the industry and the programs offered by the employer. Depending on the size and type of operation, the facility may require additional surgeries, a small clinical laboratory, a conference room, and a classroom. Certain

Figure 10.1. This occupational health facility is set up for two physicians or a physician and an occupational health nurse. Examination rooms are clustered for efficiency in busy clinical practice. The design is short on filing and conference space and lacks a combined library and conference room, which would have been a desirable feature.

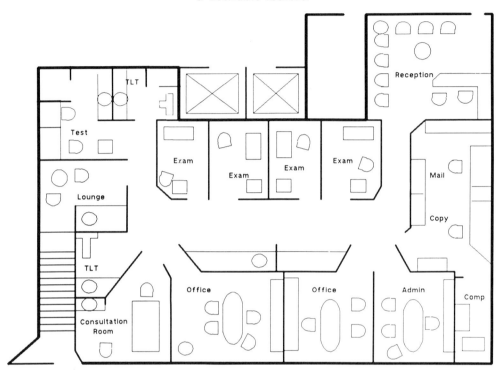

spaces can be made to serve two or more purposes: a conference room may double as a library, while a classroom may provide storage for patient education materials and, if equipped with folding chairs, may double as a fitness center for aerobics. Space for nearby industrial hygiene, safety, radiation health, and physiotherapy may be needed. These functions are often located some distance away from the main clinic area but it is desirable whenever possible to localize these functions in one general and contiguous area, in order to facilitate communication and interaction. Within the clinic area itself, special rooms for audiometric testing (including a soundproof booth), ophthalmologic examination (if eye injuries are likely and the physician is qualified to use a slit lamp), instrument sterilization, or even a small pharmacy may be considered. A small, quiet room for ill employees to lie down is very desirable. These special clinic rooms need not be clustered centrally as the basic units described in the preceding paragraph, but should be on the same floor. Custodial closets should not be forgotten when the floor plan is designed.

The interior fixtures should be appropriate for a modern clinic. The waiting area should be bright, comfortable, and relaxing. The examining rooms should be equipped

Figure 10.2. This facility sacrifices examining room space for educational and training functions. It works well for preventive and consultation purposes but would be inadequate for a busy clinical practice.

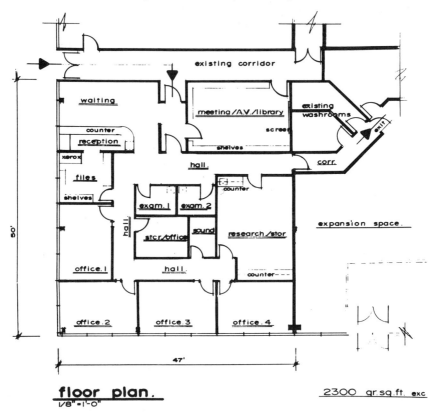

with examining tables, wall-mounted oto- and ophthalmoscopes and sphygmomanometers, vision charts, overhead lighting, sinks, and scales. The surgery room should be outfitted more completely with overhead adjustable lamps, an adjustable table, resuscitation equipment, and stools. All should have chairs, floor lamps, adequate counter space, and open shelves and cupboards clearly labelled as to their contents. All surfaces should be easy to clean and light-colored and nooks and crannies kept to a minimum. Each room in which a patient is likely to be interviewed should have a small writing desk and a prominent wall clock. Locks should be placed on all rooms or cabinets containing instruments, syringes, and drugs, even those constantly attended. (Drug and syringe cabinets should be locked after hours, even if the main clinic door is locked and bolted.) Water fountains are a courtesy that is much appreciated. Whenever possible, built-in fixtures and indirect lighting are preferred because of their convenience, appearance, and practicality. Built-in fixtures can be mounted above or below cabinets to conserve space and reduce clutter.

Interior fixtures serve many functions besides directly supporting the care given by the staff. One of these functions is communication. A clinic that looks like a modern medical facility will inspire confidence and transmit the impression that the occupational health staff is serious and dedicated. A clinic that looks like a storage cubicle or a hospital room circa 1943 will convey the impression that the health of employees is a low priority in the organization. Another function of the internal fixtures is that they help to orient employees within the facility. Even employees who are well are often anxious on entering a medical facility; this level of anxiety is greater among new employees and among the injured or ill. Nonverbal cues help to orient an individual spatially, whereas tersely worded signs alone, in the absence of visual cues, are often misread or confused by persons under stress. Color-coded rooms and printed lines on the wall (not on the floor, because the employee must then look down and will miss other signs and cues) and snappy graphics help to orient the visitor and reduce anxiety, as well as increase efficiency. A bright decor that uses soft and warm color combinations and some natural lighting will lend a more cheerful aspect to the clinic. Bold primary colors are fine for accent but are visually disconcerting when overused. Reds and yellows may even be alarming because workers associate these colors with danger signs. Pastels, on the other hand, are not usually preferred in a predominantly masculine workforce. Clinics should be neither overly trendy nor bland but should communicate familiarity and reassurance to the worker through the medium of its decor. Clinics should not experiment with unconventional or wildly imaginative interior design. However stimulating and refreshing such a decor may be to the staff, it is often disorienting, anxiety-provoking, and intimidating to an ill, injured, or nervous worker.

Equipment

The equipment needed in an occupational health center differs little from that needed in any physician's office or clinic. Table 10.1 lists commonly used instruments and devices likely to be required. Some of the common medications needed for the symptomatic relief of common occupational disorders or personal illnesses affecting employees on the job are listed in Table 10.2. Unless the clinic is remote and must function as a self-contained infirmary, it is usually not cost-effective to maintain a clinical laboratory beyond a bench centrifuge, microscope, and simple office tests, such as dipsticks and stool guaiacs. Likewise, it usually is not practical for a facility to acquire radiological apparatus unless the industry is one at high risk for serious injuries and the site is large or in a remote location. The cost of the initial investment and maintenance must be justified—usually, a local clinic or hospital can provide such services as needed at a lower unit cost with some guarantee of quality assurance.

In all cases, the proper use of equipment depends on the availability of trained and licensed professionals who keep abreast of technical developments and standards of practice and who service a sufficiently high volume to maintain their skills. The expense of equipment is so great, as is the risk of slow deterioration of skills through lack of experience that extensive equipment is unacceptable in most situations. Furthermore, where expensive laboratory and radiologic equipment is available, in-house testing frequently becomes overutilized and incorporated into a routine without critical interpretation (See Chapter 20). The end result may be excessive ordering of tests that are seldom useful in occupational health situations (such as serum electrolytes) or to the continuation by tradition of routine studies that are no longer indicated (such as annual or preplacement chest films).

Table 10.1. Equipment for an Occupational Medical Clinic

A. Furnishings
  1. Office
     Desks
     Chairs
     Bookcases
     Filing cabinets with locks
     Storage cabinets with locks
     Wall clocks
     Word processor, typewriters
     Personal business computer
     Tables
     Writing boards (blackboards or "white" boards)
     Wastebaskets
     In/Out baskets
     Desk lamps
     Bulletin boards
     Camera (35 mm) and accessories
     Calculators

  2. Clinic
     Stools, height appropriate to counter, with adjustable backs
     Chart-holders, with priority and occupancy indicators
     X-ray view boxes
     Sinks with surgical handles on faucets, towel racks
     Examination tables (see text)
     Chairs (do not leave faint or dizzy patients sitting on stools in rooms)
     Medication cabinet with locks
     Pedal-operated wastebaskets with lid and liners
     Overhead adjustable lamps (in surgery)
     Medical records filing cabinets (for color coded, side viewing)
     Opaque movable screens or curtains
     Instrument trays
     Autoclave
     Cold sterilizer (installed with appropriate venting and control procedures for ethylene oxide)
     Refrigerator

B. Equipment
  1. Major instruments
     Wall-mounted oto-/ophthalmoscope
     Wall-mounted sphygmomanometer (blood pressure cuff)
     Crash cart (cardiopulmonary resuscitation), must be fully equipped and provided with a seal to ensure that it is not opened and drugs and equipment are not used except in a true emergency
     Scales
     Electrocardiograph
     Audiometer

(Continued)

Table 10.1. Continued

    Vision screening apparatus
    Recording Spirometry
    Suction apparatus

2. Hand-held instruments
    Anoscope
    Canes, crutches, walkers
    Irrigating syringe, suitable for removal of cerumen from ear
    Assorted clamps (Halsted, Kelly, vascular, mosquito)
    Crash cart (portable pre-packed unit containing all equipment and supplies
       needed for cardiopulmonary resuscitation and stabilization for transport to
       hospital)
    Dental mirror
    Dynamometer (for measuring grip strength)
    Flashlights
    Laryngoscope (in crash cart)
    Magnifying lens
    Percussion hammer
    Proctosigmoidoscope
    Scalpels
    Surgical scissors
    Ear specula
    Nasal specula
    Vaginal specula
    Stethoscope
    Tape measures
    Thermometers
    Tuning forks
    Color vision chart (Ishihara plates)

3. Supplies, disposable
    Syringes
    Needles
    Gloves
    Vacutainers and assorted blood-drawing apparatus
    Tongue depressors
    Cotton swabs
    Gauze pads
    Assorted dressings
    Suture material and needles
    Specimen containers
    Elastic bandages, in assorted sizes
    Cold packs
    Cervical collars
    Surgical masks and hoods
    Eye patches and pads
    Cotton, in various forms
    Inflatable splints
    Finger splints
    Various types of splints, such as wrist, finger, leg, etc.

C. Special needs (variable, depending on which services are provided in-plant and which
   are referred out)
   1. Special medications to be ordered only by the physician and kept outside of the
       crash-cart

(Continued)

Table 10.1. Continued

Xylocaine (for minor surgical procedures)
Major analgesics (morphine should be kept only in crash cart)
Intravenous fluids (in order to stablize a severely injured or ill worker for transport)
Specific medications for common disorders
• Asthma
• Epilepsy
• Diabetes
Oxygen
Antibiotics (select a few appropriate to occupational injuries, e.g., dicloxacillin)
Vaccines
• Tetanus toxoid
• Hepatitis B vaccine (if hepatitis B is a hazard)
• Other vaccines for special needs (e.g., rubella in hospitals, selected vaccines
  for foreign travellers if required)

2. Physiotherapy equipment (consult with a registered physical therapist)

3. Patients and staff education aids
   Videocasette players and a monitor for viewing
   Movie projector
   Slide projector
   Portable tape recorder and players
   Library of patient education resource materials (topics should include back pain,
     smoking cessation, alcohol abuse, and others as appropriate)
   • Brochures and pamphlets
   • Books
   • Audiocassettes
   • Video cassettes
   • Movies

Table 10.2. Medications Commonly Used in an Occupational Health Service

Mefenamic acid caps 250 mg for menstrual cramps (Ponstel)
Acetylsalicylic acid 325 mg tablets (Aspirin)
Acetaminophen 325 mg tablets (Tylenol)
Actifed tablets
Chlorpheniramine maleate tablets (Chlor-Trimeton)
Dimenhydrinate tablets and suppositories (Dramamine)
Acetaminophen 300 mg + codeine 30 mg tablets (Tylenol 3)
Diazepam tablets 5 mg (Valium)
Diphenhydramine hydrochloride 25 mg (Benadryl Caps); Cream and injections 50 mg/ml
Epinephrine (Adrenalin)
Magnesia & alumina suspension (Maalox)
Kaopectate
Imodium caps 2 mg (Loperamide)
Guaifenesin syrup 100 mg/5 ml (Robitussin)
Terfenadine 60 mg tablets (Seldane)
Dequadin Lozenges
Phenylephrine hydrochloride, nasal drop ¼% (Neo-Synephrine)
Betamethasone valerate CR (Valisone V) Cream 0.1%
Bacitracin 500 unit/g ointment (Baciguent)
Dibucaine 1% Ointment (Nupercainal)
Lindane—gamma benzene hexachloride 1% (Kwell Shampoo)
Clove oil (for toothaches)
Methylcellulose ophthalmologic 0.5% used as a lubricant (Isopto Tears)
Jelonet Sterile (parafin gauze) dressing
Disposable enema

Further Reading

Howe HF: Organization and Operation of an Occupational Health Program. Chicago, Occupational Health Institute, 1975. Reprinted from J Occup Med 1975; 17:360–400, 433–440, 528–540.

Lee JA: The New Nurse in Industry. Washington DC, Government Printing Office, National Institute for Occupational Safety and Health, DHEW (NIOSH) Publication No. 78–143, 1979.

11 OFFICE PROCEDURES

The efficiency of daily operations in an occupational health facility greatly determines how clients and patients react to the services received. This chapter is a miscellany of practical recommendations for the smooth operation of the occupational health service. The three topics in office management discussed here are scheduling, billing, and clinical protocols.

Routine Scheduling

The initial scheduling of appointments and the flow of traffic once the worker arrives present a strong first impression to all those using the service, an impression that is communicated by word of mouth. A disorganized or confused procedure arouses a suspicion that the medicine being practiced will be equally confused. The procedure outlined below should help to avoid this problem.

The worker-patient must be informed, preferably in writing, of where to go and when to go there. The employer should be assured that each visit is handled expeditiously and efficiently. The staff at each station should have a schedule of appointments, so that they can direct the worker-patient and assist in keeping as close as possible to the time scheduled. Radiology and laboratory medicine departments must be educated and organized to expedite occupational medicine cases using such techniques as color coding of request slips in order to avoid unnecessary fumbling with papers. The staff should be instructed to complete their duties without delay and to make every effort to return the employee to work, if warranted, as soon as possible.

The time of departure should be recorded on the encounter form. The employer and the workers' compensation carrier must be notified promptly of the date the employee is to return to work as soon as that decision is made. If additional procedures, radiological examinations, or laboratory tests that may prolong the appointment are required, the employer's carrier or the employer should be informed of the delay and given an estimate of when the medical report will be available.

Communication by telephone with the client helps prevent a common source of friction, the lack of timely notification. At the conclusion of the appointment, or as soon as possible thereafter, the employer should be contacted by telephone and informed if there is any concern over the employee's fitness to return to work. The employer is not generally entitled to know the diagnosis, only whether the worker is fit to work at the assigned job and, if not, whether or when the worker can be expected to return to work.

Paperwork should be done within 24 hours if possible. Delay in sending out forms, bills, and reports is a principal cause of dissatisfaction among employers.

Poor morale among the clinic staff can be reflected in inappropriate behavior toward workers, especially if they are present for a seemingly minor health problem or for a routine periodic health evaluation. Comments that a person can wait because he or she is "just an industrial case" are much more common in a mixed clinic or practice than most physicians would believe, because they are always said out of hearing. Such comments are very destructive, conveying an impression to the worker that his or her case is not very important to the staff. These comments are also promptly reported back to the employer or to others in the workplace and undermine the credibility of the occupational health facility. It is therefore extremely important for the staff to be educated in the importance of providing respectful, punctual, and efficient care.

When a patient arrives with a health problem, the receptionist or nursing staff must determine as best they can whether the disorder is work-related and if the worker has authorization from the employer to be seen. A step-by-step procedure for receptionists and office staff to follow in handling patients in hospitals, clinics, and physicians' offices is provided in Exhibit 11.1. Similar procedures for check-in, treatment, referral, and follow-up might be used by in-plant facilities, but authorization would be implied and billing procedures would not apply.

Billing

Billing information should always be kept in a separate file from medical records. This expedites handling of the bill while the case is being worked up. It also keeps confidential financial information from the attention of staff dealing with the patient, and avoids unintended release of billing information, if the file is supoenaed or otherwise shared with others.

Billing for occupational health services is much like billing for any medical service. The bill should specify the patient's name, date of encounter, type of service provided, and fee. The bill should *not* specify the diagnosis, or provide any personal details regarding the worker-patient. These are confidential and the employer is not entitled to such information unless it is communicated appropriately, in a medical report, to a qualified occupational physician or nurse. Bills submitted to the workers' compensation board (WCB) should cover only occupational injuries or illnesses and should specify services for evaluating a claim under consideration. Bills for direct health care services unrelated to work should never be submitted to the WCB. Services of a preventive nature, such as fitness-to-work evaluations, are usually covered by the employer as a business cost. Again, the bill should never divulge the medical condition of the worker or any other personal information.

Exhibit 11.1. Patient Registration Procedures

1. Checking Patient In
   - Determine if the condition is job-related. If so, fill out the top of the Doctor's First Report form for reporting to the Workers' Compensation Board. [See Chapter 10.] The physician is responsible for filling out the bottom.
   - If the patient has been to this facility previously for a job-related condition, send for the chart.
   - If the patient is new, register and obtain all required information for medical and billing purposes.

2. Obtaining Authorization
   - Complete the first part of the authorization form used by the facility. (The authorization form appears as Form 11.1.)
   - Call the employer to obtain telephone authorization. If the patient has a prior authorization from the employer by note or telephone call, no call is necessary. (U.S. Federal employees will bring a special form number CA16 or CA20, which serves as both the Doctor's First Report Form and the Employer Authorization Form. If a federal employee does not bring this form, follow the standard procedure for obtaining authorization by telephone.)
   - Note the name, title, and telephone number of the person authorizing care and enter this information onto the Authorization for Medical Treatment form (Form 11.1) and the Doctor's First Report form.
   - If the clerk registering the patient is unable to obtain authorization, or if authorization is denied:
     - Note name, title, and telephone number of the person spoken to.
     - Notify the patient and explain that care may be billed to his or her personal health insurance or, in the case of uninsured patients, to the patient directly, if the employer or insurer refuses to honor the bill.
     - Complete the information on the registration form, noting the worker's status as an ''unauthorized patient.''

3. Treatment—Authorized
   - Document the authorization by recording name, title, and telephone number of employer's representative.
   - Complete the authorization form.
   - Register the patient.

4. Referrals
   - If referrals or consultations are needed, the referring physician's office must obtain authorization from the insurance carrier, or the employer, prior to scheduling the appointment.
   - The name, title, and telephone number of the person authorizing the referral must be noted on the chart.

5. Billing
   - Billing information and personal information unrelated to the health problem always should be kept separate from the medical record. The medical record can be subpoenaed and should be limited to the medical aspects of the case.
   - Complete a charge slip and insert it into the billing chart.
   - Compile all the business forms pertaining to patient, taking care to exclude medical forms, and place inside the billing chart.
   - Place the billing chart in appropriate area for administrative pick-up, and the medical chart in the appropriate area for medical records pick-up.

6. Follow-Up Appointments
   - If a patient has been treated for an occupational condition but returns to the clinic later for the same or a new problem, a new authorization must be obtained.

Form 11.1. Authorization for Medical Treatment

Date: _____ Time In: _____ Time Out: _____

To be completed by Employer

_____
Employee Name

_____
Company Name

_____
Company Address

_____
Company Phone

_____
Workers' Compensation Carrier

_____
Authorized Signature

☐ Physical Exam   ☐ Medical Services
☐ Physical therapy
Modified Work:
☐ Available
☐ Not available
☐ Call back requested

To be completed by Clinic
Treatment Administered:
☐ Office Visit—Injury Treatment
☐ Recheck or redress
☐ Medication
☐ Physical Exam
☐ Physical Therapy
☐ Refer to Specialist
☐ Return visit
   Date: _____ Time: _____
Work Status:
☐ Return to regular work
Date: _____
Modified Work Status:
☐ No prolonged standing or walking
☐ No climbing, bending, stooping
☐ No prolonged sitting
☐ No work near moving machinery
☐ Limited use: right/left hand
☐ Weight-lifting restriction

_____
_____
_____
_____
_____

Signature of Physician: _____

Billing for routine medical services, such as treatment, office visits, and laboratory tests, is highly standardized and procedures are usually automated. Medical services typically are coded by a standardized numerical coding system, such as the California Standard Nomenclature (CSN). The CSN was originally based on a system called the "California Relative Value Studies" (RVS) that assigned a "relative value" to each service. The CSN no longer assigns relative values, but the principle is still followed by practice managers and physicians when setting fees for billing and devising fee schedules. For example, a brief initial office visit by a new patient to establish a relatively simple medical problem (90000) carried a value of 5.9 in the RVS system, but a comprehensive initial medical evaluation (90026) carried a value of 17.5, and a consultation for a complex medical problem (90625) a value of 29.0. These, or similar, relative values are multiplied by a "conversion factor" (or standard fee schedule) in order to arrive at the final fee for the service to be billed to the insurance company. To continue the example, the comprehensive initial medical evaluation (90026), as billed to the California Workers' Compensation Board in 1983, would have been 17.5 (relative value) × $5.40 (conversion factor in 1983) = $94.50.

The relative values are permanent under this system but the conversion factors change annually; this allows for periodic adjustments across the board with a single rate change without the need to renegotiate every conceivable medical service, which would become an extremely time-consuming process. Surgical services carry a conversion factor that is higher than that of medical services. Relative values are intended to be consistent within, but not across, specialties in order to allow independent adjustments of each specialty category's fees. In recent years, however, the overall fee schedule for workers' compensation in California has been increasing steadily and the medical conversion factors have been slowly gaining ground compared to the other specialties. (Table 11.1 shows the California Workers' Compensation fee schedule current in 1988.)

Table 11.1. California Workers' Compensation Fee Schedule, Effective 1988.

"The 1974 Revision of the 1969 California Relative Value Studies, Fifth Edition, Revised, is hereby adopted and incorporated herein by reference as though set forth in full, including procedures, unit values and follow-up days."

"The following conversion factors are hereby adopted to be applied to the sections contained in the official fee schedule approved by the Division of Industrial Accidents, State of California:

Medicine Section	$ 6.15
Surgery Section	$153.00
Radiology Section	$ 11.20
Pathology Section	$ 1.50
Anesthesia Section	$ 34.50

The workers' compensation fee schedule may be derived by other means in other jurisdictions. Workers' compensation fees are responsive to the general level of usual and customary fees charged to insurance carriers in a state, although these usually are not quite as generous. There is great variation among states in the fee schedules payable for workers' compensation services. In Canada, the fees are tied to the provincial health plan. Services under workers' compensation are typically paid at the rate of the fee schedule for the provincial health insurance plan and for convenience may even be billed to the same provincial agency. The provincial insurance plan simply "back-bills" the workers' compensation board for reimbursement to recover the fees for services to deal with disorders identified as work-related. This system avoids the problem, common in the United States, of having an unpaid bill hang in limbo while the insurance carrier and the workers' compensation board argue over whether the injury or illness is work-related.

Most clinical services provided by occupational physicians are comparable to those already encoded in the CSN and differ only in the cognitive skills of the practitioner. Obviously, a physician trained in occupational medicine will see dimensions in a complex case that may not be apparent to another, although there would be little difference in managing an acute injury. Nonetheless, a few common services are unique to occupational medicine because they pertain to on-site plant visits, extensive consultations with employers, urgent consultations to deal with a hazardous situation, and other services that have no counterpart in personal health care. In the present CSN, these services have no identifiers but occur sufficiently enough to require a code number for billing and data management purposes. Table 11.2 presents a set of model service codes for specialized occupational health services that makes use of the gap in the numerical sequence of the 98000 series.

Under the proposed coding system, each service would be identified in the series by a five-digit number 98XXX:

Table 11.2. Proposed Numerical Codes for Specialized Occupational Health Services Provided by a Physician, Compatible With California Standard Nomenclature

Suggested Code and Relative Values	Name of Service	Description of Service
98001 (18.5)	Initial On-Site Consultation	Visit to client's location in order to ascertain client's needs, requiring approximately 1 hour.
98011 (17.5)	Initial Office Consultation	Visit by client to provider's office, in order to ascertain client's needs, requiring approximately 1 hour.
98101 (22.0)*	Consultation Visit, On-Site	Visit to client's location to evaluate a particular problem.
98131 (BR)	Routine Telephone Consultation	Telephone consultation concerning an uncomplicated problem, approximately 30 minutes in duration.
98201 (BR)	Health Hazard Evaluation	Extensive survey and evaluation of a problem, may require a team of professionals.**
98301 (26.1)	Follow-Up, Limited	Visit to plant to evaluate progress.
98302 (15.5)*	Follow-Up Evaluation	Visit to plant to assess progress in resolving a complex situation.
98401 (29.0)*	Emergency Visit, On-Site	Visit to client's location on short notice to assist with an urgent problem.
98431 (BR)	Emergency Telephone Consultation	Telephone consultation on an urgent problem not requiring presence on-site, approximately 30 minutes.
98501 (13.0)	Instructional Visit, On-Site	Visit to client's location to arrange or present a scheduled instructional program.
98921 (15.5)*	Consultation Services	Time spent in research, report preparation, or conceptualizing an approach and solution to a problem.

* Per hour
** Members of such a team may include industrial hygienists, safety engineers, epidemiologists, toxicologists, and specialized technical personnel as appropriate.
BR—By report, fees to be determined on an individual basis.

- The third digit represents *activity* (0 = exploratory discussion; 1 = consultation; 2 = health hazard evaluation; 3 = follow-up; 4 = emergency; 5 = scheduled activity such as an educational presentation; and 9 = research and literature review).
- The fourth digit represents *location* (0 = client's data bank; 3 = telephone communication).
- The fifth digit is a specific identifier. This scheme has been flexible enough to cover all situations encountered with ample latitude for expansion. The relative values assigned to the codes are multiplied by a specific fee schedule that is regularly revised.

The obsolete code 99060, "environmental intervention," should be abandoned since it is inadequate for describing occupational medicine services. Codes already exist for periodic health evaluation (90088, relative value 11.0); multiphasic health testing (99090); preparation of special reports (99080); and the administration of a programmed medical interview (99095). Except for 90088, fees for these services are all "by report," or at the discretion of the provider.

Each service, represented by a code, has a fee associated with it that is usually reviewed and updated once or twice a year. Fee schedules are usually kept in a computer file that can be easily updated. Nurses, physicians, and other medical staff keep track of the services rendered to patients on charge slips, usually by checking off the more common services from a long list and by writing in the codes of unusual services. Data from these charge slips are entered into the computer, which then automatically matches the codes with the current fee schedule and generates the bills.

It is often useful to keep track of the types of the medical services being used by employees of a particular company as a means of evaluating that company's occupational health and safety performance and identifying the employer's need for preventive services. Also, this kind of information may reveal that a company is utilizing the clinic for only a narrow range of services, such as acute care for work-related injuries. For example, a company with an unusual frequency of back injuries could be offered a back injury control program. An employer who uses only the most basic medical services could be approached by marketing personnel representing the clinic for other services, such as preplacement or periodic evaluations.

Consultation services are usually more individualized and cannot be so easily packaged as those mentioned in the last paragraph. Examples of consultation services include evaluating the validity of a workers' compensation claim; reviewing a case under litigation for medical evidence; giving testimony as an expert witness; advising on corporate policy or procedures; and designing a screening protocol for workers exposed to a particular hazard at a plant. These services do not lend themselves to the usual billing arrangement described above; one accepted format for billing for consultation services is presented as Form 11.2.

Protocols for Clinical Services

Many occupational health services are repetitive and are most efficiently performed by nurses and laboratory staff. To ensure standardization and the consistent quality of common procedures, it is important to prepare written "protocols," or step-by-step

---

Form 11.2. The Billing Format for Consultation Services

STATEMENT

(Date, Year)
Re: (Patient or Plant Name, File Number)
To: (Employer's Name)
    (Address)

Attention: (Official Responsible)
    Medical and consultative services rendered:
1. (Nature of activity), X hours at $XXX/hour $ XXX
2.   "   "
3.   "   "
(etc.)
                                                    Total $ X,XXX

Thank you for your prompt attention.

(Physician's Name)
(Social Security Number)

---

guidelines. These protocols can be used to train new staff, remind current staff to perform the procedures systematically, and check their performance for quality control.

In occupational medicine, procedures should be standardized whenever possible so that they be defensible later if a claim is questioned. As a practical matter, it is usually most convenient to write a protocol to the conduct of a particular test or procedure well in advance of the testing. Each protocol should spell out: the steps to be taken in conducting the procedure; those steps that must be documented; quality control measures; and contingencies to follow in the event of problems. Protocols should be developed with input and review from all parties concerned, including physicians, nurses, administrators, medical records personnel, and technicians. A simple but complete protocol can assist greatly in reducing confusion and can also expedite the efficient processing of patients. Protocols are absolutely necessary when many subjects are to be tested in the same way, or when testing is to be done in more than one location by different personnel.

A written protocol is also an invaluable tool that can be used for teaching new staff or for helping existing staff review procedures. Protocols can identify criteria for evaluating staff performance, as described in Chapter 14. The very act of writing a protocol forces one to think about each step in the procedure. This process helps to identify specific points at which decisions must be made and identifies opportunities for introducing efficiencies.

Exhibit 11.2 is a protocol for tuberculin skin testing, an inexpensive and reliable screen for exposure to tuberculosis. The protocol was designed to permit testing to be done in a standardized, reproduceable manner by nurses in several locations of a multi-centered medical group in compliance with accepted procedures. Most protocols will be simpler, but this example demonstrates the concept.

Exhibit 11.2. Tuberculin Skin Testing Protocol

1. *Tuberculin Skin Testing Policy*
- A Registered Nurse, Licensed Vocational Nurse, or Medical Assistant who has successfully completed a training program and guided clinical experience in the performance of skin testing may perform and interpret tuberculin skin tests upon the authorization of the physician.
- Each nurse who is to conduct skin testing will first be observed performing the procedure on two (2) occasions by a designated physician. A written statement verifying the nurse's competency in the procedure will be forwarded to the Nursing Department and permanently filed.

2. *Tuberculin Skin Test Record*
- *Original*: Kept on file as permanent record of patient visit after skin test is read.
- *Second Copy*: Employer's record, presented to patient for delivery to employer after skin test is read.
- *Third Copy*: Presented to patient for personal health records.
- *Fourth Copy*: Forward to Accounting Department at end of day skin test is read, for billing.

3. *Responsibilities of Receptionist*
NOTE: A separate appointment book will be utilized and non-contract patients notified of the prepayment fee.
- Scheduling Hours (initial and return appointments)
  Day of Appointment
  - Register patient. (Instruct patient to fill out top portion of Tuberculin Skin Test Record Form.)
  - Collect fee if appropriate. Mark "paid" and write in amount in the appropriate section on record form and sign, using your first initial and last name. Detach fourth copy and place in cash drawer.
  - Place Record Form, intact, in appropriate place for nurse.

- Scheduling Return Visit
  - Schedule return visit for Skin Test Reading as indicated on the back of the third copy of Record Form.
  - Provide the patient with an appointment card.
  - Place Tuberculin Skin Test Record Form, intact, in return visit file.

- Day of Return Visit for Skin Test Reading
  - Pull Tuberculin Skin Test Record form from the file in anticipation of scheduled arrival.
  - Upon patient's arrival, place Record Form intact, in the appropriate place for nurse.
  - Upon completion of skin test reading, when patient returns to receptionist desk, separate Record Form:
    - Original: Place in permanent file.
    - Second Copy: Private patients—present to patient to carry to Employer. Contract patient—other charges at end of day and forwarded to Occupational Medicine desk.
    - Third Copy—presented to patient for personal health records.
    - Fourth Copy: Forward to Accounting Department at end of day.

4. *Responsibilities of Nurse*
- Day of Appointment
  - Calls and greets the patient and escorts patient to testing area. This may be the examination room, if available, or nurse's station.
  - Briefly explains the procedure and asks patient the following questions:

(Continued)

Exhibit 11.2. Continued

- "Have you ever had tuberculosis or a positive TB skin test in the past?"
  NOTE: If the patient's answer is "yes"—*DO NOT TEST THE PATIENT.*
        If the patient is unsure—*seek medical (physician) assistance.*
- "Are you now taking steriods, cortisone, ACTH, cancer chemotherapy, or
  drugs to suppress organ transplant rejection?"
  If the answer is "yes"—*seek medical assistance.*

- Equipment
  Tuberculin Syringe with #27½ needle (Sterile Technique)
  Solution of *Purified Protein Derivative (5 ml. vial—use 0.1 ml.)*
  Alcohol sponge
  Felt marking pen

- Preparation and Administration
  - Withdraw (*exactly*) 0.1 ml. of PPD into a (1.0 ml.) Tuberculin Syringe with
    #27½ needle.
    NOTE: *DO NOT attempt to second-guess dead space in syringe.*
  - Cleanse the skin of the volar forearm with the alcohol sponge same side as
    the palm of the hand. *NOTE*: *Use non-dominant arm.*
  - Hold the forearm skin taut; holding the syringe with the needle bevel facing
    up, inject the full quantity of PPD into the forearm—away from the large
    veins, scars, rashes or wounds.
  - A visible bleb should rise just over the needle point of injection. If this does
    not occur, the injection was not intra-dermal, and the test is invalid.
  - Mark the location on the patient's forearm by circling the injection site with a
    felt pen.
  - Instruct the patient to return for a reading in 48 hours. (No more than 72
    hours can be allowed to elapse.) If the patient delays beyond 72 hours, seek
    medical assistance in interpreting the test.
    NOTE: *Tests cannot be read before 48 hours have elapsed.*
  - Record date performed, time, PPD strength and amount on Tuberculin Skin
    Test Record form, and sign form.

- Skin Test Reading
  - Find injection site by locating felt marker circle on forearm.
  - Ignore any redness visible at injection site.
  - Run your finger over the injection site. If you feel a *hard*, button-like, firm
    area of "induration" in the skin, note where the edges are located.
  - Utilizing a millimeter ruler, measure the diameter of the induration across the
    center, *from edge to opposite edge, perpendicular to the long axis of the
    arm.* Record this measurement in millimeters (mm).

- Interpreting the Skin Test
  - No reaction to 5 mm = Negative reaction.
  - 5 mm to 10 mm = Negative (unless there is a reason to suspect recent
    exposure to tuberculosis) *Must be questioned by the nurse.*
  - 10 mm or greater = Positive
  - 25 mm or greater; with warmth and heavy redness = Strongly positive,
    sloughing reaction.
  - All positive readings are to be checked by a designated physician.
  - If reading is 25 mm or greater, *MUST* be seen by a physician for follow-up.
  - If chest film is ordered in the presence of a positive reaction, patient must be
    registered as new patient.

(Continued)

Exhibit 11.2. Continued

- Follow-up Action
  - Negative Reaction: Advise patient and record.
  - Positive Reaction: Advise patient that medical evaluation is required without undue delay and that treatment may be required. Record that this advice was given and offer to make an appointment to follow up.
  - Sloughing Reaction: Seek *immediate* medical assistance and record. *NOTE*: Repeat skin tests should not be given for several weeks, and should NEVER be given to an individual known to have had a sloughing reaction in the past.
  - Provide patient with Record Form (intact) with instructions to proceed to receptionist's desk.

Further Reading

A Guide for the Preparation of a Manual of Policies and Procedures for the Occupational Health Service. New York, American Association of Industrial Health Nurses, 1969.

California Medical Association: 1985 California Standard Nomenclature. San Francisco, Sutter Publications, 1986.

California Medical Association: California Relative Value Studies, 1974 Revision. San Francisco, Sutter Publications, 1975.

Copeman JP, van Zwanenberg TD: Practice receptionists: Poorly trained and taken for granted? J Roy Coll Gen Pract 1988; 38; 14–16.

Doctors' Administrative Program Series. Florence KY, Medical Economics Books, 1979.

Official Medical Fee Schedule for Services Rendered Under the California Workers' Compensation Laws. San Francisco California Workers' Compensation Institute, 1980, updated annually.

12 RECORDKEEPING

No matter how small an occupational health service, recordkeeping is a necessary activity. Obviously, the service must keep administrative and billing records, but more importantly, it must maintain personal health and environmental health records that:

- Document employee hazard exposures;
- Apply employee health data to job placement (fitness to work);
- Document employee health over time;
- Provide data for use in health program evaluation; and
- Fulfill regulatory requirements.

Types of Records

Personal Health Records

The health status of each individual worker is recorded on the personal health records. These records inevitably contain personal and confidential information of special significance within the law. Chapter 4 describes the ethical constraints on physicians and nurses with regard to releasing personal information from these records outside of the facility, especially to representatives of the employer. (Obligations also apply to the maintenance and internal use of company-initiated personal health records.)

The actual record is normally the property of the employer or, in the case of an occupational health service serving many employers, whoever caused the record to be created in the first place. However, the individual worker controls the right of access to information contained in the record, and the information is held in trust by the physician or nurse who compiled it. The employer's right to this information is normally limited to the physician's or nurse's interpretation in the form of job-oriented statements of fitness to work. With certain legal exceptions, only the worker can authorize release of health information from his or her personal health record.

For maximum accuracy and medical and legal reliability, entries should be made chronologically each time the worker is seen, with each note signed by the person making the entry. Entries must accurately and completely document the care given and actions taken on the employee's behalf.

A worker's personal health record should reflect his or her health status insofar as it applies to the job. Although the content of these records may vary a great deal, the following information generally is included:

- Results of physical examinations;
- X-ray and laboratory reports (including EKG, pulmonary function results, audiograms);
- Acute care entries and progress notes (an additional separate Acute Care Register often also is kept);
- Record of immunizations;
- Occupational and medical histories;
- Hazard exposure record;
- Health programs participation record;
- Informed consent forms and authorizations for release of information;
- Documentation of refusals to undergo examination, testing, and program participation;
- Workers' compensation and insurance records;
- Progress notes for rehabilitation; and
- Consultant reports.

Current records of first aid treatment are often kept at the first aid station at each worksite. This permits accidental injuries to be recorded at the worksites where they occur, thus eliminating the need for an employee with a trivial injury to leave work and go to the clinic simply to record its occurrence. (Old records usually are stored at a central occupational health clinic in a plant.) The occupational health center or clinic should keep a record of all primary treatment it provides in an Acute Care Register.

In some locations, government regulations require that first aid records be kept. Mandated or not, such records always are important in the assessment of compensation claims and should be the responsibility of designated first aid or operations personnel. They also provide data vital to the assessment of the company's accident prevention program.

Records of employee absence and the measures taken to control absence from work are direct supervisory responsibilities. The occupational health service is not designed to police or enforce the employer's personnel regulations, but should have access to absence data in order to determine its impact on reducing health-related or -attributed absences.

Environmental Hazard Records
Environmental hazard records detail toxic or physical hazards in the job. Documents pertinent to work procedures and protective clothing may apply to a particular employee or group of employees and may be incorporated in individual health records.

Environmental hazard records include site visit reports, hazard monitoring results, worksite health and safety committee reports, and accident investigation files. These records are normally produced and maintained by the employer's safety or hygiene staff, but in a small company may be the responsibility of designated operations personnel. Personal health data should not be included in any of these records since they do not come under medical confidentiality guidelines. Access to them therefore is determined only by individual company policy and applicable legal requirements.

Miscellaneous Records

In addition to administrative records that are common to all organizations, the occupational health service may keep a number of other records, each with its own unique purpose:

- Daily log of the number of workers seen and services performed. This record is useful for assessing the impact of workplace health hazards on the workforce and also serves as a source of data for measuring the effectiveness of existing hazard controls and injury or illness preventive measures. It is invaluable in recording fitness-to-work evaluations and the impact of timely intervention on length of absence.
- Health program records and reports. These usually contain data useful for evaluating specific designated ongoing programs, such as hearing conservation, environmental monitoring, and employee assistance.
- Drug register. This is a mandatory record of all medications in stock and amounts dispensed to workers through the service. (Special procedures are required for scheduled drugs.)

If possible, the occupational health service also should maintain a regularly updated record of hazardous materials used or produced at the worksites it regularly serves, particularly in a plant or corporate occupational health facility. It also should document compliance with the worker notification and education requirements of OSHA's recent hazard communications regulation. Maintaining a file of current Material Safety Data Sheets on these materials is a useful way of keeping hazard information. However, these documents are notoriously shallow in information about long-term health effects and in the information they provide on treatment. Reference works on the clinical toxicology of commercial materials are therefore important to have on hand. Current copies of government occupational health and safety regulations, and the company's own health and safety policies and procedures also should be readily available to staff.

Recordkeeping Systems

Systems for keeping records should be economical, efficient, convenient for users, and easily retrievable, yet guard against unauthorized access. Before applying new procedures across the board, the occupational health service should try out new record forms or systems with an eye to how well they meet these criteria. In particular, the service should ensure that coding systems are compatible with existing, widely recognized systems. For example, coding for illnesses and injuries should be in accordance with either the International Classification of Diseases, Injuries and Causes of Death of the World Health Organization or Z16.2 of the American National Standards Institute. The former code is the standard system used in hospitals and epidemiological research; the latter is less refined but is widely used for administrative purposes by workers' compensation agencies. Consistent coding enables the service to compare injury and illness data with results published from other sources.

Whichever filing system is chosen, OSHA regulations require that medical and industrial hygiene records be retained for at least 30 years. This allows access to the records in the event that workers are identified as having subsequent health problems. These records must be transferred to a responsible recipient (such as a successor facility) or government agency if the employer or clinic goes out of business.

Computer storage permits automatic and very rapid retrieval of data in any combination and desired sequence. This is invaluable, not only for worker health evaluation but also for health program operations and audit. However, computer storage must be governed by strict controls that limit access to recorded personal health information.

While the service must take pains to record all relevant and necessary information, it must also guard against recording extraneous and useless data. In deciding whether to retain a particular piece of information, the service should ask:

- Is this information required by regulation?
- Will this information be used?
- Will its use justify the cost of maintaining it?
- Can the information be obtained easily and with accuracy?
- Will the process of obtaining the information contravene or compromise legislated civil rights?
- Are secure facilities available to store the records for the required retention period?

In general, a good occupational health record should allow the reader to piece together as clear and coherent a picture as possible of the worker's exposure on the job, health status, treatments, job assignment, and identity, even 30 years after the fact. Many associations between chronic diseases and occupational exposures have been made using these types of records and they are always important to maintain as legal documents.

Format of Records

Following are three forms that are useful in occupational health practice:

- A general Patient Encounter Form (Form 12.1), which provides details of the injury or illness and examination and which can be used alone for routine acute care or fitness-to-work evaluations. This form also can be used for more detailed evaluations in conjunction with the next form.
- A more detailed Individual History Form (Form 12.2), which is filled out by the patient waiting to be seen. This form is intended for medical monitoring (see Chapter 20) or in-depth medical evaluation; it is not intended for use in fitness-to-work evaluations, because the detail is not pertinent to the assessment. Form 12.2 also is designed to be used in conjunction with Form 12.1; it does not duplicate the information obtained in the earlier form but rather captures information on the worker's employment history and occupational exposures, personal health, and health-related habits. It is not sufficiently detailed to replace a careful review of systems in a complex case or to guide counselling in a detailed health assessment but it is adequate for most general purposes.
- A Release Form (Form 12.3) allowing medical records to be requested for consultation or medicolegal purposes. This legal document complies with stringent California

state laws governing confidentiality of medical records and, consequently, is possibly more elaborate than those required by other jurisdictions. Even so, in the present climate of increasing litigation, a prudent physician will obtain indisputable authorization for all transfers of confidential information. Some facilities and practitioners prefer to give themselves this additional protection against later claims by workers who did not understand that medical information might be shared in their cases.

Form 12.1. Patient Encounter Form

Name _____

Med. Rec. No. _____

Occupation, Industry _____

Employer _____

Carrier _____ Social Security # _____

Home Address _____

Home Telephone _____ Birthdate _____

Sex: M   F   Marital Status _____

Reason for Visit: ☐ Accident   Time In: _____:_____a.m.
                    ☐ Preplacement   Time Out: _____:_____p.m.
                    ☐ Periodic Examination   Date: _____
                    ☐ Other

History of Injury or Illness: _____
_____

Allergies: _____ Medications: _____

Temp: _____ Height: _____ Weight: _____ Pulse _____ BP _____ / _____

Abnormal Findings: _____

Head: _____ Eyes: R _____ L _____

Ears: R _____ L _____ Nose: _____

Throat: _____ Mouth: _____

Chest: _____ Lungs: _____

Heart: _____ Abdomen: _____

Inguinal Rings: _____ R _____ L _____

Spine: _____ Extremities: _____

Neurological Examination: _____

Mental Status: _____

CBC: WBC _____ RBC _____ Hgb _____ Hct _____ MCV _____ MCH _____ MCHC _____

Serum chemistries: _____

Urinalysis: sp. grav _____ glu _____ alb _____ blood _____ micro _____

X-ray: _____

Stool occult blood: _____

Fitness for Work: _____

Recommendation for further examination or follow-up: _____

Name of Examing Physician _____   Signature of Examining Physician   Date of Exam

(Courtesy of Sharp Rees-Stealy Medical Group, San Diego, CA)

Form 12.2. Individual History Form

Name: _____

Address: _____

Telephone: Home _____   Work _____

Date of Birth: _____   Sex: ☐ Male   ☐ Female

Social Security No. _____   Health Insurance No. _____

OCCUPATIONAL PROFILE:

Fill in the table below listing all the jobs you have ever had (even short-term, seasonal and part-time work).

Start with your present job first and go backward to the earliest. Use additional paper if necessary.

Work place/address	From To	Type of Industry/Firm	Brief Description of Job	Known Health Hazards

Do you use any form of personal protection on the job?

Face masks	Gloves	Ear plugs	Steel-tipped shoes
SCUBA respirators	Aprons	Muff-type headsets	Hard hats
Hoods/helmets	Goggles	Insulated clothing	Other

Have you ever worked at any other dusty jobs? ☐ Yes   ☐ No

If yes, please explain: _____

Have you ever been exposed regularly to any type of irritating gas? ☐ Yes   ☐ No

Other chemical? ☐ Yes   ☐ No   Noise? ☐ Yes   ☐ No

If yes, please explain: _____

Have you ever been off work for a shift or longer because of illness related to work? ☐ Yes ☐ No

If yes, please explain: _____

To the best of your knowledge have you ever worked at a job where you handled any of the following materials? Please circle if yes:

Asbestos	Cotton	Gasoline & Oil	Silica (Sand & Quartz)
Asphalt & Tar	Creosote	Lead	Powders (Please specify)

(Continued)

Form 12.2. Continued

Benzene   Dusts (Please specify)   Mercury   Solvents
Beryllium   Dyes & Stains   Paints   Welding Fumes
Coal   Fiberglass   Pesticides/Fungicides   X-Ray or Radioactive
Plastics   TDI or other Isocyanates   Materials
Other: _____

Are you allergic to anything (substances you have encountered on the job, or foods, medicines, animals, pollen, etc.)? ☐ Yes   ☐ No
If so, what are you allergic to? _____
What kind of a reaction do you get? _____
Do you smoke cigarettes? ☐ Yes   ☐ Quit   ☐ Never Smoked
If so, how many packs per day? _____ How long have you been smoking? _____
Do you use tobacco other than smoking cigarettes (pipes, cigars, snuff dipper)? ☐ Yes ☐ No
If so how?_____
How often do you use tobacco? _____ How long have you been using it? _____
Have you ever had a serious illness as an adult? ☐ Yes   ☐ No
If so, write the year in which it occurred next to the disease identified on this list. If the disease is not on this list, please write it below.

☐ Arthritis   ☐ Glaucoma   ☐ Malaria
☐ Asthma   ☐ Heart Disease   ☐ Mononucleosis
☐ Bronchitis   ☐ Hepatitis   ☐ Pneumonia
☐ Cancer   ☐ Hernia   ☐ Prostate Trouble
☐ Diabetes   ☐ High Blood Pressure   ☐ Rheumatic Fever
☐ Emphysema   ☐ Kidney Disease   ☐ Tuberculosis
☐ Epilepsy   ☐ Liver Disease   ☐ Venereal Disease
Other? _____ When? _____
Have you ever had surgery? ☐ Yes   ☐ No
If so, please list operations and give approximate year.

_____ _____

_____ _____

Are you taking any medicine now? ☐ Yes   ☐ No
If so, please list them. (Include nonprescription drugs) _____

Have you ever had any of the following: (Please circle the correct response)
Sudden or rapid weight loss without dieting? .... Yes No
Loss of appetite? .... Yes No
Unusual difficulty in being comfortable during cold weather? .... Yes No
Unusual difficulty in being comfortable during hot weather? .... Yes No
Overweight?... Yes No
A skin rash or sore which stayed for weeks? .... Yes No
Sudden changes in your vision?... Yes No
Double vision? .... Yes No
Changes in your ability to hear? .... Yes No

(Continued)

Form 12.2. Continued

Changes in your sense of smell? . . . . Yes   No
Changes in your sense of balance? . . . . Yes   No
Swelling in the armpit or groin? . . . . Yes   No
Shortness of breath? . . . . Yes   No
Wheezing when you breathe? . . . . Yes   No
A persistent cough? . . . . Yes   No
Coughing up blood? . . . . Yes   No
Pains or tightness in your chest? . . . . Yes   No
Irregularity in your heartbeat or heart "palpitations"? . . . . Yes   No
Swelling in your ankles or legs? . . . . Yes   No
Nausea or vomiting over several days? . . . . Yes   No
Pain in your abdomen? . . . . Yes   No
Loose or runny stools or diarrhea? . . . . Yes   No
Constipation? . . . . Yes   No
Vomiting blood? . . . . Yes   No
Black stools that looked like tar? . . . . Yes   No
Blood in your stools? . . . . Yes   No
Yellow jaundice? . . . . Yes   No
Swelling or lumps in your breast (women) or testicles (men)? . . . . Yes   No
Difficulty when urinating or pain when urinating? . . . . Yes   No
Heavy or irregular menstrual flow (women)? . . . . Yes   No
Loss of consciousness for any reason? . . . . Yes   No
Seizures or convulsions? . . . . Yes   No
Have you ever injured your back (enough to require: a visit to a physician,
    a chiropractor, or the need to take medicine stronger than aspirin)? . . . . Yes   No
Do you often have aching or pains in your neck, lower back or in the
    back of your legs? . . . . Yes   No
Do you have a "trick knee" or any other joint (elbow, ankle or other)
    that tends to "give out or lock"? . . . . Yes   No
Have you ever had whiplash? . . . . Yes   No
Did you play football in high school or college? . . . . Yes   No
Do you wear contact lenses on the job? . . . . Yes   No
Do you often drive without seatbelts? . . . . Yes   No
Have you ever felt, been told, or suspected that you had difficulties dealing
    with alcohol? . . . . Yes   No
Have you ever used drugs for purposes other than as medication? . . . . Yes   No

(Courtesy of Sharp Rees-Stealy Medical Group, San Diego, CA)

Form 12.3. Authorization to Receive or Release Medical Information

I hereby authorize _____

_____
(name and address of physician, hospital or health care provider)

to furnish to _____

_____
(name and address of requester)

medical records and information pertaining to the medical history, mental or physical condition, services rendered, or treatment given to:

_____
(PRINT—name of patient)

_____
(date of birth)

This authorization is limited to the following medical records and types of information:

_____

The information supplied is to be used for the following purpose(s):

_____

This authorization shall become effective immediately and shall remain in effect until: _____
(date)

I understand that the requester may not further use or disclose the medical information
unless another authorization is obtained from me or unless such use or disclosure is specifically required or permitted by law.

I further understand that I have a right to receive a copy of this authorization upon my
request. Copy requested and received: ☐ Yes   ☐ No   ☐ Initials

Signed: _____   Date: _____

Relation if not self: _____   Witness: _____
(Patient, Parent, Guardian or Legal   (name and title)
Representative of Patient)

(Courtesy of Sharp Rees-Stealy Medical Group, San Diego, CA)

Further Reading

Canadian Health Record Association: Guidelines to the Code of Practice. Canadian College of Health Record Administrators, 1980.

Goerth CR: Clarifying the verbiage of the new access to records standard. Occup Health
and Safety September 1980; 49:23–28, 74.

Guidotti TL, et al: Taking the occupational history. Ann Int Med 1983: 99:641–651.

Guidotti TL: Exposure to hazard and individual risk: when occupational medicine gets
personal. J Occup Med 1988; 30: 570–577.

Rose L: Conflicting views on the issue of accessibility. OH&S Jan. 1981; 50:33–37.

Strasser AL: OSHA and the access to records standard. OH&S Jan. 1981; 50:21–22.

U.S. Occupational Safety and Health Administration: Access to employee exposure and
medical records. Fed Reg 7 August 1981; 46(152):40490–40491.

SECTION IV
PROGRAM MANAGEMENT

13 SERVICE SELECTION AND IMPLEMENTATION

A successful occupational health service is one that is appropriate to the needs of the organization it serves, is efficiently managed, and presents many benefits for a modest cost. The programs available in the health services marketplace are virtually without limit and are heavily promoted by their sponsors. But such "packaged" occupational health programs that are for sale may be of little or no value—some may be poorly conceived or badly implemented, others may be inflexible, and still others just unsuitable to the employer's particular situation. An employer can avoid the trap of paying for a system that fails to meet its particular need through careful analysis and good planning. A successful service is rarely found "off the shelf" but a well designed existing program with a successful track record and built-in flexibility can save an employer a great deal of time and money.

In identifying and selecting service components that are appropriate to its specific situation, the employer first must determine its priority needs in occupational health. This task requires gathering information about the company and its workforce:

- Workplace health hazards in daily operations, including hazardous materials used, hazards of a physical nature, and hazardous work processes or procedures.
- The main characteristics of the employee population that would affect the response to the hazards, such as age range and average age, sex ratio, average length of employment with the company, and average educational and skill level.
- Occupational health records available for review and their reliability.
- Quality and characteristics of working life, including the nature of the work carried out by employees, conditions of work, quality of employee supervision, state of worker-management relations, the employer's existing health and safety policies and procedures, and health problems prevalent in the community at large.

If the situation is at all complex, the employer should consider hiring a qualified occupational health professional as a consultant in order to assess needs. Advice also can be obtained from external occupational health services, universities with occupational health programs, other employers, and government agencies. Analysis by external occupational health services and some consultants may be affected by a conflict of interest if they also are marketing their own services. Some employers first conduct a careful and thorough analysis and then contract with an independent consultant for advice. An objective consultant can advise on the selection of existing packaged programs and their suitability, frequently a less expensive alternative to developing a custom program from scratch. Governmental advice is free, but is often quite limited in scope and does not normally include the direct provision of occupational health services to private employers.

Once needs are identified, the employer's next responsibility is to obtain services or to implement programs. On the basis of the information obtained, the occupational health services manager can select the specific programs or delivery components the employer needs. Of primary consideration are those program elements that respond to general needs throughout industry and that serve as foundations for later development. These generally include:

- The occupational health and safety policy of the company. (See Chapter 5.)
- Acute care for illnesses and injuries. (See Chapter 17.)
- Environmental monitoring. (See Chapters 20 and 23.)
- Preplacement, periodic health, and other fitness-to-work evaluations. (See Chapter 18.)
- Industrial hygiene and other hazard control-oriented services. (See Chapter 23.)

The employer's policy heads the list because it is the keystone that supports the entire array of occupational health programs, establishing the priority given by the employer to the health of its workers and the safety of workplaces under its control. A company's occupational health and safety policy should originate with and be visibly supported by its top management. It must be more than a statement of good intent; it should include specific policy statements that pertain to: environmental hazard control, employee health monitoring and surveillance, confidentiality of personal health information, post-injury or illness rehabilitation, hazard communication, and notification of worker laboratory and medical test results. This policy statement should be accessible to all company employees. (The critical role of the policy statement is described in more detail in Chapter 5.)

There are a number of other service components, the need for which will vary with the individual plant, the workers, and the hazards faced. These include:

- Employee assistance. (See Chapter 26.)
- Health promotion and education. (See Chapter 27.)
- Special preventive programs (such as immunizations for travel, assessment for fitness to wear respirators, and institutional smoke-free policies).
- Rehabilitation for employees returning to work after injury or illness. (See Chapter 19.)
- Disaster or incident response. (See Chapter 24.)

Standards and Quality of Care

The term "standard" has two distinct, almost diametrically opposed meanings. A "standard" may be a criterion for quality or acceptability, a level of quality or performance that is sought but not necessarily achieved. A "standard" also may be the usual level of practice or the customary way of doing things. The first meaning implies that there is a test of acceptable practice that has been established by a high authority, such as a government regulatory agency, an ethical code, or the expectations of society or peers. The second meaning implies the minimum one can get away with without being perceived as conspicuously inferior, as determined by usual custom and the actual practice of even one's peers. Standards of practice may have aspects of both definitions.

Standards in occupational medicine are not as simple and direct as they are in general health care. For legal purposes in deciding malpractice cases, the criterion employed is the standard of practice in the community. The fact that a physician treats a patient in a manner similar to that used by most other physicians in a comparable area is a defense against liability for improper practice. Occupational medicine shares identical standards of clinical care for injuries and illness—but many activities fall outside the scope of a community standard of practice.

The physician in the occupational health care system is part of a much larger network that balances the legitimate interests of the five or six parties who may be involved in any case: the physician, the worker, the employer, the workers' compensation carrier, the government (OSHA or its counterpart), and, often, the workers' union. The physician's traditional one-to-one relationship with the patient is modified into a hierarchy of responsibilities in which the relationship to the patient is primary but not exclusive and which may be governed in important respects by law, government regulation, fiduciary responsibility, and obligations toward the other parties.

Quality of Care
The delivery of occupational health services is diffused in most communities, centralized only in such special institutions as industry or medical schools. It therefore is more difficult for the busy practitioner to know whether he or she is practicing at a suitable standard for services other than acute medical or surgical care. This is particularly true when occupational medicine is only a small portion of the physician's practice. In general, the medical management of an occupationally related case should be no different than that of a comparable case in general medical care. It is beyond the capability of any clinician to recall all the possible health effects of toxic exposures or the particulars of many industries. Knowing where to find this information and where to send the worker-patient for referral is a principal responsibility of any physician who deals with work-related disorders.

Frequently, the physician is faced with requests to provide services that are not medically indicated but that pose no harm to the patient, e.g., requests to perform periodic health or preplacement evaluations that are obsolete in design. The physician in this situation should generally prepare a brief letter to the employer outlining his or her reservations based on medical grounds. However, if the employer insists and there are no tests that do harm or are contraindicated, the employer's request should be honored. Screening methods in preplacement evaluations are ingrained and notoriously slow to change; most employers are reluctant to change a policy that is perceived to be successful. Physicians then should concentrate on interpreting any abnormal findings on tests and pay due attention to the principles of clinical epidemiology. (See Chapter 20.) They also should monitor the interpretation and usage of clinical tests to ensure that practices are not abused and that the unsound screening program does not unfairly penalize the worker.

The situation is very different when the physician is asked to perform a study or to employ a treatment that is dangerous or unproven. For example, absent a specific indication, low back X-rays have a very low yield of pathology, are rarely helpful in predicting whether an employee will develop back pain, and expose the subject to a significant amount of radiation for no benefit. Certain therapies, such as chelation to lower blood lead levels, are dangerous and rarely required. In these situations the physician has a duty to explain in precise, clear, and logical terms why he or she is refusing to follow the employer's request and to explain the matter diplomatically to the employee. Usually, such issues arise because an employer is following obsolete guidelines or lacks a medical consultant who has current occupational health experience.

If a physician cannot provide a service or is not knowledgeable in the area of requested care, he or she has an absolute duty either to refer the case or to acquire the necessary skill at a level commensurate with responsibilities. A physician should not, for example, accept responsibility for overseeing a screening program for asbestos-related disorders without first becoming familiar with the clinical aspects of asbestos-related diseases and the asbestos standard.

The occupational physician also must deal with questions of continuity of care. Occupational specialists may be viewed by their primary care counterparts as interlopers and encroachers; conversely, the occupational physicians may consider their primary care colleagues as lacking the specialized knowledge needed to manage many uniquely occupational problems. It is very important that such disagreements be handled in a mature and rational manner because the worker's best interest is served when the two physicians work together. In general, the occupational physician should perform or arrange for routine screening tests for three reasons:

- Primary care physicians may not have the background to interpret the implications of the findings with respect to a particular job;
- Plant physicians are in part responsible for protecting the health of employees in their plants and must be personally satisfied with the evaluations; and
- A busy practitioner is often tempted to cut corners by substituting past examinations or recent lab tests or to bend guidelines to the benefit of his or her personal patients.

On the other hand, it is often better for the private physician to handle a worker's long-term treatment, except for cases that fall outside primary care practice, such as toxicity-related problems. A personal physician who is handling the management of a case should not take offense if the plant physician routinely sees the patient or calls to monitor progress. The two physicians should consult togther following the fitness-to-work procedure, and make a joint decision to allow the patient-employee to return to work. (See Chapter 18.)

Standards of Performance

"Standards of performance" are indicators of how well occupational health services meet the needs of the workforce and the employer; they do not emphasize care of the individual worker-patient. Performance measures can be categorized in many ways; here the discussion will focus on efficiency, cost, effectiveness, and administration.

Although they are less costly than treatment of or compensation for major health problems, occupational health programs in industry are significant budget items. Whether an employer has a small-scale safety program or a complete corporate medical department, management must meet expenses associated with personnel, facilities, administrative support, and overhead (heating, maintenance, custodial services, and equipment). The manager must be able to demonstrate to the employer that a program effectively meets its goals and is run as efficiently as possible – and this in turn requires closely monitoring all costs and steering clear of unnecessary, expensive programs. From industry's point of view, this strategy is responsible and business-like and is consistent with the social purpose of industry in the first place – creating wealth and providing the goods and services needed by society.

The problem with this strategy, however, is that it is often applied too conservatively, especially in companies that are growing rapidly or that are facing financial problems. Although reasonable estimates can be made (see Chapter 15), it is often impossible to document accurately the financial benefits of employee health protection. Preventive services can only be evaluated by accounting (usually on the basis of past experience) for problems that were avoided, such as injuries that did not happen or health problems that were eliminated. Managers are usually skeptical of these estimates and tend to rely on changes from year to year. This practice is often misleading; because of the effect of other factors, such as changes in hiring or retirement policies, many health promotion activities do not make an impact over the short term. Many secondary benefits of these programs are not reflected in financial terms or in an obviously reduced risk of liability. Nevertheless, an increasing number of larger employers are taking a broader view of the health of their employees and are establishing offices to manage their human resources as well as they do their material resources. Small companies generally cannot afford such substantial outlays, one reason why occupational health services are usually weakest in small businesses. (See Chapter 5.)

Performance evaluations are even more difficult in off-site settings where occupational health services are provided through a private medical practice. The individual physician or clinic seldom serves all workers in a single plant and usually cannot easily retrieve information that is needed to judge the efficiency of the service. Employers may use as rough guides, however, certain indicators, such as the delay between the arrival of a worker for a visit and his or her release. While this is only a crude indicator of performance efficiency, it is often watched carefully by employers; excessive delays, perhaps due to bottlenecks in lab and paperwork flows, are frequent causes of complaint. First reports and supplemental reports should be filed within 24 hours – the workers' compensation system needs this information to make critical decisions on whether a worker is eligible for compensation, how long payments should last, and when a case can be closed.

Employers also need information to help them in practical concerns about scheduling work, reassigning personnel, or hiring a replacement. Too often, they are made to wait for a report when a simple – and timely – telephone call or a handwritten note from the physician or nurse would suffice. Other times, the employer may be unable to interpret a report because the information presented is vague or expressed in terms that are strictly medical. Since the quality and quantity of communication from the occupational health service can make or break the employer's impression of the service, the practitioner should strive for precise terminology and should use the telephone as freely as is necessary to clarify requests for information and to keep all parties informed.

Scheduling of return visits by workers under treatment is another common source of problems. For example, in general medical care, a patient with low back pain usually is treated conservatively and scheduled for a return visit in two weeks. This length of time for rest is now considered excessive by most authorities. In occupational medicine, however, such treatment also would be viewed by the workers' compensation carrier or the employer as evidence that the physician is not responsive to organizational needs. On the one hand, the worker-patient may be fit to return to work in one week; on the other, a second back strain a week later may have compounded the original injury, extending the temporary disability beyond the two-week period. The physician who fails to see the patient in the interim will have no knowledge of developments.

Return visits should be scheduled as often as necessary in order to monitor the course of the employee's recovery up to the point that the recovery is either complete or stable. In some cases, this may be daily, but usually it is weekly, even if the duration of the return visit is only a few minutes. Unlike general ambulatory care, occupational health care requires frequent return visits for close monitoring of even routine problems. For the workers' compensation system, the costs of additional return visits and supplemental reports are more than offset by the expenses that mount up when cases drag on without a clear prognosis or when employees do not return to work for several days despite a complete recovery. The worker also benefits from returning to a normal life at full wages or salary rather than staying off work indefinitely with an uncertain prognosis. Finally, there is also excellent evidence, particularly in the case of back strain, that prolonged time away from normal activities interferes with normal recovery.

Quality Control

As occupational health services expand, two problems arise in maintaining quality of care: controlling an increasing number of staff and managing the stress placed on the entire system by a growing caseload.

Today, quality control in occupational medicine is a major problem. In the past, the field attracted many highly questionable practitioners, and it is still overloaded with physicians who practice as if health care were a job to be done rather than a specialty and a commitment. Although developments at the leading edge of research in the specialty are progressing very rapidly, everyday clinical practice still consists mainly of routine examinations and treatment of minor trauma. The routine is subject to a deterioration in quality over time due to boredom or bad habits, particularly when the practice is isolated. Client employers are not always well informed or reasonable in their requests, and the practitioner may be tempted to take the path of least resistance and comply with ill-considered requests. Nonetheless, quality of care cannot be a variable; it must be a constant in an organization that cares for people.

Strategies for quality control among the medical staff do not have to be onerous or burdensome. Table 13.1 lists options in quality control strategies. These options are distinguished as to whether participation by the occupational health professional is voluntary or involuntary and whether the strategy used merely prevents or corrects a poor practice or actually makes a substantial, constructive contribution to improving practice. Obviously, strategies that are voluntary and constructive are preferable to those that are coercive and only corrective. Involvement in an academic program is emphasized here as a relatively painless way to promote quality control because it stimulates preparation for teaching, peer interaction, analysis of problematical cases, and chart reviews incidental to constructive purposes. It is highly appropriate for a major, diversified occupational health service to participate in training programs for occupational physicians, nurses, and mid-level health practitioners.

Table 13.1. Strategies for Quality Control in Occupational Health Services

Involuntary	Voluntary
Corrective	
Chart audits	Case discussions*
Civil claims	Continuing medical education programs*
Utilization monitoring	Board certification requirements or preference for staff positions
Legal enforcement actions	
Constructive	
Chart reviews for administrative purposes	Chart reviews for research and teaching*
	Postgraduate medical teaching*
Interviews with client employers (by marketing)	Interaction with occupational medicine physicians outside group*
	Supervising professional training*

* Activities that form part of an active academic training program.

Quality control among support staff also can be enhanced by promoting in-service training and dispensing recognition for good performance. Above all, the leaders must emphasize the attitude that occupational health is a valuable field contributing much to both workers and employers and that staff in the service are contributing substantially to the success of an important endeavor.

14 PROGRAM EVALUATION

Programs within the occupational health service not only must be chosen carefully, but also must be evaluated regularly to ensure that they are cost-effective, successful in meeting their objectives, and are managed optimally. Programs instituted to meet real needs may have to be adapted as needs change; those that are not successful or serve no real purpose should be phased out. All programs can be improved, but often a careful evaluation is needed to make constructive changes.

A methodical, objective evaluation provides management with the information it needs to select, continue, increase, or withdraw support from a program. It provides participants with a guide to their own performance and instructs them on how to improve services. It provides the client using the service with an opportunity to indicate whether or not needs are being met. A good evaluation takes planning and preparation from the onset of the program.

Goals of Evaluation

The process of evaluation is invaluable for answering important questions about the delivery of occupational health services. Evaluation allows the physician or nurse-manager to pinpoint problems and to correct them. It allows the service to adapt to change by adding equipment, staff, or space or by cutting back in some areas for more efficient operation. It permits the physician and nurse to plan for the continuing education of the staff based on the needs of the practice or gaps in their preparation. It helps reduce liability by highlighting problem areas that require better control, safer procedures, referral, or further training on the part of the provider.

The principles of evaluation are simple to know yet often difficult to apply. Programs usually are set up to provide a specific service rather than as a controlled experiment. Thus, the evaluation component is seldom an overriding consideration in the design of a program and indeed is often an afterthought. Nevertheless, at the beginning of a program, consideration should be given to the information that will be needed to evaluate it. Records and information systems then can be designed to retrieve and process the data quickly and efficiently without disrupting normal activities. An evaluation that brings a halt to operations, is disruptive, and can only be achieved at great expense will be resented by all participants and is unlikely to be carried out at all.

Programs are evaluated to answer several basic questions. These include:

- Is (or was) there a need for this program?
- Is the program meeting the need for which it was designed? Is it meeting other needs?
- Are the same people for whom the program was designed actually using and benefiting from the services being provided? If not, why?
- Is the cost of the program reasonable for the services being provided? Where are savings possible and where might more investment pay off?
- How effective and efficient is this program compared to other, similar programs?
- What changes could be made in the program to make its operation more effective and efficient in the future?
- Do the recipients of the program's services and the sponsors of the program understand its goals, feel satisfied with its services, and *like* the program? If not, why?

An informal evaluation conducted by someone involved in program implementation or operation may sometimes be very astute, but is more likely to be uncritical. A formal evaluation by an outsider who has an objective viewpoint is therefore best. The person or team performing the evaluation should be somewhat detached from program operation, especially if the stakes are high. While evaluations are always subject to bias, the extent of bias can be controlled by collecting as much objective data as needed, by recognizing potential sources of bias before conclusions are drawn, and by obtaining input from all interested parties to balance points of view.

Evaluation Methodology

The basic methodology of evaluation is to compare the program's experience against a benchmark, usually the experience of the immediate past, a comparison group, predicted results, or reasonable expectations. The experience can be expressed in quantifiable terms, such as numbers of patient visits, case fatality rate, test results positive, recovery rates, or dollars expended. The comparison between the benchmark and the program's experience is carried out against the backdrop of a set of criteria that uses statistical analysis to take into account random error and variability. These criteria are broadly classified as relating to either process (how the care was provided) or outcome (what the result of care turned out to be). For example, the evaluation may measure how frequently routine blood pressure checks were performed (process) or how well blood pressure was controlled in hypertensive patients (outcome). (A useful set of criteria to begin with is given in Appendix 1 in the form of an audit questionnaire.)

Programs that provide health services are seldom true experiments. At a minimum, a true experiment could involve an experimental group receiving a certain treatment and a control group from which treatment is withheld. While such a dichotomy is almost never possible in an occupational health program, the closer to an experimental design an evaluation method can be, the more objective and therefore less biased it is likely to be. Study designs that come close to a true experiment are called *quasiexperimental*. Quasiexperimental evaluation methods are based on comparing the experience of program participants with one of three benchmarks:

- A similar *comparison group*, which is not identical but is matched closely enough to yield useful information over the same time period;
- A *before-after comparison*, in which the group experience is compared before the program being evaluated began or in its earlier phases; or
- An *after-only comparison group*, in which the outcome of the group served by the program is compared to that of another very similar group not served by the program.

Quasiexperimental models are standard techniques in the evaluation of programs.Each, however, has serious limitations. Before-after comparisons cannot account for changes over the period that were not related to the program, e.g., changes in the incidence of a disease in the community, in education and public attitudes as the result of news media attention, and in the composition of the workforce as the result of personnel turnover. Before-after and after-only comparisons may be misleading because members of the groups may be self-selected. Individuals who cannot tolerate a job may simply quit and find another. Both the comparison group and the after-only comparison group models depend on close matching between the groups of all characteristics affecting the outcome other than the program itself.

A major limitation of the three approaches described above is that they are poorly suited to comparisons of very small groups. More versatile techniques are used to evaluate occupational health programs and the effectiveness of interventions in workplaces involving small groups. The simplest of these techniques is called *time series analysis,* which is an adaptation of the before-after comparison approach. Applied to occupational health programs, time series analysis may deal with specific organizational groups (departments or work teams), plants, or small companies. The measurement may include such variables as frequency of absence from work, reported injuries, or number of complaints of low back pain. To be valid, the changes in trends must be consistent for the different groups but the same intervention must have been introduced at different times. Comparison groups are not necessary.

Time series analysis has many advantages. It can be used for individuals or groups, and is applicable to any clinical setting in which the subject or patient can be followed over time. The technique is suitable for relatively small numbers of subjects and does not require that the intervention be instituted for all subjects at the same time. It can be used when the intervention cannot be withdrawn or is irreversible. Time series analysis does have some drawbacks, however. It cannot be used when all subjects will receive the intervention at one particular time, because the variation in the timing of the intervention is what controls for outside influences on the outcome. The technique requires repeated measurements before and after the intervention. It may not be applicable where the measurement is very subjective (such as measurement of satisfaction) or is dependent on learning or degree of training or the age of the subject, since a change may occur over time regardless of the intervention. Despite these drawbacks, time series analysis can be extremely useful for the program manager.

Selection of an appropriate method depends on the type of information accessible and the availability of a comparison group. While no model is perfect for every purpose, the most valid generally is a comparison group, followed by time series and before-after comparison. After-only comparison should be used only if no other approach is possible, for example, to evaluate a program for which no attempt has been made to collect information systematically. The validity of a model is only part of the story, however. The data also must be accurate and the measurements meaningful.

Evaluation Measures

The decision as to which variable is a good measure of the effectiveness of a program or intervention depends on the setting and the nature of the evaluation process. Basically, there are four categories of variables that allow measurements of comparisons:

- *Outcome.* Outcome measurements reflect the result of a program or intervention in terms of the actual effect on the individuals or the group. Outcome variables should be clearly associated with the intervention or program (such as blood lead in a lead control program or audiometric testing in a hearing conservation program), standardized and interpretable at the current state of knowledge (e.g., the test called "sister chromatid exchange" would not be appropriate since the relationship between the test result and actual genetic damage to humans is not fully understood), and relatively insensitive to outside factors (plant productivity reflected by overtime worked would not be useful).
- *Behavioral.* Behavioral measurements reflect the degree to which a program has changed individual behavior patterns in a way likely to affect the outcome, such as compliance with safety procedures, modifications in eating or smoking habits, self-referral to an employee assistance program, and the change in comprehension and knowledge of a problem after an educational program. Behavioral measurements can be outcome measurements if the behavior itself is of concern, but are more often process measurements because the concern is with the consequences of a health-related behavior (as in cancer and smoking, recovery and compliance with treatment, accident rates and acceptance of safety guidelines).
- *Criteria.* When a program is designed to function in a certain way, criteria can be written to describe how the process should work. The actual performance of the program then can be checked against these criteria. For example, the evaluation of an occupational hearing conservation program might include a series of questions: "Are exposure data routinely compared to hearing test results?" "Is the workplace regularly monitored every x week and when the production process is changed?" "Is a selection of personal protective devices made available to workers?" "Does the soundproof booth used for audiometric testing conform to the applicable standards recommendation?" "Does the personal hearing protection device have a Noise Reduction Rating of x or more?" To avoid bias, such criteria must never be written with an eye to the specific program being evaluated. Criteria standards are always process measures. (The criteria given in the audit questionnaire in Appendix 1 are examples of generally applicable criteria. Chapter 11 presents an example of a protocol, from which such criteria are relatively easily drawn, and Chapter 13 discusses standards of performance and quality of care.)
- *Satisfaction.* To ensure full compliance and cooperation, a program must satisfy the needs and expectations of the worker and the employer. A survey can determine

whether the user is satisfied and feels that he or she has been courteously treated, and uncover problems that have arisen. All of these are process measures, because satisfaction is not so important in itself but as a means to gain acceptance of and participation in the service being provided.

These measurements are all useful in different ways. Combined, they piece together a total picture of the program and highlight problems that can be solved through changes in the structure or procedures of the program.

Evaluation Planning

Effective evaluation depends on good recordkeeping as well as the cooperation of all concerned. Following are some practical measures for recording and keeping data on an occupational health program:

- The need for a given program should be clearly documented before a program is begun. Baseline data must be identified and appropriate measurements selected for subsequent evaluation of the program.
- The recordkeeping system should be systematic and easy to use. All pertinent data should be recorded in an easily retrievable format—whenever possible put on computer or at least noted on a standardized form that is kept in a central location. The data collected that do not directly relate to the program should be kept to a minimum in order to facilitate handling of the records.
- Criteria to be used for evaluation should be formulated by someone other than the project staff well before the evaluation is conducted. Table 14.1 presents a set of criteria developed by a special committee for evaluating the performance of an advocate presenting cases on appeal before a workers' compensation board. The success rate of the appeals was not a good guide to performance because too much depended on the merits of the case and changes in the policy of the board. Instead, the evaluation was based in this instance on process criteria applied to a review of client records.
- Subjective response in such matters as user satisfaction should be considered very carefully. Often expressions of dissatisfaction or lack of understanding signal grave problems that lie below the surface.

The information retained in the recordkeeping system allows the practitioner to construct a profile of the service. In the case of an external occupational health service, this task may involve checking appointment sheets or tracking first reports in order to determine such patterns as the frequency of new patients with occupational disorders and the distribution of cases by type of problem (for example, musculoskeletal injuries, back strain, and dermatitis); the companies that are using the service and the industries they represent; the occupations of workers who need care (e.g., whether all such patients are truck drivers or whether there is a mix); the types of services provided (acute care, consultation, fitness-to-work evaluations); and the geographic areas from which the patients are coming. With this profile in hand, the practitioner than can identify changes by comparing similar data from previous years or by continuously monitoring the utilization of the service.

Once the basic descriptive data are available, other methods of analysis can be

Table 14.1. Criteria for Performance Evaluation: Workers' Compensation Advocate

A. Case Management (based on a review of case records)
1. Clear statement of reason for encounter and the essential issues of the case involving a workers' compensation (WC) claim.
2. Assessment of client follows logically from data recorded; alternative assessments equally plausible from the data are acknowledged. Such an assessment includes: health status, level of function, mental state, and special needs.
3. Status of client as claimant in WC claim or appeal process is clearly identified and stated on chart. It is updated as it changes.
4. Referrals of client to health and social services providers are recorded, justified, and, where appropriate, given the initial and ongoing assessment.
5. Follow-up and subsequent developments are clearly recorded.

B. Services in Worker Education (based on student evaluations and a review of teaching materials)
1. The need for a particular educational program is identified and the program is designed with the characteristics of the learners in mind.
2. Opportunity for feedback from learners is provided on the quality of presentation, relevance of the material, and appropriateness to the learner's situation.
3. Educational programs are provided in a cost-effective manner, targetting larger groups and drawing sufficient numbers to justify the commitment.

applied to develop the evaluation further. For example, a sample of medical records covering representative or particular problems can be audited to determine how cases were handled and how they were resolved. Financial records can be used to ascertain whether payment was complete or whether a few cases ran up disproportionate charges. Groups with a common occupation or exposure, such as welders or asbestos workers, may be examined to determine if they are showing consistent findings and whether screening evaluations are up to date. Cases of nonoccupational problems may be reviewed to see whether consistent criteria were used in certifying absence from work or fitness to return to work.

The Evaluation Process

The evaluation process outlined in this section is designed for occupational services providing services to a number of employers. It is a general approach to the evaluation of services; Chapter 15 presents a specific approach for conducting a cost and benefit analysis.

The essential first step in designing an evaluation is to be clear on the real purposes of the exercise—to provide an accurate picture of the service and identify areas for change. The usual objectives for evaluating occupational medicine service include:
- *Effectiveness*—whether the program reduces job-related employee health problems.
- *Cost*—whether the expense of the program compares favorably with alternative ways of providing the services.

- *Acceptance and Satisfaction*—whether workers perceive the program as meeting their needs.
- *Specification*—which aspects of the program had the greatest effectiveness and at what relative cost.

The ultimate use of the evaluation is to modify the program in order to optimize Effectiveness, Acceptance, and Satisfaction by minimizing the Cost and identifying Specification.

Forming the actual yardstick for evaluation are specific goals within each objective:

A. Effectiveness
   1. To protect workers against health and safety hazards.
      - To significantly reduce the frequency of occupational injuries and illnesses in the community or among client employers.
      - To significantly reduce the severity of those occupational disorders that do occur.
   2. To provide adequate treatment to workers who have sustained occupational injuries and illnesses.
      - To significantly reduce the frequency of disability after occupational disorders.
      - To provide rapid and appropriate care to the impaired worker.

B. Cost
   1. To deliver services at a reasonable cost.
      - To hold constant or reduce the total cost to the employers of medical services.
      - To deliver more comprehensive medical services at the same cost to the employers.
      - To deliver services at a significantly smaller cost per employee than would be the case were services obtained on a piecemeal basis.
   2. To reduce the cost to the employer related to medical services.
      - To reduce employer insurance premiums.
      - To reduce employer assessments for workers' compensation.

C. Acceptance
   1. To provide services in such a way that the workers subjectively feel that their needs are being met.
      - To establish a degree of confidence in care delivered on the part of the employees.
      - To establish a sense of overall satisfaction on the part of the employees with the personal attention of the clinic staff.
   2. To ensure that workers' preferences and reactions are heard by the staff.

D. Satisfaction
   1. To provide services in such a way that the employers feel that their needs are being met.
      - To establish confidence in care delivered to their employees.
      - To establish overall satisfaction on the part of the employer as to the service's attention to the employer's special needs and desires.

E. Specification
   1. To identify those components of the program that are the most cost-effective.

- To determine those components that are the most effective by the criteria of Effectiveness.
- To determine the specific per-employee cost of each program.
2. To determine which components of the program are perceived as the most effective or desirable.
    - To determine those components of the program that are considered highest by the criteria of Acceptance by the workers.
    - To determine those components of the program that are considered highest by the criteria of Satisfaction by the employers.

Any number of other objectives could be formulated but these are the essential ones that lend themselves to measurement. The design of the evaluation then must identify outcome measurements for the objectives and compare them against one of three standards: a control or comparison group; experience prior to participation in the program; or arbitrary expectations and derived criteria.

In the real world, a company that has not contracted for services is hardly likely to release its balance sheets and offer its employees for interview. Thus, a control group is not realistic except in the case of similar companies that have chosen different programs for different groups of their employees—and this is not a common situation. Measuring company experiences pre- and post-program participation assumes that no major unrelated activities affecting health are implemented during the study period. For this reason, the study period must be kept brief, perhaps three years after entry into the program. Finally, although arbitrary criteria comprise the least desirable standard for comparison, they may offer the only option for some relatively subjective measurements, such as Acceptance.

Outcome measurements must be quantifiable and accessible. To continue the example, specific outcome measurements for each objective might be as follows:

A. Effectiveness
    1. Protection of workers
        - Reported occupational injuries and illnesses during the year preceding and the third year of participation in the program.
        - Ratings of injuries on initial clinic visit on a standard scale of disability determined during the first six months and the last six months of participation.
    2. Adequacy of treatment
        - Claims to workers' compensation and rate of awards in the year preceding and the third year of participation in the program.
        - Continuous chart audits with a medical standards review of a 5 to 10 percent sample.

B. Cost
    1. Cost of care
        - Cost to employer, per employee per component of the program (e.g., noise control, employee assistance, health hazard evaluation) and total cost by year of participation.
        - Coverage of workers as determined by the number of programs and staff hours expended or dollar cost per employee. (No direct comparison is possible with preparticipation costs but expansion of services will be obvious if present).

- Comparison of individual treatment costs with usual and customary charges in the community.
    2. Costs of coverage and liability
       - Insurance premiums before and during last year of participation.
       - Workers' compensation assessment before and during last year of participation.
C. Acceptance
    1. Employee acceptance of specific program
       - Questionnaire responses for employees using clinic program components during first six months (covering previous arrangement and expectations of new services) and last six months (covering interim experience and subjective rating of care) of employer participation during study period.
    2. Employee acceptance of program components
       - Questionnaire responses directed at determining the acceptance of each program component.
D. Satisfaction
    1. Employer satisfaction with specific program
       - Questionnaire to employers on their opinions of the program
    2. Employer satisfaction with program components.
E. Specification
       The data, tabulated by participating company and calculated per 1,000 employee-hours, then could be examined by program component and analyzed by cost-effectiveness, cost-acceptance, and cost-satisfaction.

This is a program evaluation, not a controlled epidemiologic study. Inevitably, there are practical problems in evaluating programs that exist in a competitive and political milieu. Evaluations of occupational health programs are limited by the extent to which variables can be practicably measured, and can seldom approach the ideal of a controlled study. Program evaluations do, however, solve important problems in the real world, and it is in the real world that the occupational health professional identifies and manages occupational disorders.

Further Reading

Accreditation Handbook for Ambulatory Health Care. Skokie, Illinois, Accreditation Association for Ambulatory Health Care, 1987.

Campbell DT, Stanley J: Experimental and Quasi-Experimental Designs for Research. Chicago, Rand McNally, 1963.

Hatch LL, et al: Self-Evaluation of Occupational Safety and Health Programs. Cincinnati, National Institute for Occupational Safety and Health, DHEW (NIOSH) Publication No. 78–187, 1978.

Kettering Laboratory, University of Cincinnati: Standards, Interpretation, and Audit Criteria for Performance of Occupational Health Programs. Washington, National Institute for Occupational Safety and Health, 1979.

Reeder LG, Ramacher L, Gorolnik S: Handbook of Scales and Indices of Health Behavior. Pacific Palisades, CA, Goodyear Publishing, 1976.

15 COST/BENEFIT ANALYSIS

Occupational health services are engaged by employers for a variety of reasons: the organization may believe that it has a moral obligation to provide health services to support the well-being of its employees and that there is an economic justification for such services, or may simply be complying with pertinent laws and regulations. Regardless of the employer's motivation in providing occupational health services, the program should be reviewed periodically to evaluate its contribution to the productivity of the organization.

In any analysis or evaluation, the costs of providing occupational health services are always more readily apparent to employers than the benefits derived. But any occupational health service, whether an internal department, a clinic, or a private consultant retained on a full- or part-time basis, should be able to provide a realistic financial cost/benefit analysis for the organization it serves. In business organizations, the cost/benefit analysis should be related as closely as possible to the "bottom line," since this consideration will make the greatest impression on the senior managers in the company. Other organizations, such as the government or the military, may require a different emphasis or end point for the final economic analysis. This chapter outlines an approach for the financial analysis that should support the preparation of an annual budget and the justification to management for establishing or modifying existing services. The components of the cost/benefit analysis will vary according to the size and nature of the organization and its validity will be only as good as the data upon which it is based.

Ground Rules for Analysis

The newer the occupational health service, the harder it is to do a cost/benefit analysis, since the full impact of the service's policies and programs will not be felt for several years. The effectiveness of the occupational health services will be measured according to such essential data as workers' compensation assessment costs, health insurance premiums, and days lost due to accidents or sickness. These data should be maintained on an ongoing basis by the occupational health service, dating as far back as is practical.

The operating and capital costs of an occupational health service depend upon the size and design of the facility and the specific services it provides. Ideally, the budget for a corporate or plant occupational health service should be developed and administered by the supervising occupational health professional and based on a realistic work plan that has established goals. In business, it is prepared with the help of the company's financial personnel and final approval is given by the senior company official responsible for the service.

Since construction and equipment costs vary from place to place and over time, no estimates are given here for initial or replacement capital expenses. It is important, however, that the facility and equipment chosen be appropriate to the occupational health service's own objectives and to the company's needs, policies, and financial resources. Often the best prices are obtained by using a competitive bidding process and it is prudent to seek advice from consultants knowledgeable in both architecture and occupational health before construction on or the purchase of a facility is undertaken. The capital budget will be highest when the occupational health service is first constructed and during times of major renovations. However, most organizations do not consider building or capital improvement costs in preparing a cost/benefit analysis because these are exceptional expenses that often add value to a property.

Cost Analysis

The operating budget reflects the money needed to run the occupational health service on a day-to-day basis. If the occupational health service is a department within an organization, its operating expenses eventually will be consolidated into the organization's total operating budget. Items such as rent and utilities might not be specifically identified in these cases and they would be considered part of general "overhead" costs. If the occupational health service is an external unit providing services under a contract arrangement, the employer may need to budget only for the total aggregate cost of the particular occupational health services provided. In the latter situation, the contractee, whether a health facility or an individual consultant, will need a detailed operating budget for its own internal purposes. The following general discussion emphasizes those expense elements commonly encountered in the preparation of a typical budget for an occupational health service. (A more general approach to the evaluation of occupational health services precedes this discussion, in Chapter 14.)

Compensation

Unlike management units that are staffed by many people with the same skills, the occupational health service usually employs a variety of health professionals and administrative personnel, any one of whom may be a full- or part-timer employed on either a salaried or contract basis. The level of compensation will reflect the staffer's responsibilities, experience, and qualifications. (Table 15.1 presents representative levels of compensation for various staff.) Compensation usually accounts for 25 to 60 percent of the budget.

Table 15.1. Approximate Levels of Compensation of Personnel

Position	Salary Range	Contract Fee
Occupational Physician	$70,000–$150,000	$60–$150/hr. Retainer fees vary and may be in addition to hourly or fee-for-service.
Occupational Health Nurse (Certified)	$30,000–$60,000	$15–$25/hr.
Other Staff: Technicians Psychologists Employee Assistance Counsellors Physiotherapists Nutritionists Clerks Receptionists Administrators	Equivalent to similar positions in other settings.	Psychologists and physiotherapists may have associations that can advise on recommended fee schedules.
Consultants: Epidemiologists Toxicologists Engineers Ergonomists	These positions are rarely on staff.	Varies. Best to inquire of professional associations or active practitioners regarding current professional practices.

A full-time occupational health physician generally earns a salary in the range of $70,000 to $150,000 annually; part-time physicians are paid $60 to $150 per hour. As the number of contracted hours increases, the compensation paid per hour generally falls. For example, a contract occupational physician with average skills and experience could reasonably expect to earn $100,000 per year in industry, equal to about $52 per hour based on a 48-hour week. An hourly rate of $150 per hour, while normal for a few hours of work per week, would total $285,000 annually if kept constant for the 1900 hours in a typical man-year, an amount obviously too large for the typical employer. Similarly, a part-time occupational health nurse generally earns $15 to $25 per hour, while a full-time nurse commands an annual salary in the range of $30,000 to $60,000. Local or national associations of occupational physicians or nurses and professional associations for other occupational health professions (see Chapter 1) can supply information helpful for determining appropriate compensation levels. The salaries and contract fees of other administrative and technical personnel vary greatly.

Full-time employed personnel also may receive a benefits package covering such items as disability and life insurance. The value of these benefits can amount to 20 to 30 percent of salary. Generally, contract employees do not receive a benefits package.

Employee Expenses

Personnel should be allowed and encouraged to attend conferences and courses, and the budget should provide funds to support such professional development. Reimbursement should cover transportation and living expenses incurred while attending professional development courses or meetings, as well as the cost of the course or conference itself. Additionally, the occupational health service should pay for certain license fees and memberships in professional associations for its staff. This cost element will account for 2 to 5 percent of the budget.

Rent, Utilities, and Maintenance
This element does not always appear in a budget, but if it does, it may be on the order of 20 to 30 percent of the budget. Included here are expenses for rent, light, heat, water, gas, cleaning, minor repairs, and general upkeep.

Equipment, Supplies, Telephone, and Telecommunications
Administrative supplies, clinical supplies, and small pieces of equipment not expensive enough individually to be a capital item (usually less than $1,000) should be budgeted for under this category. Depending upon the nature and activities of the occupational health service, this expense element may account for 6 to 10 percent of the budget.

Computer Services
The size of this item depends on the type of computer hardware and software used and, if a mainframe is shared, the amount of access time. It may account for 3 to 10 percent of the budget.

Miscellaneous
About 1 percent of the budget is allocated to cover items too small to be considered as separate expense elements or line-item entries.

Benefit (Cost-Saving) Analysis
While it is not possible to put a specific dollar value on the reduction or elimination of human suffering or on the absence of fines or court actions, these considerations also have a high presumptive value and always should be described in the narrative discussion accompanying the benefits analysis. "Cost savings" occur directly as a result of the reductions in direct costs, particularly in premiums for workers' compensation (WC) and aggregate health insurance (HI), including health, dental, disability, life, and any other health-related insurance costs identified. Cost savings also occur as a result of reduced indirect costs, including expenses associated with the hiring and training of replacement workers; overtime; extra supervision; material wastage; and administrative processes. Some studies have shown that these indirect costs can account for as much as 50 times the equivalent of the daily wage of the absent employee. Thus, the savings from protecting the health of employees and keeping employees on the job are considerable.

Direct Cost Savings
Following is an illustration of how cost savings may be calculated and expressed in monetary terms. This example is based on the case of an actual occupational health service serving 3,200 employees in a diversified company and with an annual operating budget of $300,000. Table 15.2 shows savings realized in workers' compensation and health

Table 15.2. Analysis of Cost Savings in Workers' Compensation (WC) and Health Insurance (HI) Example

Year of Operation	Actual WC Assessment Costs (A)	WC Cost Saving Related to Base Year (B)	Actual HI Premium Costs (C)	HI Cost Saving Related to Base Year (D)	Cumulative Cost Saving Related to Base Year E = (B + D)
Base	$1,000,000	$ 0	$1,350,000	$ 0	$ 0
1	900,000	100,000	1,300,000	50,000	150,000
2	850,000	150,000	1,250,000	100,000	250,000
3	750,000	250,000	1,200,000	150,000	400,000
4	800,000*	200,000	1,200,000**	150,000	350,000

* Premium for WC actually went back up by $50,000; there was no change in the HI costs. Therefore, the cumulative change relative to the base year fell to $350,000.
** No change in costs from previous year. Therefore, no cumulative change relative to the base year.

insurance premiums over a four-year period compared to the base year.

Calculating reductions in total workers' compensation and health insurance costs requires setting a base year as a point of comparison. Ideally this base year should be from a time prior to full operation of the occupational health service and before occupational health policies and programs were fully operative in the organization. If premiums decline over time compared to the base year absent other major changes, such as a shift in the employee population or type of work performed, the occupational health service can justifiably take some, or all, of the credit for the reduction. One must keep comparing back to the base year each year when doing this analysis because identifiable cost reductions may occur sporadically over time and are cumulative. In effect, the cost-savings analysis shows not only what has happened because of the actions of the occupational health service but also what might happen if the service is withdrawn, i.e., that costs would gradually go back to or become worse than the base level.

In the example analyzed in Table 15.2, base year costs amounted to $1 million (0.9 percent of payroll) for the annual workers' compensation premium and $1.35 million (1.5 percent of payroll) for health insurance premiums. Programs instituted by the occupational health service reduced the frequency of workers' compensation claims; accordingly, the workers' compensation and other insurance carriers granted premium reductions and rebates to the company. In the first year of program operation, these savings amounted to $100,000 (WC) and $50,000 (HI), for a total savings of $150,000. In Year 2, combined savings amounted to a further $100,000, for a cumulative total cost saving of $250,000 over the two years. In Year 3, the savings amounted to a further $150,000, for a total accumulated cost saving of $400,000 relative to the base year. In Year 4, the workers' compensation board claims experience of the company worsened and the WC premium went back up by $50,000. Health insurance claims also had levelled off, and no further cost savings occurred, thus reducing the cumulative cost savings to $350,000.

In each year, the cumulative cost savings relative to the base year give an indication of the continuing financial impact that the occupational health service is making on the employer's claims experience, as reflected in its costs for insurance premiums.

Indirect Cost Savings

The impact of the occupational health service on indirect costs can be estimated from the "hidden" expenses associated with absence, including the need for overtime, extra workers, closer supervision, etc. Studies have shown that such costs can amount to as much as 50 times the average daily wage. A very conservative approach, then, would be to figure indirect costs as a factor of 5 times the daily wage. If the average daily wage is $120, the cost of an absence per day is $600 (5 × $120).

If the records show that the actions of the occupational health service have resulted in 100 employees returning to work an average 5 days earlier (derived from absence records), the estimated indirect cost savings under these assumptions would be $300,000:

$$100 \text{ employees} \times 5 \text{ days} \times \$600 = \$300,000$$

If the company also has a health promotion program that includes fitness and smoking cessation programs, further cost savings can be achieved. These can be estimated using the same approach. Studies have shown that sedentary workers on the average miss 3 more days of work per year than those who exercise regularly. So if 100 employees who had not previously been active begin to exercise regularly because of a fitness program, the following savings can be estimated:

$$100 \times 3 \times \$600 = \$180,000$$

Smokers also are reported to lose an average of 3 days more per year due to illness than non-smokers. So, if 20 workers stopped smoking due to the occupational health services smoking cessation program the following additional savings in productivity can be estimated:

$$20 \times 3 \times \$600 = \$36,000$$

The rather straightforward assumptions used in the example show how an occupational health service helping only 220 participants prevented a company from losing $516,000 in indirect costs due to health-related absences. Assuming that these savings were achieved in Year 3 of operations of the occupational health service analyzed in Table 15.2, the total estimated direct and indirect savings due to the occupational health interventions would be on the order of $916,000 ($400,000 + $516,000).

This example uses very conservative assumptions. In reality, these numbers are likely to be much higher and the estimated cost savings even more impressive. The estimates are very sensitive to the factor chosen as the multiplier to reflect indirect cost savings. Since detailed economic studies to determine the appropriate factor are difficult and expensive, an educated guess often must be made in a given case.

Cost/Benefit Comparison

The cost/benefit analysis figures the rate of return on investment by dividing the total savings by the cost of the occupational health service. In the example, the occupational health service costs $300,000 to operate. Dividing total savings of $916,000 by $300,000 yields a 300 percent rate of return. A rate of return of this magnitude constitutes a very convincing reason for management to continue supporting the service.

In a publicly traded company, the cost/benefit analysis can be brought directly to the "bottom line," demonstrating the impact on earnings per share held by the stockholders:

- First, subtract the costs from the estimated cost savings to get the net benefit. (In the example, $916,000 less $300,000 = $616,000.)
- Then divide this amount by the number of outstanding common shares in the company. (Assuming 20 million outstanding shares, $616,000 X 100 divided by 20 million = 3.0 cents/share.) Whether expressed as earnings per share or by rate of return on investment, these calculations can make a real impression on senior management.

There are other, equally as valid, ways that an occupational health service can show its economic impact on an organization. However, this type of analysis shows an impressive return even though it focuses only on two areas — reduced health insurance costs and reduced health related absenteeism costs. Without question, a comprehensive and detailed economic analysis would document even greater savings.

Further Reading

Accident Prevention Manual for Industrial Operations: Administration and Programs. Chicago, National Safety Council, 1981.

Bird FE Jr, Loftus RG: Loss Control Management. Loganville, Georgia, The Institute Press, 1976.

DeReamer R: Modern Safety and Health Technology. New York, John Wiley & Sons, 1980.

Heinrich HW, Petersen D, Ross N: Industrial Accident Prevention. New York, McGraw Hill, 1980.

Simon RS: Is your company under surveillance? It should be! Occ Health Safety, April 1982; 51:50–54.

16 RESEARCH MANAGEMENT

The growing interest in occupational health, environmental risks, health promotion programs, management science, work psychology, and other related subjects has been paralleled by an increasing number of proposals to conduct studies within plants or specific workplaces. Often the initial reaction of plant managers and responsible corporate officers to proposals to conduct research in the plant is a simple and quick: "no way!" However, a snap reaction may overlook the considerable benefits that could accrue from this type of study.

In order to make a reasonable decision on research proposals that weighs the interests of the employer and all others concerned, the corporate officer and occupational health consultant must determine:

- Whether the study proposed is a worthwhile research effort.
- Whether the investigators are reputable and capable of conducting the research objectively.
- How the company may be able, ethically, to monitor the course of the study to ensure that it remains within agreed upon limits.
- What benefits the company may realize from participating in the study.
- What may happen if a serious problem is uncovered.

The answers to these questions will dictate how the employer should respond to the research proposal. The procedure for answering the questions is outlined here from the perspective of a manager or consultant with responsibility for advising an employer host or company in responding to a serious proposal. (While the emphasis is on studies in the field of occupational health, the same principles hold for those involving environmental hazards, work psychology, and management science.)

Evaluating the Proposed Study

The first step in evaluating a proposed study is to determine whether it asks a specific question or poses a hypothesis. Hypotheses are statements of supposition, such as

"Foundry workers have a higher rate of cancer than would be expected when compared to rates of cancer in the general population." They are meant to be tested against actual data pertinent to the problem, such as cancer rates for foundry workers from a given plant compared to rates in the local area. A research project may be designed to generate a hypothesis or to test one. A hypothesis-generating study is a preliminary, exploratory overview intended to spot possible leads that may be worthy of further research. A hypothesis-testing study is a targeted attempt to confirm or rule out a specific hypothesis. It is usually based on a previous observation, a logical extension of other research, or a previous hypothesis-generating study.

Without question, hypothesis-generating studies cause the most trouble and misunderstandings between investigators and employer hosts, primarily because chance alone may suggest a problem even when there is none. Frequently these studies make dozens of comparisons—and the traditional scientific standard for assuming significance allows a one-in-twenty chance of error. Furthermore, there is much confusion in the minds of the public and even many scientists regarding the interpretation of positive findings. Unless an association is very strong and the study is extremely well designed, hypothesis-generating studies only suggest a possible finding and rarely prove anything. Confirmation of a finding usually requires that a hypothesis-testing study be designed to look specifically at the problem of interest.

The second step in evaluating a proposal for a study is to determine whether the topic is worth studying. This task often is not as easy as it seems because a trivial-sounding project may actually be a test of a much more important general theory. (When in doubt, obtain an outside opinion from a trade association or a university.) In this situation, an astute manager also may see an opportunity to gain useful information. For example, if researchers wish to look at the health experience of employees in a specific work area of a self-insured plant, the employer may persuade them to gather data that will help in containing health care costs and in evaluating the insurance plan.

The third step in evaluating a study is to determine whether the question being asked actually can be answered by the methods the investigator chooses to employ. Research design is a very complex scientific issue, but at the very least a scientist proposing a serious research project should be able to explain what techniques will be used, how accurate they are, how many subjects will be needed to yield an interpretable result either way, and what statistical tests will be used to analyze the findings. Again, outside help may be required to evaluate the proposal.

Evaluating the Investigator

Scientists have an ethical responsibility to maintain objectivity when they conduct and report their research. A scientist who consistently publishes conclusions for or against industry may be following lines of research that actually have led in that direction or may be exhibiting bias. The best guide to determining whether an investigator is objective is what the scientist has published: Have all possible explanations for a finding been spelled out? Is industry consistently painted as the "good guy" or the "bad guy?" Is the tone of the writing thoughtful or provocative? Can the scientist separate his or her political or social feelings from the technical and scientific aspects of a problem?

The most highly respected scientists steer clear of partisan statements and make up their minds on the merits of each issue. A study by a radical activist broadly impugning industry is not likely to be taken very seriously; a study by a corporate consultant broadly asserting that no problems exist is even less likely to be viewed as credible within the scientific community.

The credentials of the scientist are also very important. Research is a serious and difficult business and those who undertake it must be well trained and competent, usually with at least a doctoral-level degree from a recognized university. In the case of a graduate student performing research for a dissertation, the credentials of the student's faculty advisor also should show evidence of substantial academic accomplishment. Unlike business, there is no "school of hard knocks" in research. An investigator's paper credentials should be complete (with no suspicious, unexplained gaps), commensurate with the scientist's age and experience, and compatible with sustained professional growth. A scientist who has not been promoted from a junior rank for many years, who has published very little recently, or who has moved frequently from one institution to another may be a bad risk. Such individuals may not be careful researchers or may feel under great pressure to blow a problem out of proportion in order to advance their careers.

The institution where a scientist now works is an important factor. Universities have the highest credibility, in part because an investigator is under scrutiny by peers and students. Private research foundations vary, from the impeccable to the fly-by-night, and should have a concrete justification for why they are involved in the work. Although there are some government research agencies that are as fine and prestigious as any university, many frequently have trouble attracting and holding the best researchers. In every case, the employer should obtain from the institution a guarantee that: confidential information will be kept private and released only in a harmless form; trade secrets will be respected; access to the plant will be limited to authorized personnel; and all findings will be divulged to the company before publication. Penalties for violating these safeguards should be spelled out in full.

If an investigator claims to have an affiliation with a university but cannot produce a university office address and telephone number, call the appropriate university department and find out the specific nature of the investigator's appointment. Adjunct, or part-time, faculty often are legitimately involved in research projects. Nevertheless, the thorough manager will ascertain where these faculty work full-time and whether there is a potential conflict of interest with any other responsibilities they may have. Case in point: sometimes individuals with only tenuous links to an institution are automatically reappointed to the adjunct faculty year after year, but do not have any substantial role on the faculty. Such persons have been known to use their courtesy appointments to lend authority to strictly personal projects. Beware of uninformative or unusual titles; the title "lecturer" (usually the lowest faculty rank in the United States and Canada, referring to a faculty member not eligible for tenure but equal to the rank of assistant professor in Europe); and strictly laboratory or administrative titles (such as "research associate" or "director"), unless the person can also show a proper faculty appointment or sponsorship of the project. The designation "in residence" usually means that a scientist supports him or herself at the university by obtaining grants that cover salary and should not in itself be cause for concern. Legitimate investigators will always welcome inquiries into their backgrounds; a questionable risk may become defensive or may present an incomplete or confusing resume or, as it is called in academic circles, "curriculum vitae" (or "c.v.").

The evaluation also should consider the source of funding for the proposed research. If the investigator already has been awarded funds by a research agency, such as the National Institute for Occupational Safety and Health, or plans to submit a proposal to such an agency, some assurance exists that the proposal will receive careful review by other qualified scientists. In particular, where direct contact with workers is involved, application to a recognized agency carries additional assurance that the proposal will be reviewed for the safe and ethical treatment of human subjects. If funds come from a private foundation or other unusual source, the manager needs to inquire as to the ultimate purpose of the work; when they come from a trade association or industry source, the manager needs to consider whether the study is likely to be accused of pro-industry bias upon release.

Finally, the investigator's attitude toward publication is important. Responsible investigators will permit the employer to review the data before the manuscript is released for publication, yet will always refuse, on ethical grounds, to allow the employer to edit the resulting paper or to block publication. Questionable applicants may compromise or hesitate on these issues, which, nonetheless, are considered fundamental to academic standards of integrity.

Employer Rights and Responsibilities

A company that allows research to be performed in its facilities has certain ethical and legal rights and obligations. The obligations are largely written into law; the rights are more vague, except in the matter of protection for trade secrets.

The participating employer has the right to stipulate that trade secrets will be kept inviolable and can seek legal redress if an investigator or a research technician steps into expressly forbidden territory. The employer is entitled to be briefed on the findings of a study, including any and all problems uncovered, prior to publication of the data. It is usually best to specify a time period, such as three to six months, between the briefing and release for publication. This allows management time to take action to resolve any major problems and to minimize adverse public relations.

The employer has a right to insist on anonymity and to remain unidentified in the published report. Where results are favorable, of course, management will want to publicize them; even when the outcome is neutral, the employer may decide that the publicity will project an image of openness and corporate responsibility.

The issue of worker participation in research studies is often troublesome for management. The employer is entitled to minimize the disruption in routine that may be caused by the study. The study protocol (procedures to be followed) should be kept as short as possible and should involve only as many employees as are necessary to answer the question.

At the same time, the corporate officer must make sure that plant managers and supervisors know the legal constraints on the employer and the ethical bounds of the researcher. Serious conflicts emerge when uninformed supervisors run afoul of ethical practices by demanding to see data that an investigator has collected before the data are statistically analyzed and all personal identification removed. Even a rumor that confidential data might be released to an employer is enough to ruin the study by destroying any possibility of cooperation by employees. Confidentiality is by far the single most sensitive issue in occupational research.

Another issue is the treatment of subjects. Studies that require direct participation by workers must be reviewed and approved by committees charged with protecting the safety and rights of human subjects in research. These studies are better received and less likely to provoke conflict when workers are informed at the very beginning about the purpose, methods, and safeguards to confidentiality of a study. This usually means making a presentation to the union or employee representatives and obtaining their approval once management has accepted the research proposal. Workers have an absolute right to their own individual results; they also should be given an explanation of the study's general findings in terms that a layman can understand. In cases where a serious problem has been uncovered, this step alone has proven invaluable in preserving labor-management relations, controlling rumors, and protecting the company from charges of cover-up.

Benefits of Participating in Research

With all the potential for problems, why should the corporate manager ever permit research to be conducted? The answer lies in the enormous benefit the employer can gain.

Most studies, of course, uncover no dramatic problems and may show exemplary conditions. Such outcomes can reassure worried employees, project an image of corporate responsibility, and provide evidence for compliance with governmental regulations.

Studies often generate information that is of great usefulness for management purposes, even when the data are collected for other purposes. For example, health data can be used to identify causes of absenteeism and controllable health care costs, while program evaluations can improve efficiency and performance.

In many cases, participation in a study may improve employee relationships. A demonstration project, such as a health promotion program, that is highly visible may boost workers' morale and sense of identification with the company. Operating here is the familiar "Hawthorne effect," in which the mere fact of being studied boosts workers' productivity by creating a sense of group identification and focusing special attention on the employees serving as subjects.

Participation in such studies provides employers with an opportunity to cement relationships with the academic community. In an era when joint ventures between academia and industry are increasingly common and are yielding profitable results, this is no small benefit. While academics are frequently accused of being too theoretical and impractical in their thinking, they cannot be otherwise if they are not allowed to participate in solving problems in the real world. A university connection provides, at reasonable cost, research to solve problems, opportunities for new product and service ideas, continuing education for technical and management personnel, and a source of qualified consultants.

The possibility of a serious health problem being uncovered is the nightmare that inhibits management from permitting research. Workers' compensation claims may increase if a problem is uncovered. Yet should this happen, the company that discovers the problem first has the advantage of time to correct it, limiting damage to both its public relations image and its finances. Cooperation in the study provides the employer with both a strong legal position that due caution was exercised and a clear defense against charges of cover-up. An employer who opts out of a study on the grounds that ignorance is bliss risks charges of neglect and duplicity at best, and screaming headlines and a cascade of litigation at worst. This is especially true if there has been some rumor or intimation of a problem prior to the proposed study. If no data are available to determine the actual magnitude of a risk, identify which workers are affected, and establish what exposures may have been responsible, a smart lawyer will parlay the resulting uncertainty into a bevy of awards for clients, including some who may not have been affected.

Managing Participation

The key to managing a company's participation in a study is understanding the research process. Management should require the investigator to submit a formal proposal detailing the work to be done. This initial proposal should be studied carefully, with the help of outside consultants in the field; a decision on whether to participate should be made only after the study is thoroughly digested and its implications thought out. A company that receives frequent proposals should establish a small standing committee to screen the studies and make appropriate recommendations. The worst way to handle a proposal is to give it five minutes in the crowded agenda of a board meeting.

A written agreement between the investigator and the company is essential. This agreement should spell out all expectations and responsibilities on both sides, the measures to be taken to safeguard trade secrets and the confidentiality of employee data, penalties for violating the agreed-upon ground rules (particularly important if graduate students are involved), and guidelines for involving workers during company time. The agreement cannot require the investigator to withhold, censor, or edit the report of the research, but should explicitly give the company the opportunity to review the findings before they are released and to respond to any problems identified or implied criticism. The company cannot control the research itself, but should manage its participation to ensure minimum disruption while the study is conducted.

While the study is being conducted, management has a right to be kept informed of progress, although it cannot obtain the data being collected. Management should assign responsibility for monitoring progress to one well prepared corporate officer. This person should stay informed about the study in some depth and be ready to respond to the results when they are presented later. Once committed to participating in a study, a company must cooperate to the end. Unilaterally cancelling a study before its completion is a disaster for all concerned and may create a public relations fiasco for the employer, complete with charges of cover-up.

Sometimes an employer inadvertently "kills" a study with kindness. To remain credible to workers, and to stay objective as a scientist, the investigator must remain an outsider. This may mean declining invitations to eat in the executive dining room or offers of clerical assistance. Depending on the situation, management should not feel rebuffed if a scientist prefers to keep some distance.

Frequently an employer will contract with consultants for assistance in resolving a problem or identifying a source of potential liability. In such cases, although the company has the right to impose more circumscribed rules on investigators, it should apply the same standards as used for externally initiated research. With the exception of product development, industry-based research has a tarnished reputation because it is susceptible or appears to be susceptible to self-serving pressure and manipulation. Academic standards for research, whatever their inconveniences and risks, have evolved precisely in order to protect the credibility of the investigator from charges of conflict of interest and coercion. If industry-sponsored research is not conducted and disseminated in keeping with academic standards, it will be unable to convincingly rebut contrary studies in the minds of the public and government regulators.

Further Reading

Cullen MR: Occupational medicine: A new focus for general internal medicine. Arch Intern Med 1985; 145:511–515.

Guidotti TL: Medicine, critical science, and the real world. West J Med 1975; 123:69–70.

Guidotti TL: Exposure to hazard and individual risk: When occupational medicine gets personal. J Occup Med 1988; 30:570–577.

SECTION V
OCCUPATIONAL HEALTH SERVICES

17 CLINICAL MANAGEMENT

Each job-related injury or illness represents a failure of the occupational health and safety system, at some level, to prevent occupational disorders – but when accidents do happen, prompt and effective treatment can save injured or ill workers from unnecessary impairment. Furthermore, an early return to work, when medically indicated, can help in their rehabilitation. Acute care in an occupational health care setting, then, has two sides: a simple service function and a safety management function. Opportunities exist to use the lessons learned from each situation to prevent recurrence of accidents.

The occupational hygienist, safety specialist, and responsible supervisors can use the pattern of incidents as a guide to identify the factors contributing to a repetition of injuries or illnesses in the workplace. The ultimate goal of an occupational health intervention, of course, is to control the hazard that caused the problem in the first place.

Acute Care of Injuries

Acute care of the injured worker is the most basic form of occupational medical care and usually involves treating straightforward injuries, primarily soft-tissue lesions, particularly strains and sprains. The occupational medical service is often involved in rehabilitation to a greater degree than general surgical or medical clinics; the nature of occupational injuries dictates that physiotherapy play a particularly important role in the early rehabilitation of injured workers. Physiotherapy may be used liberally. Frequent physiotherapy visits provide a rather inexpensive but accurate means of monitoring the progress of recovery as objectively measured by indicators of function – mobility, strength, coordination, and stability. The physiotherapist can monitor and report on a patient's progress less expensively than a physician.

Back injuries alone account for one-quarter of all occupational injuries and do present particular management problems because of their often chronic nature and subjective symptoms. All occupational health services must be prepared to deal with back injuries: medical and nursing personnel must be trained in the latest thinking on the subject and the service should consider offering preventive programs for employees, such as the so-called "back schools" that teach lifting and back care techniques. Whether on a factory floor or in an office filing room, attention must be directed toward actual work practices in order to avoid back injuries occurring through poor lifting habits or inadequate help for a given task. (Routine back x-rays, formerly a popular means of screening new hires to identify individuals susceptible to back injuries, are completely unreliable, discriminatory toward individuals with silent defects, and require an unacceptably high radiation exposure.)

Other body parts frequently involved in occupational injuries are the extremities and the trunk. Accidents to these parts usually are soft-tissue injuries or cuts that seldom result in permanent impairment, although hand and foot injuries can become management problems because of the likelihood of reinjury or difficulty in regaining function after immobilization. Eye injuries have the potential for serious impairment; anything more serious than superficial foreign bodies and conjunctivitis probably should be managed by an ophthalmologist whenever possible.

Early return to work may speed up recovery from occupational injuries in two ways: by returning the patient to familiar body movement and by resocializing the patient into a more normal life. Three months following an injury seems to be a critical point in the process of recovery; beyond this point, the more delay in returning to work, the greater probability of never returning. The level of disability seems to increase as a result of the delay itself. Psychological adjustment factors, reduced fitness, and loss of job skills influence disability levels just as much as the severity of the injury. Employers, then, should accept the injured employee back on the job whenever suitably modified work assignments are available. Unfortunately, many employers refuse to do so because they are afraid of liability for reinjury or a second injury.

Occupational Illnesses

Except where a particular industry or plant has a pattern of hazardous conditions that distorts the frequency of work-related illnesses, the distribution of work-related diseases in industry as a whole tends to follow the "rule of halves." According to this rule, the frequency of any one group of occupational disorders is half that of the preceding group. Thus, skin disorders account for approximately one-half of all occupational diseases: eye conditions (frequently related to exposures that also cause skin disorders) account for about one-quarter; lung disorders, for about one-eighth; and systemic poisonings, about one-sixteenth. Neurologic, cardiac, reproductive, hearing, and mental disorders and cancer associated with occupational exposures account for the remainder.

Occupational illnesses are usually much more difficult to diagnose and to manage than occupational injuries. (The proper medical approach to occupational illnesses is best left to a textbook on occupational medicine and is beyond the scope of this book.) Following diagnosis of and acute care for the illness, the physician should follow the patient periodically and provide supplemental reports as needed to the employer and workers' compensation board. A final report is due when the patient either is fit to return to work or reaches a permanent level of impairment from which further improvement is not to be expected.

Although the physician must use his or her judgment in deciding that a worker is fit to return to the job, determining fitness is not solely a subjective evaluation. (For a detailed discussion on fitness-to-work evaluations see Chapter 18.) Knowledge of the tasks performed on the job and the body movements and strength required for each task is important when evaluating many cases. The physician may find it most efficient to call or meet with the supervisor to explain the situation and provide an estimate as to when the worker will be able to return to work. Often in private practice there is a tendency to give the patient-employee a few extra days or even weeks off as a concealed paid holiday. This practice is to be condemned for a number of reasons: it costs the employer, slows the worker's return to a normal life, delays functional recovery, promotes without reason a poor attitude toward the employer and the workers' compensation system, and encourages the unhealthy psychological defense of retreating into a "sick role."

Problem Cases

In occupational medicine, the physician very often is concerned with workers who present with an occupational disorder due to a hazard presently in the workplace or, in cases of cancer or other chronic diseases with long latency periods, an exposure that occurred in the distant past. Conventional medical practice emphasizes the identification, evaluation, and treatment of a disorder. But in situations where a hazard persists and may affect others, correction of the underlying problem that has caused the disorder is of equal importance. (However, even with special training or expertise in occupational health, the physician is not technically qualified to recommend or advise on specific workplace corrective measures and should instead concentrate on clearly stating the nature of health problems.)

Before suggesting a course of action, the physician confronted by an occupational health problem must make the following preliminary judgments:

- Is this a serious problem for the patient? An occasional mild rash does not carry the same significance as asthma.
- Is this problem likely to affect others in the workplace with the same or more serious health outcomes? At this point the practitioner must expand the customary focus in clinical medicine on the problems of a single patient.
- Am I prepared to pursue the resolution of the problem as far as may be necessary? Some occupational health problems are easily resolved or require only short-term intervention; complex situations, on the other hand, may take months or years to resolve and involve extensive litigation. A commitment to proceed in a legal or collective bargaining action should be weighed seriously, since withdrawal later may seriously jeopardize the success of the patient's or employee group's case.
- What are my limitations as a practitioner? A reasonable clinician should be aware of his or her limitations in interpreting cases that are unusual, complex, or highly technical and in giving expert advice or testimony.

In investigating suspected health effects, the physician should try to determine patterns in the distribution of disease among workers in the particular workplace. This is a preliminary exercise in epidemiology. A clinician or several practitioners in a given area may notice an unusually large number of cases of a particular disorder among workers in a specific industry or workplace. Such patterns may be highly suggestive of an occupational association. Some occupational disorders indeed have been discovered in this way but unless the disorder in question is rare, clusters of cases are seldom strong evidence of an occupational exposure—apparent clusters of disorders without identifiable cause occur from time to time, based on chance alone. Underlying demographic features of the population also exert a powerful influence on risk factors for various health outcomes. These demographic features include age, sex, race, ethnicity, smoking habits, social class, alcohol and drug use, and family relationships. A workforce that includes a large subset from a high-risk population will be likely to reflect the health risks associated with that group.

For example, a working population consisting predominantly of black Americans is likely to have a high prevalence of hypertension and may show an elevated incidence of hypertension-related outcomes; a group of middle-aged white male employees, on the other hand, will have a proportionately higher incidence of cancer and health outcomes associated with cardiovascular disease, such as angina, sudden death, myocardial infarction, stroke, and peripheral vascular disease. The health experience of a working population, therefore, should never be accepted as evidence of an occupational exposure without careful consideration of the demographic features of the population and the expected incidence of the disease in question among individuals of similar age, sex, race, and ethnic background. Such characteristics of the population can be statistically controlled by a process known as "adjustment" of rates—the incidence of the disease in a given population is compared to that of a standard population, as if the age, sex, and racial distributions were identical. This comparison requires assistance or expertise in epidemiology, which may be available through nearby medical schools, schools of public health, and health departments.

The clinician who is excited about a possible case of occupational exposure inadvertently may overinterpret clinical findings to fit the published descriptions. For example, an inexperienced physician may consider every rash or case of acne in workers on a job with potential exposure to PCBs to be chloracne, a severe acneiform rash associated with dioxin exposure. The clinician may become convinced that these patients represent a new and significant association with a previously unrecognized occupational exposure. While many important occupational hazards have been identified in just this way—such as vinyl chloride-induced liver cancer and dimethylaminoproprionitrile-induced autonomic dysfunction— identification of an entirely new occupational association is rare and usually occurs in situations where the exposure is unique to an industry or confined to a small group of workers or has only recently been introduced. Possible associations should be investigated further only if they are convincingly plausible.

Without a working knowledge of toxicology, occupational exposures, and industrial hygiene, the physician is in a poor position to prescribe specific workplace controls to eliminate or contain hazards. This job is best left to the experts in industrial hygiene. The clinician can inform the employer of the general options available for solving the problem, but the responsiveness of the employer may depend in no small degree on the approach taken by the physician.

Whenever possible, the employer should be given an opportunity to correct the problem before third parties become involved. Proceeding methodically, on the assumption that the employer is committed to resolving the problem, is usually the best course of action—it provides the employer with a face-saving way out of the dilemma and establishes the good faith of the employee in the event of future legal actions. An open line of communication from the physician to the employer is in the best interests of the patient; the motives and commitment to protecting the worker on the part of company leaders are germane to the solution of the problem only insofar as they provide an opportunity for the physician to reason with management for the benefit of all concerned. The psychology of the relationships between labor and management is complex. The more coercive the approach, the more likely it is to provoke resistance. This is particularly true for companies that have made an initial, but inadequate, effort at developing an effective occupational safety and health policy.

Physicians who feel that they have identified a potentially significant occupational health hazard would do well to follow the procedure outlined below:

- Write a complete but concise description of the health outcome, the population that appears to be affected, and the possible occupational hazards as described by the patient. Define the problem first in medical terms and then in lay terms. If this simple step is not taken, the description of the problem may become hopelessly muddled when different terms and language are used for the various parties. Refer to this document in all correspondence and telephone conversations with the parties entitled to receive information on the case. (See Chapters 1 and 4.)
- Read the available literature on the problem critically, or refer the case to a qualified consultant. The literature must be approached skeptically and with a working knowledge of the distribution of risk factors in the population in question and the basic biology of the particular health risk. A single case report does not prove an association, nor does a case series necessarily imply a causal relationship. Likewise, an animal study of a particular toxic or physical hazard does not necessarily indicate that the effect can be observed in humans. (A paper in an obscure journal is not necessarily an undiscovered "pearl," either.)
- Establish, with employee consent, a clear line of communication with the employer. A matter-of-fact and businesslike approach works best in most cases; a confrontational, accusatory tone is invariably counterproductive in its efforts to correct the problem quickly. Enlightened management, recognizing that a problem exists, will find it in the employer's own interest to solve the problem expediently; the unenlightened employer is not likely to be moved in any case and will only resist if provoked by a confrontational manner. Contacts with all parties should be documented carefully, as they may become significant in later litigation.

In cases of work-related disease or injury, the physician is required to file a "doctor's first report" with the state or provincial agency responsible for occupational safety and health. (See Chapter 2.) This report initiates the claim for eligibility under workers' compensation and is an essential first step in the process of establishing a legally recognized association with an occupational hazard. (Furthermore, despite a lack of consistent penalties and a low likelihood of prosecution, failure to report an occupational illness or injury is technically a violation of the law.) "Supplemental reports" on the patient's progress are required by the workers' compensation insurance carrier when the patient returns for a follow-up visit, physical therapy, or other long-term treatment. The supplemental report also must provide an estimate of the most likely duration of the disability.

Conscientious communication with both the employer and the carrier by telephone and formal reports will greatly expedite the handling of the patient's case. At every step of the case, the particulars should be carefully recorded in the medical record, which is subject to subpoena. Once a claim is initiated, the recording of accurate data may profoundly affect the resolution of the case.

The physician should advise the patient of his or her rights under the Occupational Safety and Health Act (see Chapter 3) and/or the pertinent state or provincial legislation. In particular, the patient should know that it is against the law for an employer to fire an employee for refusing to work in a hazardous situation. Furthermore, the affected worker, along with two other employees or through the aid of the union, may request an inspection by the Occupational Safety and Health Administration. (The names of the employees initiating the request will be kept confidential.) Inspections are scheduled according to priority categories: (1) imminent danger, when a condition exists that might lead to death or serious physical harm; (2) fatality and catastrophe investigations; (3) investigation of complaints; and (4) routine regional programmed inspections. First priority (imminent danger) inspections are performed within 24 hours and require a tremendous effort on the part of the agency. Fatalities likewise are investigated thoroughly, although they may be less urgent after the fact. Third priority inspections are handled on the basis of severity of the complaint, the number of complaints received by the OSHA office, and the time and the resources available locally. A complete inspection of the workplace is not always made in response to a complaint, especially when the workplace has been inspected recently on a routine basis. In such cases, partial inspections are performed, focusing on the source of the complaint.

Although OSHA protects workers who complain of unsafe work practices, an employee who is perceived as a "troublemaker" may be singled out for attention and eventually may be fired, nominally for other reasons. Although the employer cannot terminate the employee for claiming a work-related injury or illness, the reality of the situation is that any employer can make life miserable for a single employee who complains.

A certain degree of judgment is required in using these rights constructively. For example, a "hazardous situation" is intended to mean a condition that could lead to serious injury, such as an unlined trench, an unstable scaffold, or a confined space in which gases may accumulate. It does not mean climbing an ordinary ladder or driving a truck, absent extraordinary circumstances. The degree of urgency with which the intervention is carried out should match the magnitude of the hazard. A company with a history of fatal accidents should be treated differently than one with an occasional spill of relatively innocuous solvents.

The employer may be contacted by telephone and advised of the magnitude of the problem but a follow-up letter is essential to document this contact. The tone should be nonconfrontational, focused exclusively on the problem at hand, and helpful in conveying the necessary information to allow the employer to address the problem. Most employers do not want trouble with the union, their workers' compensation carrier, or the government. Of course, despite one's best efforts, a belligerent or beleaguered employer may respond badly; nevertheless, management always should be treated with courtesy.

The employer can be informed of the availability of consultation services from state or federal OSHA or provincial agencies. These services provide a limited, voluntary inspection and technical advice on the specific problem and are free to the employer. Unless an imminent danger exists, the OSHA consultation service limits itself to advising the employer and does not communicate its findings to the enforcement branch. The consultation service was intended to help employers who lack the resources or technical knowledge to solve the problem themselves and cannot afford to hire outside consultants. Nonetheless, many employers remain reluctant to call OSHA under any circumstances because they fear enforcement action for what might be found.

In the United States, an OSHA consultation is a good place to start for the small or medium-sized employer. However, the technical level of OSHA consultation services usually are not high since the offices lack the facilities, time, and manpower to deal with complex problems. In such cases, the National Institute for Occupational Safety and Health (NIOSH) may also be of assistance. Certain problems are selected by NIOSH for intensive "health hazard evaluations" because of its research interest. In Canada, the Canadian Centre for Occupational Health and Safety (CCOHS) can be very helpful in providing information and advice.

The employer also may be directed to local or regional resources that can assist in providing solutions to its problems. Academic institutions and a few public agencies work on particular problems, as do numerous highly talented professional consultants. However, private consultation services in occupational safety and health are not inexpensive and the quality of services provided is often inconsistent. Academic institutions generally are more reasonable in cost while adhering to a certain standard of performance.

Further Reading

Bernstein RS, Lee JS: Recognition and evaluation of occupational health problems, in Rom WN (ed): Environmental and Occupational Medicine. Boston, Little Brown, 1983, pp. 7–19.

CEDH/ATPMF Curriculum Development/Dissemination Project in Preventive Medicine. Health Maintenance in Clinical Practice (AJ Segall and HF Vanderschmidt, eds.): Module III, Clinical Health Maintenance, v. 7: Occupational Health (TL Guidotti, author). Boston, Boston University, Center for Educational Development in Health, 1985.

Guidotti TL: Occupational Medicine: Home Study Self-Assessment Monograph 65. Kansas City, American Academy of Family Physicians, 1984.

Identification and Control of Work-Related Diseases. Technical Report Series No. 714. Geneva, World Health Organization, 1985.

Imbus HR: Clinical aspects of occupational medicine, in Zenz C (ed): Occupational Medicine: Principles and Practical Applications. Chicago, Year Book Medical Publishers, 1975, pp. 89–107.

Keogh JP: Occupational and environmental disease, in Barker LR, Burton JR, Zieve ZD (eds): Principles of Ambulatory Care, ed 2. Baltimore, Williams and Wilkins, 1986, pp. 98–111.

18 FITNESS-TO-WORK AND IMPAIRMENT EVALUATIONS

Health evaluations conducted by occupational health professionals may be grouped into four general types: fitness to work, acute care, health surveillance, and health monitoring. This chapter will describe how to conduct an objective and useful fitness-to-work evaluation appropriate for a variety of circumstances. Impairment evaluation, a special type of fitness-to-work evaluation, is addressed in the last section of the chapter.

Fitness-to-Work Examinations

Fitness-to-work examinations are objective assessments of the health of employees in relation to the specific job they hold or intend to hold. Such examinations are conducted in order to ensure that employees are able to perform a job without hazard to themselves or others. Medical examinations to determine fitness to work concentrate on the relationship between health and the demands of the job and the workplace conditions. They should not be confused with health surveillance tests for actual or potential exposure to toxic materials or harmful physical agents or with medical monitoring examinations for the promotion and maintenance of personal health.

To be fair and objective for both employee and employer, the examinations must be specifically job-related, with judgments of fitness being based upon the principle that the employee's state of health, in relation to the individual job, should not cause harm to the worker or be a hazard to others. This principle is acknowledged in various occupational research and safety acts and codes of individual rights. Fitness-to-work examinations must be conducted in a manner consistent with professional codes of ethics and be undertaken only by individuals who are familiar with the working conditions and job demands and specially trained or well experienced in occupational medicine or occupational health nursing.

In fitness-to-work examinations, the physician is asked to render an informed opinion about a person's health and functional capabilities. The physician's judgment will affect the rights and obligations of the employer as well as the worker. Given the increasing social awareness of employees, unions, and employers, these examinations must be performed with great competence and objectivity; otherwise, the concerned parties will feel unfairly treated and distrust the outcome of the examination. The physician also must bear in mind the doctor-patient relationship, which is defined by various professional codes of ethics and laws.

Fitness-to-work examinations are requested either at the initiative of the employer or voluntarily by the employee. Company-initiated examinations occur because they are required by company policy or government regulations. In performing these examinations, the occupational health professional judges the employee's fitness-to-work based upon a medical examination that is dictated by the demands of the work. A clinical opinion is reported back to the employer in the form of a fitness-to-work judgment that does not use medical terminology or reveal a medical diagnosis. Typically, the terms used are *fit, unfit,* or *fit, subject to work modifications* (the latter two categories are further qualified as *temporarily or permanently*).

At times, it may not be possible or appropriate for the in-house occupational health professional to personally perform the medical examination. The medical findings and opinions provided by outside private clinicians or consultants then must be interpreted in light of the working conditions and rendered into a fitness-to-work judgment. If an occupational health professional is not on staff, a company official must provide the private clinician or consultant with a description of the working conditions and job requirements so that the private clinician can make as accurate a fitness-to-work judgment as possible. It is not appropriate for company personnel, such as supervisors and employment office staff, to inquire after or be given specific medical findings, personal health information, or diagnoses from private clinicians and consultants.

As indicated in Table 18.1, a number of circumstances may warrant a fitness-to-work examination:

- Preplacement—In order to be useful to the employee and employer and be consistent with civil rights legislation (such as the Rehabilitation Act of 1973), preplacement examinations must be structured so that they are specific to the working conditions and job requirements. (See Chapter 19.) They must be scheduled after a job offer has been made, as an employer cannot arbitrarily deny a person a job opportunity on the basis of his or her physical or emotional impairment. However, the job offer can be made contingent on the condition that the applicant pass a job-related medical examination to determine that he or she can perform the job without endangering self or others. The prospective employee will be refused the job only if his or her health condition is not compatible with the working conditions and the working conditions and job requirements cannot reasonably be altered.

- Return to Work—Although not all organizations conduct routine return-to-work examinations, such examinations are very useful in evaluating workers following a severe illness or injury or in the face of an absence of unusual duration. Premature and unduly delayed returns to work both can cause difficulties for the employee as well as the employer. A relevant and timely examination can reduce overall lost worktime for the employee and can improve productivity for the employer.

- Continuing Impairment—Continuing impairment assessments are used when an employee remains absent from work for extended time periods or faces returning

---

Table 18.1. Reasons for Performing a Fitness-To-Work Evaluation

Preplacement
  When an employee has been offered a full- or part-time job subject to passing a relevant medical examination.

Return to Work
  When an employee is returning to work after recovery from a serious illness or injury and the person's capability of performing the original job is not known.

  When an employee has returned to work at a modified job and is still undergoing therapy, rehabilitation, or both.

Continuing Impairment
  When an employee remains absent from work and must be assessed for continuing short-term or long-term disability payment or workers' compensation.

Performance-Initiated Review
  When health reasons are identified as the cause of failing job performance and a medical review has been suggested (job not yet at risk) or required (job at risk) by the employer.

Job Transfer
  When an employee transfers to a position whose working conditions are significantly different.

Change in Working Conditions of Existing Job
  When the existing working conditions have been significantly altered.

Change in Health Status in Existing Job
  When health problems have developed that may be aggravated by existing working conditions.

---

to work with a new problem. The occupational health service can help such employees by providing rehabilitation opportunities, improving therapeutic support mechanisms, assisting private clinicians in case management, and working with the company to provide suitably modified work so as to effect a timely return to work.

• Performance-Initiated—Employee assistance programs are often the source of performance-initiated reviews, which are the most sensitive and difficult type of fitness-to-work evaluations to perform. The occupational health physician's judgment can have a profound effect on whether or not employment is continued. In such cases, the worker's health has been implicated as a cause for failing work performance; before further action is taken, the health situation must be clarified. *Supervisor-suggested reviews* may occur when job performance has not yet deteriorated to a severe degree; management only suggests that a medical judgment ought to be obtained. The employee, of course, may refuse without immediate consequence because the discipline process has not yet begun. However, if health reasons are the cause of failing work performance, a prudent employee will obtain a medical judgment to explain and to help correct the situation; absent a medical review, failing work performance will trigger the discipline process. When work performance is totally unacceptable, the employee may become subject to a *supervisor-directed review* and undergo a mandatory medical evaluation. Should the employee refuse the medical evaluation, discipline and/or dismissal will proceed without the benefit of a medical judgment.

- Job Transfer, Changed Working Conditions or Health Status—Fitness-to-work examinations also are indicated by changes in the status of an employee's health (even though the individual may not be missing work or suffering deteriorations in job performance); when working conditions have changed significantly; and when an employee transfers to a job in which working conditions are more strenuous or involve significant or different types of exposures.

Evaluation Procedure

The procedure by which fitness-to-work is judged is a process of matching the worker's health status to the job requirements. The procedure is based on objective measures that allow occupational health professionals, employers, supervisors, workers, and others to communicate effectively, adheres to professional codes of behavior, and ensures fairness for both workers and employers.

The Fitness-to-Work Record presented as Figure 18.1 records two types of information: the working conditions of a specific job (Section A) and the health standards relevant to those conditions and requirements (Section B). By comparing this information to the findings of the examination and the results of the screening tests, the physician can form a clinical opinion and arrive at an objective, ethical judgement of an individual's fitness-to-work at a particular job (Section C). Figure 18.2 illustrates this process, which can be applied to each of the circumstances listed in Table 18.1.

The form usually is filled out in quadruplicate, and copies are distributed to the employee and his or her supervisor and medical and personnel files. (Further distribution may vary according to the structure and requirements of each organization.) In order to further ensure the confidentiality of health information, Section B is completed only on the copy destined for the medical file.

The reason for conducting the fitness-to-work evaluation must be absolutely clear to the physician, the employee, and the employer. (See Table 18.1.) If the examination has been conducted at the initiation of the employer, the fitness-to-work procedure is followed and the Fitness-to-Work Record may be used.

The fitness-to-work procedure is followed only as a guide, however, when the employee voluntarily seeks confidential medical advice. In this case, the employer is not officially involved, i.e., the employee's performance is not an issue. Consequently, copies of the completed Fitness-to-Work Record would be distributed to the human resources department or the supervisor only if the physician or nurse and the employee consider this action to be in the employee's best interest.

Determining the Working Conditions (Section A)
The information recorded in this section should describe accurately and concisely the critical features of the working conditions and the manner in which the work is performed. A complete, detailed account of every aspect of the job, otherwise known as a job description, is not necessary. Specific information (e.g., work hours, stress levels, job location, and exposure to potential physical injury, noise, heat, and toxic or biologic hazards) should be recorded. In large organizations, this information is typically obtained from the employee presently holding the position, the immediate supervisor,

Figure 18.1. The fitness-to-work record, as developed by the Nova Corporation of Alberta. (The form is reproduced with permission from Nova Corporation.)

FITNESS-TO-WORK RECORD

EMPLOYEE'S NAME & NUMBER	POSITION TITLE
EMPLOYEE'S HOME ADDRESS	HOME PHONE
DEPARTMENT NAME	WORK PHONE LOCATION
SUPERVISOR'S NAME & PHONE	PERSONNEL CONTACTS NAME & PHONE

SECTION A WORKING CONDITIONS

SECTION B HEALTH STANDARDS   (FOR MEDICAL STAFF USE ONLY)

SECTION C FITNESS TO WORK   (APPLIES TO THIS JOB ONLY. IF JOB CHANGES, CONTACT THE MEDICAL STAFF)

☐ FIT   ☐ UNFIT   ☐ FIT SUBJECT TO WORK MODIFICATION

☐ TEMPORARILY   ☐ PERMANENTLY   FOLLOW-UP DATE   YY MM DD

COMMENTS

FOR MEDICAL STAFF USE ONLY

ASSESSED BY (PLEASE PRINT) M D R N	ADDRESS
ASSESSOR'S SIGNATURE	PHONE NO
	DATE OF ASSESSMENT YY MM DD

the personnel department, the occupational hygienist, the safety specialist, and the medical staff. In smaller organizations, information usually is acquired easily, since the owner-operator and employees are knowledgeable about the working conditions. The details of the working conditions that must be taken into consideration are outlined in Table 18.2, provided at the end of this chapter. Figure 18.3 is an example of a completed Section A.

Figure 18.2. The process of conducting fitness-to-work evaluations requires matching working conditions and health standards to the medical findings and clinical opinions following the examination. (Reproduced with permission from the Nova Corporation.)

SCHEME OF PROCESS FOR DETERMINING FITNESS TO WORK

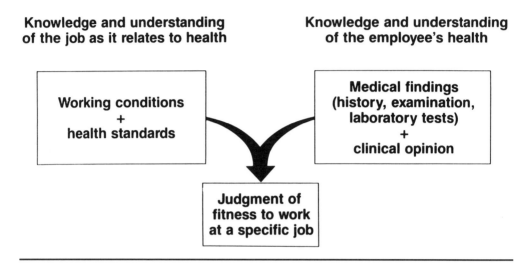

Determining Health Standards (Section B)

The health standards are determined by the physician, usually with the help of an occupational health nurse and sometimes with input from an occupational hygienist and safety professional. Standards are based on the occupational health professional's understanding of how the body may be affected by the working conditions. For example, if conditions require an employee to work for up to eight hours in isolation operating a motor vehicle, the central nervous system would be identified as one of the body systems that should be functioning within acceptable limits.

The extent of the physical examination and the laboratory tests needed to characterize the system will be determined by the specific details of the working conditions—not every body system will be examined and those that are will be investigated only to the degree indicated by the working conditions. For example, examining the cardiovascular system in one circumstance may require only that a nurse check the employee's blood pressure and pulse; in another situation, the working conditions may indicate that a physician should conduct a full review of the system, including a submaximal cardiovascular stress test.

The medical history, findings at physical examination, test results, and clinical opinions are recorded in the usual manner on the employee's medical chart and are treated as confidential health information. Through this process, the overall clinical determination is based only on those body systems relevant to the working conditions.

Table 18.3 at the end of the chapter outlines the body systems and the minimal

Figure 18.3. Fitness-to-Work Record Section A: Working Conditions. (Reproduced with permission from the Nova Corporation.)

SECTION A WORKING CONDITIONS

Office environment. Hours – 7 - 8 hour rotating shifts. Overtime occasional. Duties – handles customer requests for assistance in completing local, toll, long distance and emergency calls. 95% sitting with routine breaks. Uses a VDT, Centrex console, or cord board constantly. Must be able to differentiate between colors. Must be able to respond to emergency situations. Steady workload with heavy peaks. Minimal level of responsibility and decision making. Works under supervision. Deals with internal and external personnel and customers.

various screening methods that should be used to investigate each. The systems referred to throughout the procedure are: cardiovascular system (CVS), central nervous system (CNS), endocrine (ENDO), gastrointestinal (GI), genitourinary (GU), hearing, hematological (HEMAT), immunological (IMMUN), integumentary (INTEG), mental status, musculoskeletal (MS), respiratory (RESP), and vision. Any of the screening methods can be upgraded if the conditions warrant. For example, a history and physical examination by a nurse could be upgraded to being performed by a physician. Once the body systems and screening methods have been chosen, they are combined and listed in Section B. An example of Section B as completed for a reasonably demanding job is presented in Figure 18.4.

Unfortunately, there are few valid tests unique to the evaluation of impairment that will help an occupational health professional determine the worker's health status in relation to performing specific work. Traditional clinical examination methods and laboratory tests help the examiner form a clinical opinion but these should be applied selectively. Only those tests that are pertinent to the evaluation of a body system and relevant to the working conditions and requirements of a specific job should be used. For example, if the condition of a worker's cardiovascular system is identified as being relevant to the safe operation of a large highway transport truck, then a cardiovascular stress test might be useful as one method of assessing an employee's fitness for that job following a myocardial infarction. In other cases where the respiratory system is relevant, the health professional might consider using special pulmonary function tests, such as bronchoprovocation challenge in cases of asthma. Experience has shown that routine, nonselective use of tests is rarely if ever helpful in impairment evaluations. For example, the back x-ray has proven to be the least useful of all routine tests and is now considered to be contraindicated.

Specific and standardized clinical tests that are applicable to particular job functions, such as those that could evaluate muscle power and endurance, would be very useful in occupational health evaluations. However, much research is still needed to develop simple, reliable, and inexpensive tests that can evaluate functional capacity for

Figure 18.4. Fitness-to-Work Record Section B: Health Standards.
(Reproduced with permission from the Nova Corporation.)

SECTION B HEALTH STANDARDS   (FOR MEDICAL STAFF USE ONLY)

SYSTEMS: CVS, CNS, ENDO, GI, GU, HEARING, HEMAT, MENTAL STATUS,
            MS, VISION within acceptable limits.

SCREENING: Health history by RN; Physical assessment by RN (eye/hand
            coordination, manual dexterity, ROM); Lab – hemoglobin,
            audiogram, urinalysis 1, vision 1, color vision.

---

a wide range of jobs. (A prototype framework for developing standards appropriate to specific jobs has been formulated by the County of San Bernardino, California, and is under further development by Med-Tox Associates of Tustin, California. The military also have rigorous and explicit standards for their billets.) Until such tests become readily available, meaningful occupational health evaluations and the fitness-to-work judgments based upon them depend on the skill and motivation of the occupational health professionals and their knowledge of relevant body systems coupled with their adherence to clinical examination methods and laboratory tests that are specific to evaluations of these systems.

Judging Fitness to Work (Section C)

In Section C, the confidential clinical opinion is rendered into a fitness-to-work judgment (Figure 18.5). There are six possible judgments: fit; fit, subject to work modifications; temporarily fit, subject to work modifications; temporarily unfit; and permanently unfit.

Fit means that the employee is unequivocally able to perform the job without danger to self or others. The subcategory "temporarily" can be used for all types of medical assessments except preplacement. "Permanently" should never be used with a judgment of "fit" since physicians cannot see that far into the future.

Fit subject to work modification means that the employee could be a hazard to self or others if employed in the job as it is described or currently performed. He or she, however, would be considered fit to do the job if certain working conditions (or the way in which the work must be performed) were modified. The modifications required must be clearly described in the comments section. If they can be accommodated, the employee is considered fit for the modified job. If they cannot be reasonably accommodated, the employee is deemed temporarily or permanently unfit. "Temporarily" means that if the person's condition improves with time, the requirement for work modification may be lifted. "Permanently" means that the employee will never be fit for the job without it being modified. In either instance, follow-up visits for further reviews must be arranged in case circumstances change. The judgments at the follow-up

Figure 18.5. Fitness-to-Work Record Section C: Fitness-to-Work Judgment (Reproduced with permission from the Nova Corporation.)

FITNESS TO WORK RECORD

SECTION C FITNESS TO WORK (APPLIES TO THIS JOB ONLY. IF JOB CHANGES, CONTACT THE HEALTH STAFF)									
☐ FIT	☐ UNFIT	☐ FIT SUBJECT TO WORK MODIFICATIONS	☐ TEMPORARILY		☐ PERMANENTLY		FOLLOW-UP DATE	YY MM DD	
COMMENTS									
EVALUATED BY (PLEASE PRINT)			☐ M D ☐ R N	EVALUATOR'S SIGNATURE			EVALUATION DATE	YY MM DD	

visits should be recorded each time on a new Fitness-to-Work Record. Any employee considered fit, subject to work modification, must be fully informed of both the medical findings and any work modifications deemed appropriate.

Unfit describes the employee who is unable to perform the job without being a hazard to self or others. This judgment with the subcategory "temporarily" means that the medical condition may improve with time, thus allowing the worker to return to work or transfer to some other job. "Permanently" usually means that the employee will never be fit for the job and that no modification of the working conditions is reasonably possible or medically relevant. It may also mean the employee is unable to do any available job, with or without work modification. In such a situation a statement to this effect should be made in the comments section.

Any employee who is considered unfit, whether temporarily or permanently, must be fully informed of the medical findings. In the case of a preplacement medical assessment, no follow-up visit is required, as the applicant is clearly unsuitable for the job. In other types of fitness-to-work situations a follow-up visit must be arranged in case the health status or working conditions change.

The physician arrives at a fitness-to-work judgment by evaluating the information in Section A against a clinical opinion that is based on the medical examination dictated by the body systems and screening methods (health standards) in Section B. The fitness-to-work judgment, then, is based on the actual working conditions and the worker's current health status. While decisions must not be influenced by speculation as to what might happen in the future, they should reflect clinical acumen in detecting signs of incipient conditions. For example, a truck driver returning to work after suffering a heart attack might appear stable and well. Nonetheless, if the employee has had a particularly severe attack and has not modified bad lifestyle habits nor followed his doctor's orders, the physician would be incorrect in declaring him fit to drive a large truck.

Resolving cases in which the judgment is either "fit, subject to work modifications" or "unfit" requires close communications between the human resources department, the supervisor, and the occupational health professional. A telephone conversation or meeting may be required to supplement the Fitness-to-Work Record. Moreover, the health professional, armed with a clear knowledge of both the employee's medical status and the working conditions, must be able to provide comprehensive advice to the human resources department and supervisor without using medical terminology or giving a diagnosis. However, the employee (and any person whom the employee has designated by signing a form for the release of medical information) must be fully informed of all the medical findings and the health standards upon which the judgment was made.

If the process of developing specific health standards is based on a clear understanding of actual working conditions and the clinical opinion on a medical examination that is relevant to those health standards, a proper fitness-to-work judgment can be made. Such a judgment will be viewed as fair and valid not only by the employee and the employer but also by concerned observers, such as union representatives, proponents of individual rights, legislators, and other health professionals. Most importantly, the health professional will have acted ethically by protecting the patient's right to confidentiality of medical information; only the outcome of the process—the fitness-to-work assessment—will be revealed.

Impairment Evaluation for Work-Related Illness or Injury

A diagnosis in occupational medicine may be made at the beginning rather than the end of the evaluative process. This is particularly true for occupational illnesses due to workplace exposures and for repetitive motion injuries. Questions concerning the responsible exposure, the work-relatedness of the condition, and the worker's expected degree of impairment are sometimes more important than a precise diagnosis. On such questions often hinge decisions regarding eligibility for compensation, prognosis for rehabilitation, fitness for future work, and prevention for the protection of other workers.

Assessing the Validity of the Clinical Data

Contradictory data are common in the presentation of a work-related case. The perfectly consistent case, the one in which the patient's presentation is characteristic in every respect of a particular occupational disorder, is decidedly unusual.

The first step in clinical evaluation is to consider the validity of the data at hand. Clinical data can be validated externally, by comparing it with information collected elsewhere, or internally, by assessing its degree of agreement with other data in the case.

External validation is usually provided in a clinical setting in the form of other records from consultants, primary physicians, hospitals, company personnel, industrial hygienists, unions, and workers' compensation carriers or boards. Hygiene records are often especially useful because they may contain information about the level of exposure sustained by the worker. External evidence is most reliable when it has been gathered for reasons unrelated to the case at hand because it is then most likely to be free of bias and preconceived ideas. Statements found in a dictated summary, historical summary, or other secondary sources (especially regarding such critical matters as smoking habits) are often unreliable. The physician should try to corroborate them by comparing at least two independent sources in which the parties responsible for recording the information had no contact.

The internal validation of data is often more practical in a clinical setting. The physician should consider whether the data are reasonably consistent by comparing the stated chief complaint with the review of systems and the findings on physical examination with the patient's own description of the problem. The physician should be alert to major inconsistencies in a patient's history of the present illness, bearing in mind that minor lapses or changes in the history are only human. When contradictions fall beyond the range of usual clinical experience, the physician must consider as possible explanations whether the patient:

- Is upset or distracted;
- Does not believe that the clinician is taking the problem seriously enough and is exaggerating to get the point across;
- Is experiencing a true compensation neurosis without intent to deceive the physician and does not realize that the story given is contradictory;
- Is a poor historian and simply is in error;
- Is mentally ill; or
- Is malingering.

Simple errors in recall and minor inconsistencies in findings tend to be random and relatively trivial. However, when all of the mistakes point in the same direction there should be a high index of suspicion for intentional or unintentional distortion of the history.

Deriving a Clinical Impression from the Findings

The most intuitive step in the process of evaluating a patient is the jump from the clinical picture to the diagnosis, which in turn leads to considerations of causation and work-relatedness.

The process of arriving at a diagnosis is the essence of a clinician's cognitive skill, combining deductive logic, intuition, pattern recognition, and judgments on probability. Clinicians reach a diagnosis most often through pattern recognition, which tends to work most reliably on common problems. The use of deduction, which is the way clinicians are "supposed" to work, is usually reserved, in practice, for complex cases. Nonetheless, a pattern encountered frequently in a common disease also may be repeated in an uncommon disease or exposure situation, misleading any clinician who does not consider the possibility of an occupational etiology. For example, some variant forms of occupational asthma resemble intrinsic asthma, and the two forms of fume fever (metal fume fever and polymer fume fever) resemble influenza. Experienced clinicians may err by assuming that a familiar pattern represents a familiar disease. Generally, the process of diagnosis is no different in occupational medicine than it is in medical practice, but occupational medicine places more of a premium on deduction because of the complexity of many cases.

In occupational medicine, complex problems frequently involve several organ systems. The physician faced with a new and complex case may find it helpful to arrange the patient's complaints and the clinical findings into problems, as in the problem-oriented medical record, and then to categorize these by organ system. Another useful approach is to think in terms of structure and function. For example, are the abnormalities seen on the chest film compatible with the deficit on spirometry?

In occupational medicine, the process of deductive reasoning usually begins with a differential diagnosis that includes both occupational and nonoccupational disorders.

A relatively common example of this process applies to pulmonary interstitial fibrosis, which may arise from a number of occupational exposures besides having a wide range of nonoccupational causes.

The deductive pathway to diagnosis requires sequential testing to rule out alternative diagnoses. The clinician first considers all the conditions that are likely to produce the clinical picture and the possibility of other conditions that may rarely present in this way. The list of diagnostic possibilities is the differential diagnosis. Until the correct diagnosis is found, the deductive process proceeds by eliminating the various possibilities by special tests, by observing the clinical course of the disorder, or by a therapeutic trial. Since most clinical tests are not absolutely specific for a given disease, the deductive process more often involves ruling out conditions because of their incompatibility with the clinical findings than confirming the diagnosis with a specific test.

Facilitating the process of deductive reasoning in occupational medicine are the many special toxicologic tests for detecting toxic substances and their metabolites (for example, urinary free benzene and phenol in the case of benzene exposure). A growing role also is being assumed by biological monitoring tests for the early detection of physiologic and biochemical changes induced by toxic exposure (for example, plasma and red blood cell cholinesterase levels for the organophosphate and carbamate pesticides). However, these special toxicologic tests are only useful when the occupational exposure is considered in the differential diagnosis. Thus, it is extremely important that the index of suspicion for occupationally related disorders be high. Since the nonspecialist cannot be expected to remember the details of the many occupational illnesses, some of which are quite infrequently seen, he or she should consult authoritative reference works or obtain consultation by telephone.

Identifying Causation

The distinction between a diagnosis and the identification of an etiology is important to occupational medicine. A diagnosis implies recognition of a known disease, which may or may not have a known etiology. When a number of etiologic agents or exposures produce an identical clinical picture but different prognoses, the diagnosis is incomplete without the etiology. For example, "interstitial fibrosis" is not a diagnosis; "usual interstitial pneumonia, resulting from diffuse alveolar damage from recurrent or chronic exposure to a toxic gas" would be a diagnosis without a clear statement of the etiology. The specific toxic gas, such as nitrogen dioxide, would be the etiology.

Causation in occupational medicine implies an understanding of the etiology of the disorder, the circumstances of exposure, and the predisposing conditions of the patient. In the case of a camera repairman with painful lower-extremity paresthesias and diminished sensation, the causes may be multiple, involving diabetes, alcohol abuse, and transdermal absorption of mildly neurotoxic solvents. Toxic exposures are not always occupational. For example, in a clear case of lead intoxication, a patient initially presumed to have experienced exposure on the job turned out to have been exposed much more heavily from stripping lead-containing paint off the walls of an old house he was renovating.

A judgment regarding causation is the interpretation, in a specific case, of the most probable direct cause of the disorder. Because the question of causation in an individual case is sometimes impossible to prove beyond doubt—particularly in the case of a chronic illness with a long latency period, such as cancer—the clinician must often play the odds by relying on the epidemiology literature. A plausible statement of causation must specify what the offending agent was, when and where the individual was exposed, and why this particular patient developed the disorder while another worker in the same workplace did not.

Identification of causation in an occupationally related case is critical. If the causation is work-related, identification may establish the patient's entitlement under workers' compensation as well as force correction of the problem, if it still exists. The resolution of causation leads naturally to the assessment of work-relatedness.

Judging Work-Relatedness

When an employee falls off a ladder at work and sprains his foot, work-relatedness is obvious. However, assessing work-relatedness in cases of chronic disease and in contested workers' compensation cases is sometimes difficult. Many disorders that are known to have occupational causes may also occur for other reasons; a worker may have a history of multiple exposures, each associated with a particular health outcome. This is particularly common in cases of bladder cancer, asthma, hearing impairment, and osteoarthritis.

After establishing the diagnosis and making a presumption of causation, the physician must follow a three-step process to verify work-relatedness:

- First, document whenever possible that the patient actually did sustain the presumed exposure. Consider the case of a worker in a cement factory who smoked and who developed squamous cell bronchogenic carcinoma at only 40 years of age, much earlier than would have been anticipated from just smoking. The presence of pleural plaques on his chest film was convincing evidence that he indeed had been exposed to asbestos, which was added to the cement used in manufacturing sewer and water pipes.

- Second, rule out associations having nothing to do with work. Skin rashes, hepatitis, fever, aplastic anemia, purpura, nausea, and many other problems that may appear to be work-related in fact may be caused by medication. Employers, of course, are not responsible for problems that arise from avocational activities— hobbies, volunteer service, or domestic chores that may expose the patient to hazards without any relation to gainful employment. Many people engage in hobbies at home that carry some risk of serious exposure, such as making jewelry or stained glass, building model airplanes, constructing ceramics, and refinishing furniture. Broadly speaking, these activities are occupational, but they are not work-related in the context of workers' compensation entitlement.

- Third, rule out deception. Occasionally, a patient injured at home will go to work and claim that the injury occurred on the job. Although it may be impossible for the clinician to know the truth, many cases of fraud can be detected from inconsistencies in the history or uncovered by communicating with the employer about the patient's work assignments. Sometimes a patient will claim a serious injury is work-related because the worker is afraid that otherwise disability coverage will not be available. There is no acceptable reason for a worker to fraudulently submit a claim to the workers' compensation board: the practice is, of course, illegal, and benefits are available under employee health insurance plans or, where applicable, through state disability compensation.

Assessing Disability

Disability is the diminished ability, resulting from the effects of an injury or illness, of a worker to compete on the open labor market in the occupation for which he or she is trained and otherwise well suited. The extent of disability depends on the degree of the worker's functional impairment, training and skill, the condition of the labor market in the worker's occupation, and the availability of alternative gainful employment for someone in the same condition.

The physician does not bear responsibility for judging the level of a worker's disability under workers' compensation, social security, or state disability programs. The role of the clinician is to supply accurate information on two important determinants of disability: impairment and prognosis. Although these determinants are very important in any given case, they do not define disability—this is done by adjudicators and review boards in the responsible agency, using criteria that include the claimant's education and the job market. The clinician cannot possibly have the detailed knowledge of local and regional labor market conditions for a wide range of occupations needed for such judgments. Furthermore, since clinicians see the process from only one side and hear the complaints of many disgruntled applicants, they may easily develop a distorted view of the system when a judgment does not match their expectations or those of the patient. Often, there is a tendency on behalf of the physician to write an evaluation that exaggerates (or sometimes minimizes) the worker's impairment in order to benefit the patient. However, attempts to manipulate the system by over- or underestimating impairment only introduce more confusion into an already imperfect system and may hurt the worker.

A disability may be categorized as temporary or permanent, partial or total. Temporary disability exists when the injured worker is recovering but cannot yet return to work. Disability becomes permanent when no further change is expected and the patient's capacity for work will persist at that level for the remainder of his or her economically productive life. Total disability does not mean a total incapacity to do any meaningful work but rather an inability to compete in the labor market, as defined by the skills necessary for the job. (Loss of manual dexterity from any cause might not be totally disabling to a longshoreman, for example, but would be to a surgeon.) Partial disabilities are rated on a percentage basis. For example, in California a back injury that precludes heavy lifting carries a standard disability rating of 30 percent. This standard rating then is adjusted for each occupation: the same back injury would be rated 44 percent disability for a structural steel worker and 23 percent for a lawyer. In each case, an additional adjustment is made by age.

Clinicians aiming at the most practical approach to correctly evaluating impairment should take advantage of the many resources available: obtain guidelines from each of the workers' compensation and disability insurance programs most likely to be encountered in practice (including Social Security) and follow the *AMA Guides to the Evaluation of Permanent Impairment*. Workers'compensation boards require from the clinician a clear, unambiguous statement in quantitative terms of what the patient can and cannot do compared to the patient's capabilities before the disorder. When a succession of injuries has occurred, a clear statement is needed describing how each has progressively limited function. Any deterioration in function should be documented or quantified whenever possible by objective measurements, such as range of motion, grip strength, visual acuity, forced expiratory volume in one second, or distribution of sensation.

The clinician is frequently asked to speculate on the percentage of the patient's impairment that may have been due to a given exposure or accident or the percentage of the causation that might be attributed to a given exposure. This is relatively easy to do when the patient's condition can be compared with a previously measured and recorded "baseline." When the patient's own baseline is unknown, it is customary to use population-derived averages that serve as estimates (e.g., expected pulmonary function based on age, sex, and height). The objective is to determine what proportion of the loss of function may have been due to the accident or illness, and what proportion may be due to other work-related disorders, previous personal illness, or other causes. This is referred to as "apportionment," and can only be an informed judgment in the absence of a baseline evaluation.

In general, the apportionment of causation is virtually meaningless. One can never conclude with certainty that a given condition was caused by certain exposures in a particular proportion. For example, speculating that a given case of lung cancer was 50 percent due to smoking and 50 percent due to asbestos is no better than guessing. Such statements are not accepted by most workers' compensation appeal boards. Apportionment of impairment, on the other hand, is feasible and useful. In this case, the apportionment is a judgment regarding the proportion of the observed impairment that has arisen due to the disorder. Apportionment of impairment contributes significantly to a workers' compensation case. Accurate apportionment of impairment depends on accurate baseline data, which may be found in preplacement or earlier periodic examinations.

Chronic diseases and health effects that cannot be attributed to just one employer are increasingly recognized and accepted by workers' compensation boards under the legal doctrine of "cumulative injury." This concept is used to refer to conditions that have arisen as the result of countless minimal injuries on the job; it allows the apportionment of coverage among insurance carriers on the basis of the duration of exposure a worker sustained at each place of employment. Such apportionment is particularly important in cases of noise-induced hearing loss and when workers move from job to job within the same industry.

Increasingly, insurance carriers, workers' compensation boards, and disability review boards are demanding objective clinical measurements and are discounting subjective clinical impressions. Unsupported judgments are no longer taken very seriously.

Table 18.2. Working Conditions to be Detailed in Section A of the Fitness-to-Work Record

1. *Short Description of the Job Function*
   - Write a short but precise statement of the job function.
   - Record percentage of time spent on specific duties (e.g., 50% cleaning and servicing furnaces and air conditioners, 20% snow shovelling and gardening, 30% unloading supplies and moving furniture).

2. *Location*
   - Record approximate percentage of time in:
     - Office/field/lab/computer center/plant/service center.
     - Offshore rigs and other isolated locations.
     - Expatriate (foreign country).
     - Indoors/outdoors.
     - In transit; specify form of transportation.

3. *Hours of Work*
   - Shifts: 12-hour, rotating.
   - Lunch breaks: scheduled, unscheduled.
   - Overtime: may be described as:
     - excessive (daily and/or weekends).
     - frequent (2–3 times/week).
     - occasional (one time/week).
     - rare (one time/month).
     - periodic (episodic), emergency call, on-call duty.

4. *Occupational Safety Hazards*
   - Safety (Acute Traumatic Injury)
     - Machinery: specify type of equipment used, indicate whether working near (within 3 feet) or operating moving or dangerous machinery.
     - Working in tanks and vessels.
     - Working at heights.
     - Walking over rough terrain and/or slippery surfaces (more than 3 times/year).
     - Other.
   - Ergonomic (Chronic Traumatic Injury)
     - Lifting, carrying, pushing or pulling; record the amount of weight involved.
     - Bending, stooping, twisting, pushing and pulling; record how much or how often.
     - Climbing to heights; record how high and how often.
     - Working in awkward positions or cramped quarters.
     - Standing, walking, sitting; record percentage of time spent at each.
   - Using repetitive motions.
     - Using equipment: VDT/word processor, hand tools.
     - Performing office functions.
     - Other.

5. *Occupational Health Hazards*
   - Physical Agents
     - Thermal: temperature, humidity.
     - Radiation: ionizing, non-ionizing, ultrasound, ultraviolet, infrared, radio frequency.
     - Sound: continuous (greater than 85 dB), intermittent, impulse.
   - Vibration.

(Continued)

Table 18.2. Continued

- Atmospheric pressure.
- Other.
- Chemical Agents: List any actual or potential chemical agent exposures.
- Biological Agents
  - Bacteria, molds, fungi.
  - Other.

6. *Special Requirements*
   - Operating mobile equipment: driving heavy equipment or trucks, servicing or flying company planes, driving company vehicle.
   - Participating in offshore survival training and working in an offshore environment.
   - Participating in fire-fighting training.
   - Responding to emergency situations.
   - Travel requirements: plane, helicopter, car, truck, all-terrain vehicles.
   - Special tasks or conditions: requiring color vision; performing detailed, precise work; working near or directly with food; conducting aerobic fitness classes; working with laboratory chemicals, etc.
   - Personal protective equipment required.
   - Isolation (record percentage of time): use geographical statement such as offshore, meter station; working alone.

7. *Psychosocial Demands*
   - Level of decision-making and responsibility, e.g., minimal, moderate, high.
   - Dealing and working with others, e.g., frequently, by telephone, in person, etc.
   - Workload: intensive, moderately intensive, peaks, steady deadlines to meet, whether critical, frequent, occasional.
   - Other.

Table 18.3. Health Standards to be Specified in Section B of the Fitness-to-Work Record

Working Conditions	Minimal Health Standards	
	Body Systems	Screening Methods
1.0 JOB FUNCTION Short description		
2.0 LOCATION Office/field/lab/service center/plant/service center, indoors/outdoors Offshore rigs/supply boats. Expatriate	The specifics of the job and the location in combination will indicate the system to be assessed.	These are listed elsewhere under specific working condition sections.
3.0 HOURS OF WORK Shifts: rotating shifts, overtime 12-hour shift, on call or emergency call out	CVS, CNS, ENDO, GI, GU, HEMAT, MENTAL STATUS, MS	Health History by R.N. Physical assessment by R.N. BP, pulse, Lab • Hemoglobin • Urinalysis 1
Lunch Breaks: unscheduled meal hours	ENDO, GI	Health History by R.N. Lab: Urinalysis 1
4.0 OCCUPATIONAL SAFETY HAZARDS		
4.1 *Safety* Working near (within 3 feet) or operating moving equipment	CVS, CNS, ENDO, HEARING HEMAT, MENTAL STATUS, MS, VISION	Health History by R.N. Physical assessment by R.N. BP, pulse, balance, eye/hand/foot coordination, manual dexterity, ROM Lab: • Audiogram • Hemoglobin • Urinalysis 1 • Vision 1, peripheral vision and depth perception
Working in confined spaces	CVS, CNS, ENDO, HEARING HEMAT, MENTAL STATUS, MS, RESP, VISION	Health History by R.N. Physical assessment by R.N. BP, pulse, balance, eye/hand/foot coordination, facial structure assessment for use of breathing apparatus, flexibility, ROM Lab: • Hemoglobin • Audiogram • Urinalysis 1 • Vision 1, peripheral vision • Pulmonary function
Working or climbing to heights	CVS, CNS, ENDO, HEMAT, MENTAL STATUS, MS, VISION	Health History by R.N. Physical assessment by R.N. BP, pulse, balance, eye/hand/foot coordination, ROM (Continued)

Table 18.3. Continued

| Working Conditions | Minimal Health Standards | |
	Body Systems	Screening Methods
		Lab: • Hemoglobin • Urinalysis 1 • Vision 1, depth perception and peripheral vision
Walking over uneven terrain and/or slippery surfaces (more than 3 times/year)	CVS, CNS, MS, RESP, VISION	Health History by R.N. Physical assessment by R.N. BP, pulse, balance, eye/hand/foot coordination, ROM, strength and endurance Lab: • Vision 1, depth perception • Pulmonary function
4.2 *Ergonomics* Lifting, carrying, pushing and pulling objects over 20 lbs.	CVS, CNS, HEMAT, MS, RESP, VISION	Health History by R.N. Physical assessment by R.N. BP, pulse, balance, eye/hand/foot coordination, flexibility, ROM, strength and endurance Lab: • Hemoglobin • Vision 1 • Pulmonary function
Bending, stooping, twisting, pushing and pulling (more than 1 hr./day)	CVS, CNS, HEMAT, MS, RESP	Health History by R.N. Physical assessment by R.N. BP, pulse, balance, eye/hand/foot coordination, flexibility, ROM, strength and endurance Lab: • Hemoglobin • Pulmonary function
Working in awkward positions or cramped quarters	CNS, MENTAL STATUS, MS, VISION	Health History by R.N. Physical assessment by R.N. BP, pulse, balance, eye/hand/foot coordination, flexibility, ROM Lab: Vision 1
Prolonged periods of continuous sitting (more than 4 hours)	MS, CNS	Health History by R.N.
Prolonged periods of continuous standing (more than 2 hrs./day)	CVS, CNS, MS	Health History by R.N. Physical assessment by R.N. BP, pulse, balance, endurance
Prolonged periods of continuous walking (over 1 hr./day)	CVS, CNS, HEMAT, MS, RESP, VISION	Health History by R.N. Physical assessment by R.N. BP, pulse, balance, eye/hand/foot coordination, ROM, strength and endurance (Continued)

Table 18.3. Continued

Working Conditions	Minimal Health Standards	
	Body Systems	Screening Methods
		Lab: • Hemoglobin • Vision 1 • Pulmonary function
Using repetitive motions	CNS, MS	Health History by R.N. Physical assessment by R.N. eye/hand or eye/hand/foot coordination, manual dexterity, strength and endurance Lab: Vision 1
Using equipment • VDT/word processor (continuous use over 1 hr./day)	CSN, MS, VISION	Health History by R.N. Physical assessment by R.N. eye/hand foot coordination, manual dexterity, ROM Lab: Vision 1
• Hand tools	CNS, HEARING, MS, VISION	Health History by R.N. Physical assessment by R.N. eye/hand/foot coordination, manual dexterity, strength Lab: • Vision 1 • Audiogram
Performing office functions	CNS, HEARING, MS, VISION	Health History by R.N. Physical assessment by R.N. manual dexterity, ROM Lab: • Vision 1 • Audiogram
5.0 OCCUPATIONAL HEALTH HAZARDS		
5.1 *Physical Hazards* Exposure to: Extremes of temperature • Cold	CVS, CNS, ENDO, INTEG, MS, RESP	Health history by R.N. Lab: Urinalysis 1
• Heat	CVS, CNS, ENDO, INTEG, MS	Health history by R.N. Lab: Urinalysis 1
Humidity	INTEG, RESP	Health history by R.N.
Radiation (Ionizing)	ENDO, HEMAT, INTEG, VISION	Health history by R.N. Lab: • CBC and Diff. • Urinalysis 1 • Vision 1
Sound > 85 dBA • Continuous • Intermittent • Impulse	CNS, HEARING	Health history by R.N. Lab: Audiogram

(Continued)

Table 18.3. Continued

Working Conditions	Minimal Health Standards	
	Body Systems	Screening Methods
Vibration	CNS, MS	Health history by R.N. Physical assessment by R.N.
Increased Atmospheric Pressure	CNS, CVS, ENDO, GI, HEARING, HEMAT, MENTAL STATUS, MS, RESP, VISION	Health history by M.D. Physical examination by M.D. Lab: • Audiogram • CBC and Diff, SMA 12 • Electrocardiogram • Pulmonary Function • Urinalysis 1 • Vision 1 & 2, depth perception, peripheral vision
5.2 *Chemical Hazards*	Depends on the specific action or characteristics of the agent exposed to and the route of exposure—inhalation, skin, or eye contact, ingestion and injection.	
5.3 *Biological Hazards* Exposure to: Bacteria, Molds, Fungi	IMMUN, INTEG, RESP	Health history by R.N. Physical assessment by R.N. Lab: Pulmonary Function
6.0 SPECIAL REQUIREMENTS		
6.1 Operating Mobile Equipment • Driving heavy equipment or trucks (larger than one ton) • Servicing or flying company planes	CVS, CNS, ENDO, GI, GU, HEARING, HEMAT, MENTAL STATUS, MS, RESP, VISION	Health history by M.D. Physical examination by M.D. Lab: • Audiogram • CBC and Diff, SMA 12 • Electrocardiogram • Urinalysis 2 • Vision 2, depth perception peripheral and color visions
• Driving car or truck (less than one ton) while on company business	CNS, CVS, ENDO, HEARING, HEMAT, MENTAL STATUS, MS, VISION	Health history by R.N. Physical assessment by R.N. eye/hand/foot coordination, ROM Lab: • Hemoglobin • Audiogram • Urinalysis 1 • Vision 1, peripheral vision • depth perception
6.2 Offshore Survival Training and work in an offshore environment	CVS, CNS, ENDO, GI, GU, HEARING, HEMAT, IMMUN, INTEG, MENTAL STATUS, MS, RESP, VISION	Health history by M.D. Physical examination by M.D. (Continued)

Table 18.3. Continued

Working Conditions	Minimal Health Standards	
	Body Systems	Screening Methods
		Lab: • Audiogram • CBC, SMA 12, GGT • Electrocardiogram • Urinalysis 1 • Vision 1 and 3, depth perception, Peripheral vision • pulmonary function
6.3 Fire-Fighting Training	CNS, CVS, ENDO, HEARING, HEMAT, MENTAL STATUS, MS, RESP, VISION	Health History by R.N. Physical assessment by R.N. BP, pulse, balance, eye/hand/foot coordination, facial structure assessment for use of breathing apparatus, flexibility, strength and endurance Lab: • Hemoglobin • Audiogram • Urinalysis 1 • Vision 1 and 2 • Pulmonary function
6.4 Respond in emergency situations	CVS, CNS, ENDO, HEARING, HEMAT, MENTAL STATUS, MS, RESP, VISION	Health History by R.N. Physical assessment by R.N. BP, pulse, eye/hand/foot coordination, ROM, strength Lab: • Hemoglobin • Audiogram • Urinalysis 1 • Vision 3 • Pulmonary function
6.5 Travel	CNS, CVS, ENDO, GI, GU, HEMAT, MENTAL STATUS, MS, RESP	Health history by R.N. Lab: • Hemoglobin • Urinalysis 1 BP, pulse
6.6 Special Tasks: • Differentiating between colors	VISION	Lab: color vision
• Performing detailed, close-up work	CNS, MS, VISION	Health History by R.N. Physical assessment by R.N. (eye/hand coordination, manual dexterity Lab: Vision 1, phorias
• Working directly or closely with food	CNS, INTEG, MS, RESP, VISION	Health History by R.N. Physical assessment by R.N.

(Continued)

Table 18.3. Continued

Working Conditions	Minimal Health Standards	
	Body Systems	Screening Methods
		(eye/hand coordination, manual dexterity, personal hygiene, ROM) Lab: • Chext x-ray (within the past year) • Nasal swab for C & S • Stool culture for C & S • Vision 1, depth perception
• Conducting aerobic fitness classes	CNS, CVS, ENDO, HEARING, HEMAT, MS, RESP, VISION	Health history by M.D. Physical examination by M.D. Lab: • Audiogram • Electrocardiogram and submaximal stress test • Hemoglobin and complete blood count • Pulmonary function • Urinalysis 1 • Vision 1 • SMA 12
6.7 Personal Protective Equipment: • Regularly wearing a breathing apparatus or mask	CVS, CNS, ENDO, HEARING, HEMAT, INTEG, MENTAL STATUS, MS, RESP, VISION	Health History by R.N. Physical assessment by R.N. BP, pulse, eye/hand coordination, facial structure assessment for use of breathing apparatus, ROM, strength and endurance Lab: • Audiogram • Hemaglobin • Pulmonary function • Urinalysis 1 • Vision 1
• Wearing a breathing apparatus only in an emergency situation	CVS, HEARING, MENTAL STATUS, MS, RESP, VISION	Health History by R.N. Physical assessment by R.N. BP, pulse, eye/hand coordination, facial structure assessment for use of breathing apparatus, ROM and strength Lab: • Audiogram • Vision 2

(Continued)

Table 18.3. Continued

Working Conditions	Minimal Health Standards	
	Body Systems	Screening Methods
6.8 Isolation:		
• Works in an isolated geographical location	CNS, CVS, ENDO, GI, GU, HEMAT, MENTAL STATUS, MS, RESP, VISION, HEARING	Health History by R.N. Physical assessment by R.N. BP, pulse Lab: • Hemoglobin • Urinalysis 1 • Vision 1 • Pulmonary function • Audiogram
• Works alone	CNS, CVS, ENDO, HEARING, HEMAT, MENTAL STATUS, MS, RESP, VISION	Health History by R.N. Physical assessment by R.N. BP, pulse Lab: • Hemoglobin • Audiogram • Urinalysis 1 • Vision 1
6.9 Working with laboratory chemicals	CVS, CNS, ENDO, GI, GU, HEMAT, IMMU, INTEG, MENTAL STATUS, RESP, MS, VISION	Health history by M.D. Physical assessment by M.D. Lab: • Complete blood count with differential • SMA 12 • Urinalysis 2 • Vision 1 • Color vision • Pulmonary function
7.0 PSYCHOSOCIAL DEMANDS		
Moderate/high level of responsibility and decision making	CVS, GI, MENTAL STATUS	Health history by R.N.
Very high level of responsibility and decision making	CVS, ENDO, GI, HEMAT, MENTAL STATUS	Health history by M.D. Physical examination by M.D. Lab: • CBC and Diff, SMA 12 • Electrocardiogram • Urinalysis 2

DEFINITIONS

Audiogram—an audiometric test that establishes pure-tone, air-conduction thresholds at 500 to 8000 Hz for each ear.

CBC and Differential—a venous blood test that includes hemoglobin, hematocrit, total white cell count and white cell differential count.

Chest X-ray (CXR)—a standard Posterior Anterior (PA) film.

(Continued)

Table 18.3. Continued

Electrocardiogram (ECG)—a resting, standard 12 lead.

Electrocardiogram (ECG)—Submaximal Stress Test—an exercise electrocardiogram performed while the subject exercises until the target heart rate is reached.

Target heart rate range = 70 to 85% × (220 − age) beats/min

Health History—a thorough history relating to the designated body systems outlined on the Fitness-to-Work Form. Any positive response to the health history taken by the nurse must be referred to the physician for further clarification.

Hemoglobin Test—a finger prick blood test measured by using a Hemoglobinometer.

Mental Status—an examination that includes observation of general appearance and behaviour, mood and affective reactions, thought flow and content, fears, perceptions, orientation, memory (recent and remote), intelligence, judgment, and insight.

Physical Examination—a minimum examination includes measurements of height, weight, blood pressure, and pulse rate.

Pulmonary Function Test—a spirometric testing including FVC and FEV_1.

Range of Motion (ROM)—appropriate range of motion for each joint under consideration.

SMA 12—an automated multiple biochemical blood analysis that usually includes: total protein, cholesterol, spot blood sugar, BUN, calcium, phosphorous, uric acid, bilirubin—total and direct, alkaline phosphatase, LDH and SGOT levels.

Urinalysis 1—an Ames multistix or other similar reagent test.

Urinalysis 2—a laboratory urinalysis that includes microscopy.

Vision 1—a test of visual acuity in both eyes with or without corrective lenses. Minimal expected standards: near—20/30; far—20/40 corrected.

Vision 2—a test of visual acuity in both eyes without corrective lenses. Minimal expected standards: far—20/100 in one eye.

Further Reading

Battigelli MC: Determination of fitness to work, in Zenz C (ed): Occupational Medicine: Principles and Practical Applications. Chicago, Year Book Medical Publishers, 1975, pp. 109–116.

Bond MB, Messite J: Preplacement medical evaluation and recommendations, in Zenz C (ed): Developments in Occupational Medicine. Chicago, Year Book Medical Publishers, 1980, pp. 131–138.

California Workers Compensation Institute: Cumulative Injury in California: The Continuing Dilemma. San Francisco, California Workers' Compensation Institute, 1978.

Campione KM: The pre-employment examination: An evaluation. Ind Med Surg 1972; 41:27–30.

Canadian Medical Association: Basic Principles for the Provision of Occupational Health Services. Ottawa, Canadian Medical Association.

Canadian Medical Association: Code of Ethics. Ottawa, Canadian Medical Association, 1984.

Chamber of Commerce of the United States. Analysis of Workers' Compensation Laws. Updated annually.

Cowell JWF: Guidelines for fitness-to-work examinations. Can Med Assn J 1986; 135:985–988.

Cowell JWF: Organization and management of occupational health and safety programs. Occup Health Ont 1985; 6:75–86.

Engelberg AL (ed): American Medical Association Guides to the Evaluation of Permanent Impairment (ed 3). Chicago, American Medical Association, 1988.

Gadian T: Health monitoring in industry: Medical considerations. R Soc Health J 1980, 100:130–132.

Goldman RH, and Peters JM: The occupational and environmental health history. JAMA 1981; 246:2831–6.

Guidance on Ethics for Occupational Physicians (ed 2). Faculty of Occupational Medicine, Royal College of Physicians, London, 1982.

Guidotti TL: Occupational health monitoring and surveillance. Am Fam Physician 1985; 31:161–169.

Guidotti TL, et al: Taking the occupational history. Ann Int Med. 1983; 99:641–651.

Health and Welfare Canada: Task force on health surveillance of workers. Can J Pub Health 1986; 77:89–108.

Hogan JC, Bernacki EJ: Developing job-related preplacement medical examinations. J Occup Med 1981; 23:469–476.

Human Rights: We're All Responsible. Guidelines on the Application of the Individual's Rights Protection Act to a Person with a Physical Characteristic in Employment, Alberta Human Rights Commission, Edmonton, Apr 1984.

Individual Rights Protection Act, RSA 1980, as am S 7(1), 8(1).

Kanner RE: Impairment and disability evaluation, in Rom WN (ed): Environmental and Occupational Medicine. Boston, Little, Brown, 1983, pp. 43–47.

Key MM, et al: Occupational Diseases: A Guide to their Recognition. National Institute for Occupational Safety and Health, 1977.

Kusnetz S, Hutchison MK (eds): A Guide to the Work-Relatedness of Disease. National Institute for Occupational Safety and Health, 1979.

Lerner S: Development job-related preplacement medical examinations [E]. Ibid: 475–476.

Levy B, Wegman D: Occupational Health. Boston, Little Brown, 1983.

Nylander SW, Carmean G: Medical Standards Project: Final Report (ed 3). San Bernardino, California, County of San Bernardino, 1984 (2 volumes).

Occupational Health and Safety Act and Regulations for Industrial Establishments, RSO 1980, S 23(3) (a), (b) and (c).

Periodic Health Examination Monograph. Report of a Task Force to the Conference of Deputy Ministers of Health (cat no H39-3/1980E). Minister of Supply and Services, Ottawa, 1980.

Rothstein MA: Medical Screening of Workers. Washington DC, Bureau of National Affairs, 1984, pp. 8–22, 121–129.

Sackett DL: Screening for early detection of disease: To what purpose? Bull NY Acad Med 1975; 51:39–52.

Schilling RSF (ed): Occupational Health Practice. London, Butterworths, 1981.

Schussler T, Kaminer AJ, Power VL, et al: The preplacement examination: An analysis. J Occup Med 1975; 17:254–257.

Wald MS: The current status of preplacement health evaluations. San Bernadino County Med Stand News 1984; 1(6):3–5.

19 EQUAL ACCESS AND OPPORTUNITY FOR THE HANDICAPPED

In 1973, the United States Congress passed the Rehabilitation Act, setting forth the civil rights of individuals with physical and mental handicaps. Sections 503 and 504 of the Rehabilitation Act are of particular interest to employers and physicians providing occupational medical services to employers because they concern the employment rights of handicapped persons. Section 503, an affirmative action provision that promotes employment of people with physical and mental handicaps, applies to contractors and subcontractors of the federal government (primarily private industries) with contracts totalling more than $2,500. Section 504 is an antidiscriminatory provision that applies to institutions benefitting from federal assistance, including nonfederal governmental institutions, not-for-profit organizations, hospitals, and universities. Close to half of all private businesses in the United States are covered by Section 503; nearly all governmental and not-for-profit institutions are covered by Section 504. In addition, most states have passed legislation that extends the antidiscrimination provisions to cover situations in which the Act does not apply. All U.S. citizens are covered by the intent, if not the letter, of the Act. Physicians who provide employment examinations for employers should be governed by the intent of the Act and by its implications for the conduct of medical examinations.

Coverage of the Act

The Rehabilitation Act does not provide a medically precise definition of "handicap," but it does specify who is covered by the Act. A person is "handicapped" if he or she has:
- A physical or mental impairment that substantially limits one or more of the person's major life activities;
- A record of such impairment; or
- Grounds to show that he or she is regarded as having such an impairment.
    The Act also defines several terms that are important in interpreting the intent of the law:

- "Major life activities," as used in the Act, include seeing, hearing, speaking, breathing, walking, learning, performing manual tasks, and caring for oneself. The definition encompasses socialization, education, vocational training employment, transportation, and adaptation to available housing.
- "Substantially limits" pertains to the degree that an impairment affects employability. A handicapped individual who is likely to experience difficulty in securing, retaining, or advancing in employment would be considered "substantially limited."
- "Physical and mental impairments" include impairments of organ systems, mental retardation, organic brain syndrome, emotional or mental illness, and specific learning disabilities. In some instances, they include alcoholism and drug addiction. (Recently, the Supreme Court added active tuberculosis to this list, an action involving an infectious disease that may have major application to other conditions, such as AIDS. See Chapter 21.) Furthermore, a person may be considered handicapped even if there is no actual impairment—the individual need only have a past history of impairment, or a history of having been regarded as having an impairment, with the result that he or she has had difficulty securing, retaining, or advancing in employment.
- A "qualified handicapped individual" is a handicapped person who is capable of performing, with reasonable accommodation to the handicap, the essential functions of the job or jobs for which he or she is being considered. "Reasonable accommodation" refers to any changes or modifications that can be made in the structure of a job or in the manner in which a job is performed without imposing an undue hardship on the way the business is conducted. Such accommodation may include modifying the workplace facilities or restructuring the job itself, and often can be done at little or no cost to the employer.

Partially as a result of the stipulations of the Rehabilitation Act, the term "preemployment medical examination" is an anachronism. It implies that a normal medical examination is a prerequisite to employment. The term "preplacement" examination is now preferred; the medical examination is given only after an individual is offered employment based on other qualifications. Placement in the job applied for is contingent on the physician's confirmation that the candidate is medically qualified to travel to and from the job, be at the job, and perform the duties and tasks assigned. The employer must provide a thorough description of the job so that the examining physician can determine the kinds of physical and mental abilities that will be required of the applicant. (See Chapter 18 on fitness-to-work evaluations.)

All preplacement examinations must be tailored to the job, not to any one individual. The equal rights provision of the Act dictates that individual candidates cannot be singled out for examination; if one is asked to submit to an exam, then all applicants otherwise qualified for the job, whether handicapped or not, must be examined medically for the job.

Obligations of the Employer

Under the Act, the employer is restricted as to the manner of determining whether a person is medically qualified for a job. Although an applicant may be required to provide medical documentation of an impairment, the history of an impairment alone cannot be used to disqualify an individual from obtaining a job. Nor can a person be disqualified on the basis of physical or mental conditions that do not bear on the safe performance of the job. In general, an employer must show the worker's present inability to perform a job safely and effectively. The risk of *future* injury to self or others may be used as a criterion for denying employment, as long as the assessment of the risk is not merely speculative.

Finally, the employer must make a reasonable attempt to accommodate the individual. What is "reasonable" is an administrative and, if contested, a legal decision rather than a medical one, although the physician may offer suggestions.

"Reasonable" accommodation need not be an expensive undertaking. It may be as minor as substituting handles for round doorknobs, or it may require only an administrative change, such as allowing a handicapped individual to work on the ground floor or to travel to and from work at non-rush-hour times. If a reasonable accommodation could be made but the employer has reason to anticipate that an applicant may be absent from work in excess of allowable sick leave, management is entitled to regard the individual as incapable of filling the position.

Responsibilities of the Health Professional

The physician has a number of responsibilities to both the employer and the individual worker. For the employer, the physician must make a number of determinations:
- Is the individual capable of performing the functions of a job?
- Does the individual have a health condition that represents a clear hazard to others in the workplace?
- Does the individual have a health condition that places him or her at high risk of suffering serious adverse health consequences as a result of performing the functions required by the job or being exposed to the environment of the workplace?

In identifying an individual as being at high risk for serious health consequences, all of the following considerations should apply:
- The examination, test, or procedure upon which the employment decision is based must be job-related.
- The examination, test, or procedure must have a high predictive value and must be the most appropriate and feasible test for use in clinical evaluation.
- The examination, test, or procedure must indicate that the individual has a strong likelihood of developing a serious injury or illness in the not too distant future and that the individual's likelihood of injury or illness represents a significant variation from that of the general population of workers.

Only the physician may determine types of medical procedures and examinations that should be included in a health assessment of a prospective or current employee. In most cases, however, the employer will request or expect a specific test, usually on recommendation of a medical advisor or management's own medical director. The physician should supervise the collection of health information about an individual to ensure that appropriate procedures are followed.

The physician also has the responsibility of ensuring that the employee's health is protected and maintained. The physician must inform the individual of any medical care that is required to protect his or her health or the health of others in the workplace and must communicate to both the employer and the employee any restrictions on working conditions necessary for the safety of the employee or his co-workers. The physician or nurse has the further responsibility to tell the worker of any significant observations about his or her health status and to recommend further study, counselling, or treatment as needed.

The physician must exercise independent medical judgment in conducting employment-related health assessments, regardless of the nature of his relationship to the employer requesting the assessment. To do this effectively, the physician should have direct knowledge or a detailed description of the workplace to which the worker will be assigned.

In the presence of certain medical conditions, the occupational physician also may become involved in managing and monitoring personal health problems. Two prime examples are the management of brittle diabetics and the treatment of essential hypertension. The occasional attention of the occupational physician or occupational nurse at the worksite may prevent subsequent problems and complications that otherwise would lead to absenteeism or loss of work time. While individual patient management at the worksite should not be a substitute for care by the personal physician, it can be an effective complement to personal medical care, providing the patient-worker with the best opportunity to remain productive on the job while ensuring that health care needs are met. This type of commitment does place some creative strain on an occupational medicine service, requiring it to accept responsibility for providing routine health care and maintaining liaisons with the worker's personal physician.

All occupational health professionals have an absolute responsibility to treat as confidential information obtained through an employment-related health assessment. Unless required by law or requested in writing by the individual, the physician should not release medical information to any third party. (See Chapter 4, on ethics.) Although management may be informed that the individual needs medical treatment, no specific health information, such as the diagnosis, may be revealed to the employer; the physician should provide only summary statements about an individual's health status and fitness-to-work. Finally, clear and accurate medical records must be maintained and procedures established to protect the confidentiality of those medical records.

Physicians and other health care personnel play crucial roles in the process of ensuring equal opportunity and access to employment for all qualified workers. By building up their knowledge base of medicine with training in ergonomics and vocational rehabilitation, health professionals can provide significant assistance to impaired individuals seeking employment and to employers wishing to offer them jobs. Physicians must understand, however, that they are consultants. They must avoid being placed in the position of approving or disapproving a person for a job. Employers should never ask physicians whether they should give an applicant a job. Management itself must decide the answer to this question.

Resources

The President's Committee on Employment of the Handicapped (PCEH) operates a Job

Accommodation Network (JAN), based at West Virginia University in Morgantown, WV. This free service can be reached by a toll-free number (1-800-JAN-PCEH). JAN consultants search data bases and provide employers with recommended accommodations based upon the information they receive by telephone or in writing. These data bases include information on technologies that may not be generally known, such as alarm systems that convert auditory signals into unique vibration patterns so that a hearing-impaired person can feel and discriminate among a set of alarms. In a survey of employers assisted through the service, JAN found that 31 percent of the accommodations it recommended were made at no extra cost to the employer; another 57 percent cost less than $1,000. The respondents to the survey also reported that 86 percent of the accommodations had a dollar benefit of $1,000 to $30,000, attributable to such factors as increased productivity, job satisfaction, and ease of performance. Overall, the benefit-to-cost ratio was $9 to $1.

Also available are systems that are designed to help employers assess and describe the abilities required for individuals to perform particular jobs. The task-specific "functions" of a job are what determine whether a person will be eligible or ineligible for a job, even before the individual's abilities are considered. An "ability" is not task-specific in the sense that it must be learned by formal training, education, and experience. Rather, an ability is a general function of the body and mind that develops in childhood and that requires no special training. Examples include static strength (the ability to use muscle force to lift, push, pull, or carry objects) and dynamic strength (the degree to which muscles do not fatigue when they are exerted in repeated or continuous movements). The County of San Bernardino, California, developed a physical abilities assessment system for its employees, ranging from office workers to firefighters. Other organizations that provide similar systems are Med-Tox of Tustin, California, and Advanced Research Resources Organization of Bethesda, Maryland. (Fitness to work is discussed more fully in Chapter 18.)

20 HEALTH MONITORING AND SURVEILLANCE

Rapid advances in the field of occupational medicine have produced some confusion as to the meaning of certain terms, particularly the distinction between health "monitoring" and "surveillance" and how they are distingushed from "screening." Surveillance is the strategy used to determine the experience of a group of workers when the risk of a particular disease is known to be increased in a particular industry. Monitoring is the strategy for observing the overall health experience of the individual or group without regard to any particular outcome. Monitoring is the more general term, and surveillance activities are, in a sense, a subset of monitoring activities. Used without qualification, however, monitoring implies a more general approach. Although the two terms, monitoring and surveillance, often are used interchangeably, there are differences between them that are important in occupational health theory and practice.

Monitoring focuses on the overall health experience of the individual or group. The strategy may be applied to individual workers, as in the case of voluntary periodic health evaluations, or to groups, as in special research studies to determine the health risks of certain workplace exposures or certain jobs. In general, monitoring programs are more extensive and more costly to establish than surveillance programs. These programs usually are limited to key employees or executives as a means of protecting the employee and the company from unexpected losses due to illness. As such, they are primarily intended for individual health care and not for population monitoring, and seldom cover high-risk groups unless they are arranged as part of a research study. Monitoring lends itself more readily to the physician's efforts to discover previously unrecognized health problems in an individual, to reduce absence from non-occupational illnesses, or to identify previously unsuspected health effects. When the experience of a group of workers is followed over time, patterns of illness may appear that suggest either unusual characteristics of that working population or exposures requiring identification and control. Monitoring programs often are performed by physicians in private practice who also are family physicians for the workers. The principal challenge facing individual physicians conducting voluntary monitoring programs is maintaining a high level of attention while examining many, mostly healthy, individuals.

Surveillance is a strategy to determine a group experience with a particular disease outcome. Surveillance is applied when the diseases in question are associated with a particular industry, such as asbestos-associated lung disorders. Although increasing numbers of employers in high-risk industries are providing surveillance programs at company expense in excess of regulatory requirements, surveillance is usually restricted to high-risk groups. The law requires that employers provide surveillance at company expense to workers exposed to specific hazards covered by Occupational Safety and Health Administration standards or other regulations involving, for example, asbestos, noise, or lead. OSHA presently is considering a generic standard for health surveillance covering all workers in high-risk occupations.

The design of monitoring and surveillance programs is advancing rapidly— occupational health professionals screening for early detection of abnormalities may select from among a number of tests depending on the degree of sensitivity, specificity, and predictive value required, given the prevalence of the abnormality in the population of workers. Physicians involved in these programs must understand the rationale of these tests and the biological characteristics of the disease in order to make sense of the results.

The terms "health surveillance" and "medical surveillance" or "medical monitoring" and "health monitoring" are often used interchangeably. Ideally, medical surveillance and medical monitoring should refer only to programs or actions undertaken by physicians; health surveillance and health monitoring are more general terms referring to programs or actions undertaken by a variety of occupational health professionals, including physicians, nurses, and health technicians.

Principles of Screening

The selection of a screening test is based on three variables: the sensitivity and specificity of the test and the prevalence of the disease in the community. Exhibit 20.1 describes the essential concepts that apply to any tests used in detecting disease.

Sensitivity refers to the proportion of diseased persons in the population who are identified by the test. The higher the sensitivity of the test, the more likely it will identify the diseased individuals.

The specificity of a test refers to the proportion of nondiseased individuals in the population who are identified by a negative test result. The higher the specificity of a test, the more reliably it will exclude nondiseased individuals. The ideal is a combination of high sensitivity and high specificity; most tests in clinical use fall well short of the ideal.

A test with low sensitivity but high specificity will detect only a small fraction of diseased individuals, but a positive result will more reliably indicate that the disease is present in an individual. However, a negative test result will not reliably rule out the disease. A test with high sensitivity and low specificity will correctly identify most true cases but will also yield positive results for many individuals who, in fact, do not have the disease. In other words, an insensitive but specific test may yield many false-negative results, whereas a sensitive but nonspecific test may give many false-positives. If a disease is rare in the population, the false-positive results of a sensitive but

---

Exhibit 20.1. Definitions, Adapted from *A Dictionary of Epidemiology*, Last JM (ed), New York, Oxford University Press, 1983.

Sensitivity and Specificity (of a screening test). Sensitivity is the proportion of truly diseased persons in the screened population who are identified as diseased by the screening test. Sensitivity is a measure of the probability of correctly diagnosing a case, or the probability that any given case will be identified by the test (Syn: true positive rate).

Specificity is the proportion of truly nondiseased persons who are so identified by the screening test. It is a measure of the probability of correctly identifying a non-diseased person with a screening test (Syn: true negative rate). The relationships are shown in the following table, in which the letters a, b, c, and d represent the quantities specified below.

Screening Test Results	True Status		Total
	Diseased	Not Diseased	
Positive	a	b	a + b
Negative	c	d	c + d
Total	a + c	b + d	a + b + c + d

a. Diseased individuals detected by the test (true positives).
b. Nondiseased individuals positive by the test (false positives).
c. Diseased individuals not detectable by the test (false negatives).
d. Nondiseased individuals negative by the test (true negatives).

$$\text{Sensitivity} = \frac{a}{a + c} \qquad \text{Specificity} = \frac{d}{b + d}$$

$$\text{Positive predictive value} = \frac{a}{a + b} \qquad \text{Negative predictive value} = \frac{d}{c + d}$$

$$\text{Prevalence} = \frac{a + c}{a + b + c + d} \qquad \text{Accuracy of test} = \frac{a + d}{a + b + c + d}$$

Predictive Value. . . . (T)he probability that a person with a positive test is a true positive [or that a negative test is a true negative] . . . The predictive value of a screening test is determined by the sensitivity and specificity of the test and by the prevalence of the condition for which the test is used.

---

nonspecific test may outnumber the true positives, requiring additional diagnostic tests to confirm a positive result in any individual. The diagnostic efficiency of a test is called its predictive value. (Chapter 25 demonstrates how to calculate the predictive value of a test in reference to an evaluation of a drug screening program; Exhibit 20.2 illustrates a screening test applied to a group of workers in apparently normal good health.)

Studying the specificity and sensitivity of diagnostic tests and calculating their diagnostic yield in a population with a given prevalence of a disease comprise one aspect of clinical epidemiology. When physicians order diagnostic tests for their patients, they are applying these same concepts but the diagnostic yield is higher because the predictive value of a test is much higher—diagnostic tests are used in a small population of persons selected for testing precisely because they have presented with suggestive symptoms. However, when used for surveillance or monitoring, tests have a low predictive value because most individuals tested are normal or, at least, do not have a clinical disorder.

Exhibit 20.2. Illustration of the Application of a Screening Test to Identify the Presence or Appearance of a Disorder in the Population Under Study.

In this example, assume that a two-hour postprandial blood sugar level is being used to screen for diabetes. A value is chosen to make it unlikely that many cases will be missed because the sponsors of the test believe in early recognition and tight control. At 100 mg/dl, this test is known to be 89% sensitive and 70% specific. (See Exhibit 20.1 for definitions.) Its predictive value will vary with the prevalence of the condition in the population.

Case 1. The test is performed on a group of people seen in clinic for complaints of frequent urination, thirst, and visual changes. Half of the these people do, in fact, have diabetes. The results of the test are as follows:

		Diabetic		
		Yes	No	Totals
	Yes	45	15	60
Test Positive				
	No	5	35	40
	Totals	50	50	100

Prevalence of disease in population = 50%
Predictive value of a positive test = 75%
Predictive value of a negative test = 88%
Accuracy of the test = 80%

The appropriate interpretation is that although this test is not very accurate in an absolute sense, it satisfactorily discriminates between those who do and those who do not have diabetes in a group of people selected for a high likelihood of having the disease. If one of these patients has a positive test, the odds are 3:1 (75% probability) that that patient has diabetes.

Case 2. This test is performed as a screening test for 1,000 workers concerned about their health, as part of a health promotion program. None have complaints, but 1% actually have a subclinical case of diabetes, the prevalence among otherwise healthy people in this community. The results of the test are as follows:

		Diabetic		
		Yes	No	Totals
	Yes	9	297	306
Test Positive				
	No	1	693	694
	Total	10	990	1,000

Prevalence of disease in population = 1%
Predictive value of a positive test = 3%
Predictive value of a negative test = 99.9%
Accuracy of the test = 70%

Screening tests incorporated into surveillance programs therefore should conform to certain standards of use. As enunciated by Fletcher, et al., these include the following:
- The test should be sensitive and specific.
- The test must be simple and inexpensive.
- The test must be very safe and avoid causing more harm than good by subjecting a very large number of normal people to a small but real risk.

- The test must be acceptable (i.e., not inconvenient, time-consuming, uncomfortable, or unpleasant) to the subjects and to those conducting the test.

These standards are most often violated by compromises in acceptable sensitivity and specificity, absent alternative practical tests. The Canadian Task Force on Periodic Health Surveillance of the Healthy Worker, after evaluating many tests that are in common use, has concluded that some tests (e.g., x-rays of the lower back to predict future risk of injury and back pain) are ineffective and potentially harmful. Other tests (e.g., sputum cytology to detect early lung cancer) also have been found ineffective in providing benefits to the subject. The majority of common screening tests are lacking in both sensitivity and specificity. Fortunately, a new generation of clinical tests is being introduced (largely as a result of the advances made in biotechnology and biochemistry) that promise greater diagnostic accuracy in the future. These tests are described later in this chapter in the section on biological monitoring.

For reasons of cost and reliability, occupational health surveillance programs tend to be simple, use a few well established tests, and be rigid in their requirements. For example, the OSHA-mandated surveillance program for noise-induced hearing loss is designed for workers who are exposed to high noise levels and relies on an annual audiogram covering the prescribed frequencies. Annual testing must be performed by certified personnel with specialized training and equipment meeting prescribed specifications.

Periodic Health Evaluation of Persons at Low Risk

Medical professionals are re-evaluating skeptically the scientific basis for and cost-effectiveness of strategies for periodic health evaluation. The application of such strategies as the "annual physical," multiphasic screening, and the "executive physical" is controversial but their practice is preserved through long tradition. Medical practice slowly is changing in response to new data and informed opinion regarding optimal screening schedules.

Employers are concerned about the fitness of their key personnel, whose death or incapacity would deprive them of special skills and knowledge and would result in disruption of work during a replacement period. Consequently, most large and many small companies provide periodic evaluations for their key managers and their executives. These evaluations are usually in the form of an "annual physical." Some employers set up screening for groups of workers during the off-season in their particular business; others conduct screening programs throughout the year, scheduling these examinations on the anniversary of a worker's employment or reassignment.

Although now considered obsolete as a screening strategy by most authorities, the annual physical examination has been sanctioned by years of tradition in industry. It has been a traditional function of occupational medicine practice and is deeply entrenched among the services customarily provided. The annual physical examination enjoys the force of law in certain OSHA standards, the acceptance of industry, and the tradition of an executive perquisite in the form of the "executive physical." A consensus is emerging, however, that individualized periodic evaluations are likely to yield more useful health information and are more likely to result in effective interventions. The American College of Physicians, the Canadian Task Force on the Periodic

Health Examination, and the U.S. Preventive Services Task Force all have recommended substituting for the annual physical examination another form of periodic health evaluation for the asymptomatic patient.

One alternative to the annual physical examination is multiphasic health screening, in which a battery of standard tests is performed at periodic intervals. Multiphasic health screening is often provided for nonexecutive personnel but its effectiveness is limited in practice because it is seldom integrated into the patient's personal health care by the family physician receiving the information.

Lifetime Health Monitoring

A more sophisticated strategy is the lifetime health monitoring program (LHMP) developed by Breslow and Somers. This form of health monitoring schedules certain tests, examinations, and health education interventions at different times according to the patient's age and known risk factors. The LHMP offers a medically sound approach to periodic health evaluation that is unlikely to miss preventable diseases or conditions identifiable by the screening elements selected. Properly performed, the LHMP requires personal health and risk factor information with absolute guarantees of confidentiality. A personal health problem uncovered in a periodic evaluation must be communicated in confidence to the worker. Where appropriate, the occupational physician should be prepared to advise the worker as a patient apart from the occupational context and to suggest follow-up by the worker's own physician or referral to a specialist.

For optimal effect, the lifetime health monitoring program should be combined with a program of health promotion that enhances fitness and encourages self-help measures. LHMP is designed to create opportunities to provide educational and preventive services—it continues on from suitable health promotion programs implemented at younger ages and extends into retirement years. In brief, the strategy is intended to be a segment of a true lifetime program rather than a self-limited periodic health evaluation program covering only the working years. Interruptions in the continuity of the program due to changes in employment may be avoided if a successor employer continues the LHMP on schedule rather than reverting to the traditional annual physical. Combining the LHMP with an employer-sponsored or -supported health promotion program also provides an opportunity for encouraging periodic health examinations beyond retirement age. Despite its advantages, however, the LHMP has not been offered on a large scale in industry.

All periodic health evaluation formats are to some degree arbitrary and subjective in formulation, based as they are on interpretations of data from many sources. The LHMP chart presented in Form 20.1 aims at founding the periodic health evaluation on a rational basis that considers the cost-effectiveness of program elements, the biology of the diseases and conditions to be ruled out, and the characteristics of the population to be evaluated.

In constructing a LHMP for a specific population, the occupational medicine professional should use the known risk profile of the individual to modify screening recommendations adopted for the general population. Table 20.1 presents factors that should be taken into account in modifying the LHMP to individual needs.

Form 20.1. One suggested format for the lifetime health monitoring program as applied to adults in low-risk managerial positions.
(Guidotti TL. Adaptation of the Lifetime Health Monitoring concept to defined employee groups not at exceptional risk. J Occup Med 1983; 25:731–736, reprinted with permission and modified to incorporate more recent recommendations of the American Medical Association.)

Lifetime Health Monitoring Program

Entrance into Program

	30	31	32	33	34	35	36	37	38	39	40	41	42	43	44	45	46	47	48	49	50	51	52	53	54	55	56	57	58	59	60
Complete History	□									□										□					□						□
Alcohol Intake History	□				□					□					□					□					□						□
Tobacco Use History	□				□					□					□					□					□						□
Emotional & Sexual History	□				□					□					□					□					□						□
Physical Activity & Exercise History	□				□					□					□					□					□						□
Nutritional History	□				□					□					□					□					□						□
Occupational History	□				□					□					□					□					□						□
Complete Physical Examination	□									□					□					□					□						□
Blood Pressure	□		⊡		□		⊡			□		□	□		□		□	□		□		□			⊡	□	□		□		□
Weight and Height	□		⊡		□		⊡			□		□	□		□		□	□		□		□			⊡	□	□		□		□
Vision	□				□					□					□					□					□						□
Hearing	□									□					□					□					□						□
Oral Examination	□		⊡		□		⊡			□		□			□		□			□		□			□		□				□
Breast Examination	□		⊡		□		⊡			□	□	□	□	□	□	□	□	□	□	□	□	□	□	□	□	□	□	□	□	□	□
Pelvic Examination	□	□	⊡		□		⊡			□	□	□	□	□	□	□	□	□	□	□	□	□	□	□	□	□	□	□	□	□	□
Rectal Examination	□				□					□	□	□	□	□	□	□	□	□	□	□	□	□	□	□	□	□	□	□	□	□	□
Stool occult blood	□				□					□		□			□	□	□		□		□	□	□	□	□	□	□	□	□	□	□
Complete blood count	□				□					□					□					□					□						□
Serum glucose	□				□					□					□					□					□						□
Serum lipids (cholesterol and triglycerides)	□				□					□					□					□					□						□
Urinalysis, chemical (dipstick)	□				□					□					□					□					□						□
Urinalysis, microscopic	□									□										□		⊡			□			⊡			□
VDRL	□				□					□					□					□											□
PPD	□									□																					
Tonometry	□									□										□					□						□
Spirometry	□									□										□											□
Electrocardiography	□									□										□					□						□
Pap smear	□		⊡		□		⊡			□			□		□		□		□		□		□			□					□
Proctosigmoidoscopy	□									□										□					□			□			
Mammography						⊡				□		⊡		⊡		⊡		⊡		□	□	□	□	□	□	□	□	□	□	□	□

Identifying Workers at High Risk

Environmental monitoring is the measurement on a periodic or continuous basis of the potential exposures in the workplace. Such measurements provide information on the potential exposure received by an individual or group of employees; medical monitoring or surveillance indicates the effect. If an association exists or is suspected between a given exposure and a disease outcome, the data from environmental monitoring and either medical monitoring or surveillance can be used to construct an exposure-

Table 20.1. Conditions that May Modify Elements of the Lifetime Health Monitoring Program in Healthy Subjects*

Procedure	Factor	Modification
Complete history	Family history of cancer in several members; possible genetic risk	Increase frequency of history and physical examination to annually if appropriate
History of alcohol intake	Family history of alcoholism, pattern of heavy use	Increase frequency of history of alcohol intake; refer for education or counseling (see Chapter 26)
History of tobacco use	Heavy smoker	Increase frequency of history of smoking; use spirometry as opportunity to counsel patient on cessation
Sexual history	Multiple partners; homosexual life style	Evaluate frequency of Papanicolaou smear, VDRL, rectal examinations. See Chapter 21 on AIDS and HIV interactions
Occupational history	Exposure on job to hazardous substances, continuing or antecedent	Increase frequency of occupational history, considering appropriate surveillance strategy
Complete physical	Family history suggestive of elevated risk	Modify frequency of screening elements accordingly
Blood pressure	Race—black; family history of essential hypertension	Increase frequency to annually and every visit in-between
Breast examination	Family history of breast cancer; female	Increase frequency to annually before age 40; reinforce need for self-examination
Pelvic examination	Family history of malignancy	Increase frequency to annually before age 40; see Papanicolaou smear
Rectal examination	Family history of malignancy; male homosexual life-style	Consider increase in frequency
Stool occult blood	Family history of malignancy	Increase frequency to annually before age 50
Serum glucose	Family history of juvenile-onset diabetes	Increase frequency to annually
Serum lipids	Family history of cardiovascular disease	Consider increasing frequency; emphasize cardiovascular examination
VDRL	Homosexual or heterosexual life-style with multiple partners	Consider increasing frequency
Papanicolaou smear**	Multiple sexual partners; proclivity to noncompliance	Consider increasing frequency to annually
Proctosigmoidoscopy	Family history of malignancy	Increase frequency

(Continued)

Table 20.1. Continued

Procedure	Factor	Modification
Mammography	Family history of breast cancer, female	Consider increasing frequency before age 50; emphasize need for breast self-examination
HIV Antibody	Men who have sex with other men, intravenous drug users, partners of those in high risk groups	See Chapter 21

* These recommendations apply only to asymptomatic individuals. Positive findings, known pre-existing conditions, and unusual exposure opportunities alter the subject risk profile and impose additional requirements for surveillance or monitoring.

** The American Medical Association recommends periodic Pap smears for women starting at age 18 or at time of first sexual intercourse.

response relationship. The demonstration of a strong exposure-response relationship is powerful evidence in support of a suspected association.

Monitoring the environmental levels of hazards is one of the most important functions of an occupational health service. Environmental monitoring can be completely preventive—finding dangerous levels may enable the service to take corrective action before harm comes to employees. Environmental monitoring data from industrial hygiene surveys must be disclosed to the worker and should be made available to the worker's physician.

Unfortunately, certain hazards (of which mental stress is one example) do not lend themselves to the monitoring methods used by the industrial hygienist. Moreover, the fact that workplace hazard levels may be found to be within "safe" or acceptable limits does not necessarily mean that workers will be unaffected.

Employee populations are not homogeneous and certain members will be particularly vulnerable or at greater risk than others. These high-risk populations include employees who are:

- New to a hazardous job;
- Undergoing on-the-job rehabilitation after injury or illness;
- Under severe emotional or psychological stress from any cause;
- Displaying a condition or illness that can be adversely affected by the workplace hazard (e.g., a pregnant worker using materials potentially detrimental to the unborn child or a sensitized painter spraying an isocyanate-containing urethane paint); and
- Working with very hazardous substances or whose work process itself is very hazardous.

Providing workers at high risk with the highest possible degree of protection requires identifying them as early in employment as possible. Preplacement examinations (see Chapter 18) afford the ideal opportunity for identifying workers at risk because of personal health characteristics. This examination also allows the employer to document workers' health status before exposure for purposes of later comparisons, providing a "baseline" evaluation. Others at risk due to injury or illness should be identified as such on their return to work. By identifying an employee as being at special risk, the service can provide appropriately timed periodic medical examinations, biological monitoring, and additional preventive measures, as needed.

Ideally, surveillance of the high-risk employee should continue until the abnormal level of risk has ended; unfortunately, some occupational diseases do not produce signs until many years of exposure, or many years after exposure, have passed. Employees may leave a company, change their line of work, or even retire. How long should surveillance continue in these circumstances and how should it be paid for? The occupational health service can advise management on a policy of continued medical surveillance, but the decision is one that ultimately must be made by employers, employee associations, workers' representatives, and governments.

Surveillance of Populations at High Risk

When a specific health outcome is known or suspected, the task of observing a population's health experience is much simplified. Surveillance programs are targeted to specific high-risk groups as defined by workplace assignment, known exposure history, and previously collected environmental monitoring data.

Several standards promulgated by OSHA specify surveillance procedures for workers exposed to certain hazards. Surveillance procedures required by regulation are termed mandated surveillance. The National Institute for Occupational Safety and Health has issued voluntary surveillance recommendations that apply to a larger number of exposures.

Surveillance programs are multifaceted. Their primary function is to ensure adequate workplace protection by identifying cases of occupational disease that occur despite proper industrial hygiene measures. A surveillance program that identifies no disease outcome despite suitable screening procedures suggests that the exposure in question is adequately controlled and therefore should be judged a success. (However, the existence of previous cases and a lack of extensive control measures should raise suspicion that new cases are being missed because the surveillance program is inadequate.)

A secondary function of surveillance is to identify new cases as early as possible in order to prevent the disease from progressing. Because surveillance programs are highly visible, they have sometimes been proposed as alternatives to workplace exposure controls. This, however, is an unacceptable compromise—the mere detection of a disease is not a substitute for its prevention.

Surveillance programs may be conducted in-plant or by an outside medical facility or physician under contract or agreement with the employer. The tests to be conducted and the frequency of screening must be clearly specified, and the referral process for individuals found to have a disorder, as well as the employer's response to these individuals, should be spelled out in advance.

A new surveillance program, even when mandated by law or contract, should have the approval and understanding of all the workers involved, through their union or, in unorganized workforces, through direct worker education programs. The education program should explicitly delineate the purpose of the surveillance, the measures being taken to control workplace exposures, the steps that employees can take to minimize personal exposure and to reduce the risk of the outcome in question, and the right of an employee to withdraw from a voluntary program.

Testing Procedures

A surveillance program must be built around the best testing procedures currently available. Tests that are very controversial or difficult to interpret will lead to considerable confusion and may delay prompt action. The OSHA-mandated surveillance procedures in widespread use therefore are based on relatively simple and straightforward tests. For example, the lead standard is based on determining the blood lead levels, the noise standard on audiometric screening, and the asbestos standard primarily on the chest film and spirometric testing.

A surveillance program may incorporate an experimental test. However, when a new screening test is validated and introduced as a replacement for an older test of less reliability, both tests should be performed for a period of several years so that the findings can be compared and trends will not be obscured by the transition.

The frequency of testing in a surveillance program depends on the pattern of exposure and the biological characteristics of the disease. Most surveillance procedures are repeated annually, merely because one year is a convenient interval of time. The noise standard, for example, requires annual audiometric screening for workers exposed to 85 dBA or more of noise. There is nothing inherent in noise-induced hearing loss that makes annual testing optimal, but with less frequent testing hearing loss could deteriorate without being detected. Furthermore, testing on an annual basis makes the inadvertent omission of tests less likely. On the other hand, audiometric testing more often than once a year would be very expensive and unlikely to identify a significantly higher proportion of new cases of hearing loss.

To be useful in surveillance, a screening test must detect an exposure-related abnormality as early as possible. The particular test used must directly reflect the entry of the hazardous substance into the body, the chemical change it may undergo, its effect on body tissue, its route of excretion, or its place of storage in the body. "Shotgun" screening or testing for multiple unrelated variables is wasteful and the results usually present more questions than answers. Ideally, this kind of a test would detect an adaptation to the exposure well before subclinical impairment develops. Such tests fall into two categories:

- Biological monitoring, which encompasses techniques to determine the magnitude of the exposure's effect on the body without directly measuring the toxic substance (e.g., measuring serum and red cell cholinesterase levels after low-level exposure to organophosphate insecticides, and determining free erythrocytic protoporphyrin levels after exposure to lead).
- Toxicological screening, which involves tests that determine, by direct measurement, the levels of a toxic substance or its residues in tissue body fluids or excreta (e.g., testing for blood lead levels, a common example of this more traditional approach). The term "biological monitoring" often is used to incorporate toxicological screening, but this usage is technically incorrect and obscures a useful distinction.

The intent of both biological monitoring and toxicological screening is to detect potentially toxic exposures before their effects become manifest. However, disease caused by hazardous exposure often cannot be detected during the subclinical phase; some, because of their natural history and biologic characteristics, are already in an advanced stage by the time detection is possible, and a targeted intervention to change the outcome is fruitless in all but a handful of cases. Unfortunately, such is the case in screening for lung cancer with sputum cytology and chest roentgenography. These tests should be considered screening techniques for case-finding and diagnosis. If the disease being sought is infectious, as in the case of tuberculosis, secondary infection (the spread to others) can be prevented.

The final section of this chapter illustrates a surveillance program for high-risk workers using the common example of asbestos exposure.

Issues in Surveillance

Health surveillance at the workplace is a controversial topic—the passions it inflames alone constitute ample justification for using a high degree of discrimination in selecting the tests to be performed. Requiring employees to undergo testing may be a condition of employment, but it must be accompanied by adequate worksite hazard monitoring and control and by employee health hazard information and education.

Mandatory surveillance has the advantage of ensuring that all workers at risk are regularly screened. Whenever abnormal results occur, appropriate action can be taken at the earliest possible time. Mandatory or employer-required surveillance also enables the occupational health service to collect sufficient health data on the hazard so as to compile a complete and unbiased record of the effectiveness of its preventive program. With a voluntary system, on the other hand, a significant number of exposed workers may never be monitored, and the service may find it impossible to draw valid conclusions about the condition of the population of workers who are at risk. Do acceptable levels found in volunteered samples indicate that *all* workers at risk are remaining healthy? Did the workers who agreed to be monitored do so because they are by inclination conscientious and safe? Are those who declined more slipshod in their approach to personal health, or are they afraid to reveal what possibly could be significant absorptions of the hazardous substance? Are they just taking a stand on a personal belief that their health is their own business? Absent a valid opinion survey, the service will never know for certain what the answers to these questions might be.

Voluntary surveillance may avoid one major drawback to mandatory testing—labor unrest caused by the workers' perception that management is unilaterally imposing its will on employees. Of course, in situations where the hazard is such that regulatory authorities require regular monitoring of all exposed workers, the situation is resolved for all concerned: the employer, the occupational health service, and the workers.

Deciding whether or not to start a surveillance program is one problem; closing down an existing program is another. Occasionally, surveillance that has been carried on for some time, possibly for many years, is judged to provide no real return on investment. The occupational health service may find that over the course of years the program has uncovered so few positive results, relative to the number of samples analyzed, that the cost in time and dollars to detect those few cases is unreasonably high. Furthermore, there now may be better methods available to monitor workers, or a work process or equipment introduced since the program began may have significantly decreased the hazard. However, the workers, now well accustomed to being monitored, feel reassured by the program and appreciate that the positive results that were obtained resulted in timely action. The workers may well question whether the service can justify, on the basis of a few dollars in savings, cutting off a program that has prevented some of them from becoming ill due to unhealthy workplace conditions.

Deciding whether or not to monitor, absent a regulatory requirement to do so, is a difficult choice and one in which no solution will be acceptable to both the employer and the workforce. Naturally, local circumstances do come into play, but there are definite criteria that always should be considered before acting on a particular surveillance program. Following are criteria for making an informed decision on starting or discontinuing a surveillance program:

- The information obtained must be of demonstrable importance to the health or safety at work of the employee being tested.
- The test should not be a substitute for eliminating or controlling the hazard.
- The test results should be applied for the purpose of improving the health and safety situation at the worksite and maintaining or improving the health of the individual tested.
- If the test is to determine absorption or intake of a substance, it should be specific for that substance or the family of substances involved.
- If the test is to anticipate an effect, it should detect early signs of absorption at an early stage.
- The employee's baseline level for the substance, before exposure in the workplace, should be known in order to permit later comparison and interpretation.
- The test must be acceptable to the employee; a test that is painful beyond drawing blood or very uncomfortable or inconvenient must be clearly justified and agreed upon by the workers subjected to it.
- The advantages of using a particular method to identify cases of excessive exposure should be greater than the advantages of using alternative measures.
- Each employee should be informed of his or her individual and group test results and their meaning and of the health implications of the results.

Example: Asbestos Exposure Surveillance Program

Rationale

Asbestos is thought to be the most common occupational carcinogen and the most common and widespread occupational hazard conferring a substantial risk for the development of cancer. Although the health effects of asbestos were well described in Europe in the early part of this century, it was not until the 1960s that these health risks were recognized widely in the United States. According to current estimates, approximately 3.5 million workers in the United States have sustained significant exposure to asbestos. Very few of these workers are involved in the process of mining and milling asbestos; most are exposed by using asbestos-containing products and processing asbestos materials into these products. The single largest group, numbering approximately 2 million workers, are engaged in automobile service and repair. A large group of workers also has been exposed to asbestos in the shipbuilding industry.

During the second World War, many hundreds of thousands of workers sustained heavy exposure to asbestos; the experiences of this group make up a large proportion of the current epidemic of asbestos-related lung cancer. Plumbers and pipefitters, insulation workers, construction workers, cement pipe manufacturing operatives, and workers handling hot metal objects (such as welders and foundry workers) all have had significant asbestos exposure, particularly in the past. A number of other occupations also have been exposed to asbestos, but at relatively low levels, and such exposure may not be immediately apparent without close examination of the work processes.

Asbestos is associated with a number of serious illnesses, primarily asbestosis, a disease of pulmonary parenchymal fibrosis leading to a profound restrictive defect that ultimately may result in respiratory failure. Asbestosis also is associated with increased susceptibility to infection and a high risk for lung cancer. Asbestos exposure has been linked to three forms of thoracic cancer: bronchogenic carcinoma of the epithelial type, adenocarcinoma of the lung, and mesothelioma. Mesotheliomas may be pleural or, on occasion, peritoneal or pericardial and are exceedingly rare in the absence of a history of exposure to asbestos. Both forms of lung cancer, particularly bronchogenic carcinoma, are synergistic with cigarette smoking; neither mesothelioma nor asbestosis, however, are known to have a relationship to cigarette smoke exposure. Other health outcomes associated with asbestos exposure include pleural fibrosis (frequently difficult to distinguish from mesothelioma), benign pleural effusion (also frequently resembling mesothelioma), Blesovsky's syndrome (invaginated or in-folded lung parenchyma creating an atelectatic mass resembling a tumor), and asbestomas (which appear on the lung as solitary nodules and on the skin as asbestos corns). The variety of conditions tentatively associated with asbestos exposure include gastrointestinal malignancies, laryngeal carcinoma, lymphomas, and ovarian carcinomas. The relationship of these conditions to asbestos is still uncertain.

Regulation

The asbestos health surveillance program is an important example of an occupational health surveillance program for high risk workers. Every jurisdiction in North America requires by law occupational health surveillance programs for workers exposed to asbestos. Asbestos exposure surveillance programs should monitor workers exposed currently to asbestos in their present occupation or in their past work. The intent of such programs is to detect as early as possible adverse health effects occurring as a result of exposure so that future exposure can be controlled and disability limited.

In California, the management of surveillance programs for asbestos-exposed workers is covered in the General Industry Safety Orders of Title Eight of the California Administrative Code, Section 5208. At the time of writing, this regulation specified a permissible exposure level of two fibers (longer than five microns) per cubic centimeter as an eight-hour time weighted average and a peak exposure level of ten fibers per cubic centimeter. The standard is likely to be reduced to one-half fiber in the near future. The method of determination specified is the phase contrast illuminated microscope examining a membrane filter at 400–450 times magnification. The regulation specifies work processes for handling asbestos products, emphasizing wetting and prompt cleanup of spills, and, with certain exceptions, prohibits spraying of asbestos-containing material. The regulation stipulates that asbestos is to be disposed of in sealed bags and treated as a hazardous waste.

Other provisions of the regulation specify that personal protective equipment is to be used in the absence of feasible engineering controls, although engineering controls are preferred, and require that employers provide special clothing for workers. Work clothes cannot be worn home and must be kept separate from street clothes by the use of separate lockers and laundering facilities. (This provision is amply justified by demonstrations that spouses and children of asbestos-exposed workers have indeed contracted asbestos-related diseases, some fatally, because of their passive exposure to asbestos brought home on work clothes.) All employers using asbestos must evaluate employee exposure on a semiannual basis and following any major change in the industrial process. Employers also are required to maintain complete and accurate records of monitoring for at least 30 years, to label asbestos-containing materials, and to post warning signs where asbestos is present.

The standard also requires that employers establish programs for medical surveillance of workers at risk for asbestos exposure, train employees in the safe handling of asbestos, and notify workers when exposure has occurred. The protocol provided in Exhibit 20.3 is designed to satisfy surveillance requirements. The asbestos surveillance flow sheet provided as Form 20.2 facilitates recording the results of the screening program described in Exhibit 20.3 and interpreting trends and identifying key signs. This flow sheet is structured so as to do more than provide a simple record of test results over time—rather, it guides the physician to consider the significance of the various signs. The intent of this format is to prompt the physician to think in terms of health outcomes and their early identification rather than treating each test result piecemeal.

The concepts and rationale behind the California asbestos exposure standard and the asbestos surveillance program suggested here illustrate the legal requirements that are common to all surveillance programs. Details on the specific requirements of mandated surveillance for particular exposures covered by U.S. regulatory standards are available from state or federal OSHA. In Canada, the specifics are available from provincial occupational health agencies. Many standard reference works detail reasonable protocols for recommended surveillance programs, and NIOSH has outlined suitable programs for a number of exposures not now covered by mandated surveillance standards. The swelling movement within the United States to review and revise many of the current OSHA standards may lead to changes in mandated surveillance requirements in coming years.

Exhibit 20.3. Surveillance Protocol for Asbestos Exposure
(This protocol is designed to satisfy California state requirements for
medical surveillance of workers exposed to asbestos.)

1. Preplacement and termination examinations: To be performed within 30 days of initial assignment to a work place in which asbestos is used and within 30 days of termination of employment, if a periodic examination has not been performed within the preceding year.
   - A comprehensive medical history emphasizing respiratory and gastrointestinal symptoms and conditions.
   - Physical examination emphasizing thoracic and gastrointestinal findings.
   - Chest films, to include the following views: posteroanterior (PA), right anterior oblique, left anterior oblique.
   - Spirometry, with forced vital capacity and forced expiratory volume at one second entered into the record.

2. Periodic evaluation for younger employees with relatively brief exposure histories: To be administered to employees who are younger than 40 years of age and who have had a duration of potential exposure to asbestos of less than 10 years. This evaluation is to be repeated every three years.
   - Interim medical history emphasizing respiratory and gastrointestinal symptoms covering the previous three years.
   - Physical examination emphasizing thoracic and gastrointestinal signs with notation of changes occurring during the three-year intervals.
   - Chest film, PA view only, with notation of changes occurring over the three-year interval.
   - Spirometry with comparison of forced vital capacity and forced expiratory volume at one second with the results of the previous triannual evaluations.

3. Periodic examination for older employees and employees with a longer duration of potential exposure to asbestos: To be administered to employees 40 years of age or older or any employee of any age who has been exposed to asbestos for more than 10 years. The initial exposure does not necessarily have to be with the current employer. This examination is to be repeated annually except as noted.
   - Interim medical history, emphasizing change in status from the previous year.
   - Physical examination, emphasizing changes in physical signs from the previous year.
   - Chest film to include the following views at the frequency specified: PA annually, right and left anterior obliques every three years.
   - Spirometry, emphasizing changes in pulmonary function from the previous year and establishing trends in the decline of pulmonary function with adjustment for the age of the employee.
   - Rectal examination as part of the physical examination, to be performed annually.
   - Stool guaiac for occult blood, to be performed annually.

Form 20.2. Asbestos Surveillance Flow Sheet

NAME:
ADDRESS:
EMPLOYER:

+ = Present   − = Absent

Conditions now known or strongly suspected to be associated with asbestos exposure: asbestosis*, benign pleural effusion, asbestoma, pleural plaques*, Blesovsky's syndrome, mesothelioma*, bronchogenic carcinoma*, laryngeal carcinoma*, lymphomas.

* Probably most common

	Year of Assessment							
FINDINGS	19	19	19	19	19	19	19	19

	FINDINGS
Indices of Exposure	History of continued exposure
	CXR: pleural plaques
Rule out benign asbestos-associated disease	Dyspnea, dry cough, tachypnea
	Clubbing, with/without cyanosis
	Rales on auscultation
	CXR: interstitial fibrosis
	CXR: asbestosis criteria
	CXR: pleural effusion
	PFT: restrictive defect
Rule out malignant asbestos-associated disease	History of exposure years previously
	Clinical symptoms compatible
	Stool guaiac positive
	CXR: solitary nodule
	CXR: pleural effusion
	CXR: infiltrating mass

Follow-up investigations:
1. _____
2. _____
3. _____
4. _____
5. _____
6. _____
7. _____

Further Reading

American Cancer Society: ACS report on the cancer-related checkup. CA 30:194–239, 1980.

A New Perspective on the Health of Canadians. Ottawa, Health and Welfare Canada, 1974.

AOMA Conference on Medical Screening and Biological Monitoring for the Effects of Exposure in the Workplace: J Occup Med (Part I) 1986; 28(8), (Part II) 1986; 28(10).

Brandt-Rauf PW: New markers for monitoring occupational cancer: The example of encogene proteins. J Occup Med 1988; 30:399–404.

Breslow L, Somers AR: The lifetime health-monitoring program: A practical approach to preventive medicine. New Engl J Med 1977; 195:601–608.

Canadian Task Force on the Periodic Health Examination: The periodic health examination. Can Med Assn J 1979; 121:1194–1254.

Charap MH: The periodic health examination: Genesis of a myth. Ann Intern Med 1981; 95:733–735.

Dales LG, Friedman GD, Collen MF: Evaluating periodic multiphasic health checkups: A controlled trial. J Chron Dis 1979; 32:385–404.

Dept. of Clinical Epidemiology and Biostatistics, McMaster University Health Sciences Centre: How to read clinical journals: II. To learn about a diagnostic test. Can Med Assn J 1981; 124:703–710.

Fletcher RH, Fletcher SW, Wagner EH: Clinical Epidemiology: The Essentials. Baltimore, Williams and Wilkins, 1982.

Frame PS, Carlson SJ: A critical review of periodic health screening using specific screening criteria. J Family Practice 2:29, 123, 189, 283, 1975.

Frank AL: Identification and surveillance of individuals at high risk. Cancer Detect Prev 1986; 9:429–434.

Froines JR, Dellenbaugh CA, Wegman DH: Occupational health surveillance: A means to identify work-related risks. Am J Pub Health 1986; 76:1089–1096.

Gadian T: Health monitoring in industry: Medical considerations. R Soc Health J 1980; 100:130–132.

Guidotti TL: Adaptation of the lifetime health monitoring concept to defined employer groups not at exceptional risk. J Occup Med 1983; 25: 731–736.

Guidotti TL: Exposure to hazard and individual risk: When occupational medicine gets personal. J Occup Med 1988; 30:570–577.

Guidotti TL: Occupational health monitoring and surveillance. American Family Physician 1985; 31:161–169.

Guinan P, et al: What is the best test to detect prostate cancer? CA 32:141–145, 1981.

Halperin WE et al: Medical screening in the workplace: Proposed principles. J Occup Med 1986; 28:547–552.

Health and Welfare Canada, Task Force on Health Surveillance of Workers: Health surveillance of workers. Can J Pub Health 1986; 77:89–108.

Howe HL: Social factors associated with breast self-examination among high risk women. Am J Pub Health 71:251–255, 1981.

Inkeles S, Eisenberg D: Hyperlipidemia and coronary artherosclerosis: A review. Medicine 60:110–123, 1981.

Institute of Medicine: Preventive services for the well population: Healthy people. Washington, D.C.: US DHEW, 1978, pp 1–22.

Last JM (ed): A Dictionary of Epidemiology. New York, Oxford University Press, 1983.

Lynch HT, et al: Hereditary cancer: Ascertainment and management. CA 29:216–232, 1979.

Medical Practice Committee, American College of Physicians: Periodic health examination: A guide for designing indiviualized preventive health care in the asymptomatic patient. Ann Intern Med 95:729–732, 1981.

Mintz BW: Medical surveillance of employees under the Occupational Health and Safety Administration. J Occup Med 1986; 28:913–920.

Office of the Surgeon General: Healthy People: The Surgeon General's Report on Health Promotion and Disease Prevention. Washington, D.C.: DHEW publication (PHS) 79-55071, pp 3–18, 53–69, 152–154.

Periodic Health Examination Monograph. Report of a Task Force to the Conference of Deputy Ministers of Health (cat no. H39-3/1980E). Minister of Supply and Services, Ottawa, 1980.

Prevention '82. Washington DC, U.S. Dept. of Health and Human Services, DHHS (PHS) Publication No. 82-50157. Updated biennially.

Romm FJ, Fletcher SW, Hulka BS: The periodic health examination: Comparison of recommendations and internist's performance. Southern Med J 1981; 74:265–271.

Sackett DL: Screening for early detection of disease: To what purpose? Bull NY Acad Med 1975; 51:39–52.

Spirtas R et al: A Conceptual Framework for Occupational Health Surveillance. Washington DC, US Government Printing Office, National Institute for Occupational Safety and Health, DHEW (NIOSH) Publication No. 78–135, 1978.

U.S. Centers for Disease Control: Guidelines for evaluating surveillance systems. MMWR 1988; 37(suppl. S-5):1–18.

Yodaiken RE: Surveillance, monitoring, and regulatory concerns. J Occup Med 1986; 28:569–571.

21 AIDS IN THE WORKPLACE

Reason, not panic, should be the response of management to the question of AIDS in the workplace. While AIDS is not an occupational disease, except in a very few situations, there are important issues that must be discussed if concern over AIDS in the workplace is to be dealt with in a rational manner. This chapter provides essential information at a level of complexity suitable for managers and workers.

The Disease and Its Transmission

The medical condition known as AIDS (acquired immunodeficiency syndrome) is a terminal illness with no presently known cure. It is caused by a family of human immunodeficiency viruses (HIVs) that affect the body's immune system and, commonly, the central nervous system. The virus attacks the cells responsible for maintaining immunity and actually invades their genetic material permanently. As a result, the body's defense mechanisms can no longer fend off certain disease-causing organisms and some rare cancers that otherwise would be easily repelled. These so-called opportunistic infections and cancers are the direct cause of the infected person's death. AIDS-related complex (ARC) is a medical condition also caused by HIV infection that is characterized by swollen lymph nodes and systemic symptoms. While AIDS itself is characteristic in its symptoms and progress, ARC's symptoms resemble those of many other diseases. About 20 percent of persons infected with HIV develop ARC within five years; of these, 15 percent develop AIDS itself in five years, according to the U.S. Centers for Disease Control. Scientists currently do not know what percentage of persons infected with HIV ultimately will develop ARC or AIDS over the years.

When the virus enters the body, it stimulates a slow and ineffective immune reaction. This immune reaction usually produces specific antibodies (small bits of protein that attack elements of the virus in a vain effort to destroy it). These antibodies appear weeks to months, even years, after initial infection. They do not seem to protect the person against any of the effects of the virus nor do they stop the virus from being produced and shed by the body. However, they do act as a marker indicating whether a person has been infected in the past. Unfortunately, because only 95 percent of persons infected with HIV develop these antibodies, the test is not absolutely reliable in detecting infection by HIV. (See Chapter 20 on principles of surveillance and screening tests.)

HIV is not easy to transmit. It is spread from one person to another only through sexual contact (by vaginal secretions and, especially, semen) and through direct entry into a person's blood (by, for example, the sharing of intravenous needles or during the pregnancy of an infected mother, when the fetus and neonate are at risk). Prior to 1985, HIV's ability to spread through blood and certain blood products caused the infection of patients who received blood transfusions and hemophiliacs who received blood products from infected donors. In North America, however, this problem now has been virtually eliminated by programs that screen each blood donation for antibodies to HIV. Contact with normal skin poses no risk; the virus must actually enter the bloodstream of the recipient before infection can occur.

HIV is a very fragile virus outside the protected environment of the body. It survives for only a short time once exposed to air and dry conditions, and can be killed by virtually any disinfectant, including common household bleach, and by soap and water. It cannot be spread through the air like the common cold or with the relative ease of other sexually transmitted diseases. It is not even spread as easily as other viruses, such as hepatitis B, for which existing guidelines have been proven effective. It should be apparent, therefore, that if entry of a quantity of virus into the blood of the recipient is necessary to establish an infection, HIV cannot be spread by casual contact, by mere proximity to an infected person, or by touching.

Occupational Risks

Since the AIDS virus is not spread by casual contact or by contaminated food, only workers who come into contact with bodily fluids and particularly blood—primarily health care professionals—are at risk for potential infection. Nurses or laboratory personnel who handle blood from infected people might be exposed to HIV in such a way that the virus either is directly introduced into their blood or tissue or comes into contact with a direct portal of entry. Such exposure could only come from a needlestick, for example, with actual injection of some amount of blood, or contact between contaminated blood and an open wound on the worker's body of such prolonged duration that the virus directly enters the worker's bloodstream. These types of circumstances actually have occurred, but both are extremely unusual and are completely preventable by following the guidelines for dealing with highly infectious materials that are recommended for all hospitals and laboratories. Barbers, morticians, policemen, prison guards, ambulance attendants, and other workers who conceivably could come into contact with blood may wish to take some precautions, but simply using standard hygienic practices will keep the risk extremely low. On the other hand, there is no evidence for or likelihood that sharing a respirator or face mask could transmit HIV. Concern over the possibility that respirators and face masks might spread HIV has emerged time and again among fearful workers. Such a misconception is dangerous, particularly since it could lead a worker to refuse to use personal protective equipment under hazardous conditions or in an emergency.

The fact that AIDS is not transferred through normal everyday casual contact obviates any need in the general workplace to routinely identify an HIV-antibody positive (infected) person or even a person with AIDS. Most of the estimated 1.0 to 1.5 million Americans infected with HIV (and who are antibody-positive) are unaware of their infection, and are in apparently normal health. Mandatory mass screening of workers for the HIV antibody is completely unnecessary. The screening test is not perfect, and a certain small percentage of positive results are false; actions or diagnoses based on an unsubstantiated screening test can lead to serious legal and ethical problems. The only justification for doing any sort of employment-related medical test in the workplace is to determine whether the person in a particular job is a hazard to self or others. This does not apply to the otherwise healthy and fit applicant who may or may not be antibody positive; antibody status is not relevant to the question. Routine HIV antibody testing in the general workplace cannot be justified on the basis of a need to isolate AIDS patients or healthy HIV antibody-positive persons because they are a hazard to others or are unable to do their jobs.

Workplace Issues

AIDS is primarily spread by unsafe sexual practices and by shared needles, as occurs commonly among drug users during illicit intravenous drug use. Such practices generally occur off working time and outside the confines of the workplace.

Nevertheless, while the risk of spreading or contacting HIV infection is virtually nonexistent in the general workplace, AIDS does pose some real issues for management. The most important are ensuring fair employment practices for workers infected with AIDS or other HIV disorders and establishing an AIDS awareness program in the workplace so that employees learn the facts about the disease and how to prevent its spread.

Employees with AIDS

AIDS is a serious disease; it affects individuals in much the same way as any other chronic, debilitating, and eventually fatal disorder. However, the person with AIDS also faces discrimination and the potentially high cost of medical care and hospitalization. Like any other serious disorder, AIDS should be covered by the employer's policy on medical leave and disability. A separate AIDS policy should not be needed; this tends to perpetuate the idea that people with AIDS should be singled out as different.

Fitness-to-work determinations (Chapter 18) evaluate the health of the worker according to the requirements of the working conditions of the job. A test for HIV antibody might be considered as part of this medical evaluation if the examining occupational health professional clearly sees that the worker is ill or for some reason suspects he or she is dealing with an AIDS or an ARC patient. Otherwise, the test is not appropriate as a routine screen. The health professional also must obtain the consent of the patient before performing the antibody test, and should provide appropriate counselling before and after the test.

Ascertaining the HIV status of a worker in some situations is important because of the risk of infection to persons with AIDS. The immune system of the AIDS patient appears to be unable to handle many common infections that may be widespread in a normal workplace. Furthermore, the prognosis in a given case may be such that the worker could not reasonably be expected to master a job or complete an assignment. However, a person with AIDS should not be handled differently from any other person who suffers from a serious disease—and the employment rights of the AIDS patient may be protected by human rights codes that outlaw discrimination on the basis of physical disability. (See Chapter 19.) An employed AIDS sufferer enjoys the same protection from wrongful dismissal for health reasons as would anyone else. On the other hand, a worker who is discovered to suffer from AIDS during a preplacement evaluation could be legitimately declared unfit for the position if in fact the working conditions are demonstrably unsuitable or too hazardous for the worker's condition. The status of a person who is infected with HIV but who is not symptomatic with AIDS is not as well defined as that of persons covered under equal opportunity legislation, but logic and ethics suggest that in matters of employment they should be accorded the same protection as would be extended to those with any potentially disabling condition.

AIDS Education

AIDS should be treated at the worksite just like any other disease. Employers have an obligation to provide information on how AIDS is spread and how AIDS is not spread.

So noted the Surgeon General of the United States, Dr. C. Everett Koop. Certainly it makes sense for an employer to educate employees in order to avoid problems and misunderstandings and provide for the workers' own protection. AIDS is a serious epidemic and preventing its further spread is the responsibility of all in positions of influence and authority. An AIDS awareness program that draws on the many resources now available in the community should be extended to the workplace. The objective of such a program is to help educate workers in making reasonable decisions about appropriate individual health-related behavior. AIDS awareness programs should not present management's views on morality and personal conduct. AIDS awareness programs serve to put the situation into perspective by reassuring workers that they have no real risk of contracting the disease or becoming infected with HIV in their workplace.

The emergence and rapid spread of AIDS and the discovery of HIV as the transmissible cause created fear and much anxiety. Here and now is a time for correction, reasonable adaptation, and accommodation. Except in workplaces where there is a real risk of exposure to contaminated body fluids, a specific AIDS policy is simply not necessary and has the unfortunate effect of unintentionally promoting discrimination. What is necessary is a two-fold program of (1) fairly determining fitness to work in a way that treats AIDS objectively and (2) educating employees on the facts of AIDS.

Further Reading

AIDS–The Workplace Issues: AMA Management Briefing. New York, American Management Association, 1985.

Bayer R, Levin C, Wolf SM: HIV antibody screening: An ethical framework for evaluating proposed programs. JAMA 1986; 256:1768–1774.

Burke DS, Brandt BL, Redfield RR, et al: Diagnosis of human immunodeficiency virus infection by immunoassay using a molecularly cloned and expressed virus envelope polypeptide. Ann Intern Med 1987; 106:671–676.

Cowell JWF: Fighting fear with reason. OHS Canada 1988; 4:14.

Elliot C, Saxe S: AIDS in the workplace: A lawyer's point of view. Employment Law Rep, Jan 1986; 7(1):1–2.

Information on AIDS for the Practicing Physician. Chicago, American Medical Association, 1987.

Meyer KB, Pauker SG: Screening for HIV: Can we afford the false positive rate? N Engl J Med 1987; 317:238–241.

Tremayne-Lloyd T (ed): Report of the Canadian Bar Association Ontario Committee to Study the Legal Implications of Acquired Immunodeficiency Syndrome (AIDS). Toronto, 1986.

U.S. Centers for Disease Control: Additional recommendations to reduce sexual and drug abuse-related transmission of human T-lymphotropic virus type III/lymphadenopathy-associated virus. MMWR 1986; 35:152–155.

U.S. Centers for Disease Control: Recommended additional guidelines for HIV antibody counseling and testing in the prevention of HIV infection and AIDS. Atlanta, Georgia: US Department of Health and Human Services, Public Health Service, 1987.

U.S. Centers for Disease Control: Tuberculosis provisional data–United States, 1986. MMWR 1987;36:254–255.

U.S. Centers for Disease Control: Diagnosis and management of mycobacterial infection and disease in persons with human T-lymphotropic virus type III/lymphadenopathy-associated virus infection. MMWR 1986; 35:448–452.

22 ABSENCE MONITORING

Absence from work is a difficult management problem: it introduces considerable uncertainty into scheduling work and staff assignments, is an important cause of lost productivity, and very often precipitates labor-management conflict and misunderstandings. Indeed, the topic of unauthorized absence from work has given rise to an elaborate mythology featuring the "lazy worker," the "selfish and inflexible boss," and the "manager who phones in sick from the golf course." Because people from different cultural backgrounds view absence from work very differently, the issue is laden with prejudice, misperceptions, and hidden hostility. In no other area of working life are the rigid, quasi-religious expectations of the work ethic more likely to conflict with notions regarding personal freedom and flexibility. There are also few areas of working life where abuse of privileges so directly undermines the relationship between manager and worker.

Absence often triggers an emotional response in both worker and manager. This emotional response is reflected in the value-laden term "absenteeism," which will not be used here. This discussion uses the term "absence," meaning simply that the worker is not present at his or her assigned job. The term absenteeism has connotations of a recurrent condition, a tendency to be absent, or a type of illness; none of these connotations contributes positively to a discussion of absence from work. Indeed, there are many valid reasons why a worker may not report to work on a given day, some of which may benefit the employer by preventing future absences or preserving the worker's health and productivity.

Attempts to control unauthorized absence often make matters worse by introducing measures that workers may perceive as arbitrary, authoritarian, and unresponsive to their needs. Human resources personnel often persuade management to take a more "objective" approach by treating the problem as one of validation and documentation. Much of the total absence experience in industry is due to sickness. Even more is claimed to be sickness. From management's point of view, therefore, it is only logical to try to reduce absence through medical means by requiring employee health evaluations, screening to identify workers likely to be frequently absent, medical certification of claimed illness, and investigation of individual cases. Some employers expect an in-house occupational health service to monitor absence directly as one of its principal responsibilities. Unfortunately, these measures work no better than other tactics and have the potential to destroy the overall effectiveness of the occupational health service.

This chapter will discuss the role of the occupational health service in dealing with issues related to absence, technical aspects of absence monitoring (with an emphasis on issues that tend to involve the occupational health service), and the certification of sickness absence by physicians.

Role of the Occupational Health Service

Transferring responsibility for absence monitoring and control from the personnel or human resources department to the occupational health service converts an administrative problem into a medical nightmare. It may succeed in getting the human resources department off the hook but presents the occupational health service with a fundamental dilemma quickly perceived by workers and even more quickly exploited by some managers. As discussed earlier in this book, the corporate or in-plant occupational health service balances employee trust and responsibility toward management. However, involving the service in routine monitoring and control of absence destroys this delicate balance, even if the service is able to reduce absence due to worker incapacity. Under these circumstances, the occupational health service becomes the personnel manager—and when workers view it as the means by which management reviews their attendance and singles them out for discipline, cooperation and goodwill promptly evaporate and are seldom, if ever, regained. The physician in such a position becomes labelled as just another management functionary and medical judgments from the occupational health service are viewed as being untrustworthy and prejudicial against the worker. Furthermore, having taken the occupational health service this far down the road, insensitive managers may then press even further for the physician to become a "team player," siding with management in violations of confidentiality. (See Chapter 4.)

Although the occupational health service should never accept absence monitoring and control as an operational responsibility, it can positively affect the absence experience of an employer to the mutual benefit of both employer and worker. Means of effecting positive results include:

• Evaluating employees who come voluntarily to the service or who are directed to come by their supervisors because of frequent or prolonged absences due to apparent health problems. The process for these evaluations is described in the fitness-to-work procedures. (See Chapter 18.) A private, confidential interview and examination may have a number of beneficial outcomes. Besides uncovering a treatable illness, such an examination may suggest a means by which the patient could be treated at work conveniently and without disruption to the work schedule (see Chapter 19) or a minor modification in the work environment or job responsibilities that would allow the worker to stay on the job (see Chapter 18). The exam may identify a worker who has emotional or substance dependency problems that might benefit from a referral to an employee assistance program (see Chapter 25 and 26). In all of these cases, the emphasis for the occupational health service should be on fitness-to-work and the well-being of the worker, not on policing compliance with the employer's policy on sick leave.

- Dealing with personal health problems. Although occupational physicians are primarily concerned with the work-health relationship, they frequently are confronted with the difficulty of assessing a person's ability to work in the presence of a personal health problem. There are many circumstances (e.g., hypertension) in which a personal health problem is better managed and monitored in the worksite. The occasional attention of the occupational physician at the worksite may also prevent subsequent problems that otherwise would lead to loss of work time, as in the management of brittle diabetics. These kinds of individual patient management at the worksite should not be considered competitive but rather complementary to management by the worker's personal physician in that they provide the worker with the best opportunity to remain on the job while ensuring that the worker's health care needs are met.
- Identifying and evaluating individuals with personal health behaviors that are self-destructive and that interfere with work performance. The occupational physician engaged in providing employee assistance services, either directly or more commonly through supervising the referral of troubled employees to outside services, quickly realizes the degree to which personal health problems play a role in employee satisfaction and performance.
- Promoting healthy lifestyles. Health promotion programs in the workplace are one clear means by which occupational medicine can address nonoccupational factors determining health. As noted in Chapter 27, employee participation in such programs may reduce absence in many ways. The program should never lend itself to management attempts to accumulate personal health data as a means of validating or predicting sickness absence or to evade responsibility for workers' compensation claims that are submitted later or for occupational health conditions.
- Providing simple assessment of and treatment for minor illnesses at the workplace for the convenience and comfort of workers. While such care should not replace personal health care provided by the worker's own physician, it can keep an employee who would otherwise stay home because of minor symptoms safely on the job. Occupational health services are seldom equipped for sophisticated treatment and diagnosis, however, and must limit their involvement in personal health care to avoid overextending their limited resources and to ensure that occupational health problems take priority. Nonetheless, a service that provides simple dispensary care for the common cold and other minor ailments can be a real convenience.

The occupational health service itself can benefit from pursuing a role of limited involvement in personal health care and recording personal health-related information on workers. Occupational health physicians must have a working knowledge of personal health problems that are prevalent among the group of workers for whom they have responsibility in order to be able to discern whether newly recognized health outcomes are occupationally related. One of the major criticisms of occupational epidemiology, for example, is that data on smoking habits are rarely available for occupational groups under study and the absence of data on this possible confounding factor often calls into question the conclusions of an otherwise rigorous study. As occupational medicine becomes more sophisticated and prevention-oriented, the need to sort out occupational from nonoccupational risk factors becomes even greater, requiring an appreciation of the personal health of workers as well as their occupational experience.

Although there are general measures that may have a positive effect on absence in the workplace, there is no way to predict individual absence with any reliability, and screening programs for this purpose are not very effective.

Absence Monitoring and Control

There are only two possible ways to keep track of absence: recording attendance at work or recording incidents of absence, assuming employee attendance unless notified otherwise. For a variety of reasons that have much to do with assumptions regarding social class and behavior, attendance recording is normally used for blue-collar and manual labor occupations. Absence recording, on the other hand, is usual for professional, white-collar, and most office workers, who are more often paid on a salary basis and whose productivity is judged primarily by qualitative standards of individual performance. Absence recording is inherently less accurate but the implicit assumption is that the professional and white-collar workers for whom it is used need only to justify their output to prove their worth to the employer. At higher levels of management responsibility, the freedom to take time off whenever one's schedule permits is tantamount to an executive perquisite, or "perk." However, the socialization process of executives is such that the option is provided with the expectation that it will not be exercised very often; the executive role dictates that the serious senior manager demonstrate commitment to the employer by assuming the compulsive behavior that, at an extreme, characterizes the workaholic. By contrast, the blue-collar worker or laborer is assumed to have less commitment to a career path with a given employer, to require constant supervision, and to be essentially interchangeable with other workers. Thus, the mere recording of attendance or absence, as symbolized by punching a time clock or by possessing the liberty to play golf on a weekday afternoon, raises sensitive issues and suggests that measurement of absence is not a simple matter.

Measuring Absences

Absence is usually measured in terms of either days or "spells" since these are the most convenient and universal units to record. However, there are other measurements more useful for certain purposes. Hours or, more often, shifts lost reflect loss of productivity more directly since some workers may leave at midday or work double shifts at other times. Recording time lost addresses only part of the problem, however—presence at the worksite represents the opportunity to be productive, not the worker's actual level of productivity. For example, a worker in a creative field may find inspiration at any time of the day, on or off the job, and may spend relatively little time actually producing a tangible product. On the other hand, an office worker in a large and complex organization, assigned ambiguous or poorly defined responsibilities, may sit at a desk daily for years without making any substantial output. For most jobs, however, time put into the task bears some relationship to productivity.

The frequency of "spells," or identifiable continuous episodes of a worker's absence due to the same or related causes, may reveal a pattern that suggests a medical or a behavioral cause. For example, binge drinkers not uncommonly lose a day or so preceding or following weekends or holidays. Their pattern of absence in single days lost can be frequent but the time spent drinking or the loss of productivity following a binge may not be reflected in the numerical count of days of work lost. An individual with a severe, chronic illness may lose many days but on recovery may only have a few spells of illness per year.

Once counted, absence can be compared and monitored by the calculation of summary measures, each of which has its own limitations:

- Frequency rates report the number of "spells," or episodes of absence, per year, and may be calculated for a particular person or as the total or average for a group. They may include all episodes of absence, short-term absence only, or only absence lasting more than a few days, depending on the purpose for which the statistic will be used.
- Severity rates are based on the number of days (or shifts or hours) lost per year, either for an individual worker or the average for a group. These are sometimes expressed as the percentage of total working time lost due to absence.
- Prevalence rates are calculations of the percentage of employees absent on a particular day. Unlike the other two types of measurements, prevalence rates cannot be calculated for individuals because any one person is either there or not there. They are valuable for estimating or evaluating manpower needs and are commonly used in departments of human resources.

In practice, employers use many different systems to calculate and express absence. Except for the crude measurement of days lost, there is little consistency in the systems used among companies or between private corporations and public agencies. The crude nature of absence counting and the questionable validity of its classification in practice makes elaborate statistical analysis pointless, except in unusual situations. Meaningful comparisons are very difficult to make. No absolute standards have been developed by which to compare one employer's experience with others in the same industry or community. Measures of absence should not be confused with epidemiologic measures of the frequency of illness, such as morbidity, incidence, point prevalence, and period prevalence, each of which has precisely defined meanings. Absence measurement is just that and cannot be readily converted into measurements of morbidity without additional information, which is rarely available in practice.

Absence Classifications

Absence can be categorized in many ways. One simple system that appears to be the most satisfactory recognizes five basic categories:

- Sickness absence. Absence that is attributed to incapacity due to illness or injury that is not work-related.
- Personal leave. Absence for personal reasons that have nothing directly to do with incapacity.
- "Time-lost" occupational injuries or, much less commonly, illnesses. By definition, these are reportable under workers' compensation regulations and therefore are closely monitored.
- Pregnancy and child-care leave. By its nature, this type of absence is planned and preauthorized under the employer's policy.
- Partial absence. An unscheduled absence during part but not all of the work period. As suggested in Table 22.1, each of these categories has further subcategories and

Table 22.1. Categories of Absence

Sickness absence:
    Certified by physician (up to maximum allowed by sick leave policy)
    Uncertified (up to 3–5 days usually permitted), or "self-certified"
    Prior authorization (e.g., for a physician's appointment for an ongoing problem)

Personal leave (with or without pay, with or without authorization):
    Personal business
    Family illness
    Bereavement
    Jury duty

Occupational injuries and illness ("time-lost")

Pregnancy, family, and child care leave:
    Antenatal and confinement
    Postpartum and early child care
    Paternal
    Family illness (worker attends to member of family)

Partial absence:
    Late arrival
    Early departure
    Prolonged absence from post

nuances of measurement. Sickness absence and personal leave are discussed here in greater detail.

The definitions of "sickness absence" and "time-lost" occupational disorders are problemmatical in that neither satisfactorily identifies conditions that are aggravated by, but not otherwise caused by, working conditions, such as preexisting hernias, back strain, bursitis, asthma, skin rashes, and other problems made worse on the job. In practice, these types of conditions are usually counted under sickness absence, even though the loss of productivity associated with them stems in large part from the work environment.

A further problem related to the monitoring of absence is that often the employer as well as the employee finds it advantageous to misclassify particular kinds of absence. A worker may call in sick, rather than using his or her allowed vacation time, in order to take advantage of paid sick leave. An employer may count a real illness that is inadequately documented against an employee's vacation time in order to avoid paying wages for the time off. Abuses of the monitoring system occur in every industry and in almost every workplace; a perfect system has yet to be devised.

From the manager's point of view, the primary classification problem is differentiating sickness absence from unauthorized personal leave. Employers may require a physician's "certification" of an illness as verification of the employee's declaration of illness. However, this process leads to its own problems and complications, as will be discussed in the final section of this chapter.

Patterns of Absence
Absence rates vary greatly from place to place, employer to employer, industry to

industry, and reflect socioeconomic factors such as the state of the economy and available sick leave benefits. There are no generally accepted "normal" absence rates that can be used as a standard of comparison. However, it is true throughout the developed world that absence rates have slowly risen over the last 30 years.

There are some generalities regarding patterns of absence. In general, smokers are absent more often with minor illnesses than nonsmokers. As mentioned previously, abusers of alcohol are often absent sporadically, typically on the days following weekends and holidays and often without notice. Women are absent from work, on average, about twice as often as men, even discounting absences for pregnancy. Women use health services more often than men, but not enough to fully account for the difference in absence. More importantly, women in general have greater domestic responsibilities and are also more likely than men to be employed in lower status occupations where timekeeping is rigidly enforced, hours are inflexible, and advance scheduling of time off is more difficult to accomplish. Women do not seem to have more severe illnesses, on average, than men, and are less likely to work in hazardous occupations. The difference in absence rates thus appears to have more to do with social and employment patterns than with health and commitment to work or career.

Despite these general trends, there is no accurate way of predicting absence for individual workers. Workers with chronic illnesses frequently are among the most reliable employees because they not only are committed but also have learned to be adaptable. Normal, healthy workers may be absent for reasons that have very little to do with health or other characteristics that can be assessed in advance. The only reasonable predictor of absence in any individual case is the worker's own history of absence. Even then, a person's pattern can often change, either for the better or for the worse.

Control Measures

Controlling absence has been a major challenge to human resource managers in all industries. While few universally successful strategies have been identified, some useful approaches have emerged. The use of personal leave may reduce unauthorized leave masquerading as sickness absence by introducing flexible hours or permitting a certain number of days off per month or year in which workers can attend to personal business, subject to prior notification. This minimizes both disruptions caused by individuals' needs to attend to pressing personal errands and appointments that occur during regular working hours and the incentive to claim paid sick days.

A sensible sick leave policy can reduce incidents of absence abuse that arise when workers take time off to "get back" what they may feel is owed them. A policy might require that the worker provide medical certification of illness after three days' absence and that he or she communicate regularly with the supervisor by telephone for as long as the episode lasts. In this way, management demonstrates some degree of trust in the employee yet minimizes the opportunity for flagrant abuse.

The most effective control measure, however, seems to be an overall improvement in the relations between labor and management and the parties' attitudes toward each other. Worker absence is often affected by personal factors: attitudes toward the employer, identification with group performance and objectives, interest in the work, and self-respect. A general sense of personal satisfaction and identification with the objectives and success of the employer may remove some of the temptation for abuse. A sense cf personal involvement also may motivate workers only somewhat inconvenienced by minor complaints to come to work.

Absence is determined in large part by attitude. Persons who have similar levels of illness and discomfort may vary considerably in their adoption of "sick" behavior, with one stoically carrying on and another taking to bed. Some of this difference is cultural, some is due to family attitudes and upbringing, some is due to such circumstances as other stresses in the worker's life, and some is due to individual patterns of strength and weakness. There are always a few individuals in any large group who are immature and who seize on any inconvenience as an excuse to avoid work. However, these people are in a small minority and treating all workers in the same manner as the immature few antagonizes the dependable majority. Most employees not only accept work as a responsibility to be met with varying degrees of commitment but also use their working environment as an opportunity to make friends, engage in social interaction, and develop a social support system. Through group identification, some workers may even come to work when they should otherwise stay home. The task of the human resources manager is to put into place human resource policies that are effective but also humane. These should allow the worker who is ill to take time off without harassment but at the same time motivate the worker who is well or only slightly inconvenienced to come to work. However, personnel policies are the responsibility of personnel officials, not of the physician or the occupational health service.

Certification of Sickness Absence

One of the most common duties of a physician is to certify that a patient has missed or will miss work due to illness. This function places considerable responsibility on the physician, who rarely has had any training in sickness certification. In obvious cases physicians are seldom hesitant to excuse their patients from work or to certify return to work. However, the job of reviewing job requirements and matching them to documented capabilities requires more familiarity with human factors and occupational demands than most physicians possess. By becoming involved in approving workers' return to work and certifying their time off, the occupational physician establishes a clear commitment to understand a worker's personal health problems in relationship to the working conditions. Unfortunately, this commitment is rarely recognized as such and many physicians continue to treat medical certification very casually.

In fairness to the practicing physician, patients frequently ask for medical certification or a "note from the doctor" after the fact or for complaints that are impossible to confirm or deny. A busy physician is not likely to spend much time on this seemingly administrative task. (Nonetheless, the discussion in Chapter 18 should suggest that this task is actually a less structured variation of the fitness-to-work evaluation and therefore is less involved than is usually appreciated.) The implications of certifying sickness absence are significant and the physician is obliged to accept the act as a serious responsibility. When a question arises, the physician should communicate with the employer, either by telephone or in writing in the format suggested in Form 22.1. This type of communication is easily conducted in workplaces with an in-house occupational health service. The physician can communicate directly with the employer's occupational

---

Form 22.1. Medical Leave of Absence Certification

I have examined _____ and have
                                      (employee name)
determined it is medically necessary that he/she be given a medical leave of
absence from _____ to _____.

It is physically difficult or not medically desirable for him/her to work during this
period because: [Do not enter a diagnosis or any personal information.]

_____

_____

_____

_____

Check if applicable:

☐ If sitting or otherwise physically limited work may be available for this worker, I
recommend such assignment until the worker is certified as fit to return to normal duties.

☐ I will be seeing this patient again on _____ and will inform you
of changes in fitness to work at that time.

SIGNED: _____ DATE: _____

PHYSICIAN'S TELEPHONE NUMBER FOR FURTHER INFORMATION: _____

---

health nurse or physician and can be much freer in discussing confidential matters, such as the specific diagnosis. Usually the occupational health service can facilitate the worker's reentry into the workplace.

There is no excuse, however, for a physician to knowingly comply with a false certification or extend a worker's leave period beyond the time when he or she is fit to return to work. Physicians are often urged by the patient to stretch the time off work, particularly if there is a holiday, long weekend, or social event ahead. The pressure may be great if the physician treats the patient's family, has many other patients who know the insistent patient, or has close ties with the community and will inevitably and constantly run across the patient and his or her close associates. In such situations, it may seem only a small matter to bend on what appears to be an administrative issue. However, to do so is neither good medical judgment nor good occupational health practice. Undue extensions of sick leave are very costly to the employer and further delay the return of the worker to a normal life, which is part of the recovery process. The patient should return to work when he or she becomes fit to work—certainly not before then but also not long after.

The alert physician, whether in a corporate setting or in community-based practice, may spot a pattern in absence from work that leads to the identification of a health problem. In interpreting the illness pattern of an individual worker, the physician should consider the following possible factors:

• Alcohol or substance abuse;
• Depression;
• Incomplete recovery, followed by subsequent absence or reinjury;
• Covert illness, such as dementia, associated with inability to do or sustain work;
• Stress and emotional distress, whether personal or job-related, as in the case of "burnout"; or

- Abuse of sick leave, which may predict poor compliance or lack of cooperation in other situations.

The medical certification form presented as Form 22.1 is modified from a standard document developed by the Employers' Health Cost Coalition, a council with representatives from business and medicine formed in San Diego, California, in 1982 in an effort to contain rising health insurance costs. It represents an attempt to standardize the granting of medical leave by explicitly documenting the worker's duration of absence and the reason for certifying that the employee is unfit for work. It is reproduced as an example for physicians to use in communicating with employers.

Further Reading

Brown JAC: The Social Psychology of Industry. New York, Penguin, 1954.

Hendrix WJ, Taylor GS: A multivariate analysis of the relationship between cigarette smoking and absence from work. Amer J Health Promo 1987; 2(2):5–11.

Hilker RRJ: Problem employees, in Zenz C (ed): Occupational Medicine: Principles and Practical Applications. Chicago, Yearbook Medical Publishers, 1975, p. 902.

Soderfeldt B, Danermark B, Larsson S: Social class and sickness absence. Scand J Soc Med 1987; 15:211–217.

Taylor P: Aspects of sickness absence, in Gardner AW (ed): Current Approaches to Occupational Medicine. Bristol (UK), John Wright and Sons, 1979, pp. 322–338.

Taylor PJ, Pocock SJ: Sickness absence—its measurement and control, in Schilling RSF (ed): Occupational Health Practice (ed 2). London, Butterworth, 1981, pp. 339–359.

Workers' health—occupational or personal? Lancet 1984; 1:1390–1391.

23 HAZARD EVALUATION AND CONTROL

The average workplace seldom presents many uncontrolled hazards—but any that are present must be identified, assessed, and dealt with. When an enterprise is very large or contains several operations or workplaces, this may seem an impossible task. However, grouping hazards into a few basic categories facilitates this effort.

Workplace health hazards can best be described as belonging to one of four groups:
- Physical hazards—those involving forms of energy or having a mechanical or gravitational basis.
- Chemical hazards—those produced through the actions or reactions of chemical substances.
- Biological hazards—those caused by living organisms or their products.
- Psychological hazards—those related to stress, the emotional reaction to the environment, or interpersonal relations.

Identifying Hazards

Hazards may be identified in many ways. Common means of identification are:
- Worker health complaints. A worker may present to the occupational health service with a disorder that is suspected of being caused by a hazardous exposure. Since the ill effect has already taken place, this is not the most desirable means of identifying a hazard. A harmful exposure may in fact have continued for months or years with the effects only recently becoming evident.
- Literature, product descriptions, and MSDS information. Workers or supervisors may become aware of the presence of a hazardous substance in their workplace through information disseminated in the media or on a Material Safety Data Sheet (MSDS) provided by a supplier or by the employer. The MSDS can be a valuable source of information for not only the worker but also the occupational health service. Figure 23.1 gives an example of an MSDS. Every MSDS is required by law in the United States and Canada to contain information under the headings shown.

Figure 23.1. A Material Safety Data Sheet (MSDS)
(courtesy Amoco Corporation, Chicago, Illinois, Reprinted with permission).

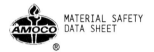

MATERIAL SAFETY   PANASOL AN-2K
DATA SHEET

MANUFACTURER/SUPPLIER: EMERGENCY HEALTH INFORMATION: (800) 447-8735
Amoco Chemical Company   EMERGENCY SPILL INFORMATION: (800) 424-9300
200 East Randolph Drive   OTHER PRODUCT SAFETY INFORMATION: (312) 856-3516
Chicago, Illinois 60601

IMPORTANT COMPONENTS: Xylene (CAS 1330-20-7) ACGIH TLV 100 ppm, 150 ppm (STEL),
                        OSHA PEL 100 ppm.
                        Naphthalene (CAS 91-20-3) ACGIH TLV 10 ppm, 15 ppm (STEL),
                        OSHA PEL 10 ppm.
                        Catalytic reformer petroleum distillate (CAS 68477-31-6).
                        Cosolvent: trade secret.
                        No exposure limit established.

WARNING STATEMENT: Warning! Combustible. Causes skin irritation. Can be harmful if
                     high concentrations are inhaled. Harmful if aspirated into the
                     lungs.

HMIS/NFPA CODES:(HEALTH;2)(FLAMMABILITY;2)(REACTIVITY;0)

APPEARANCE AND ODOR: Clear yellow liquid, aromatic odor.

───────────────────────────── HEALTH HAZARD INFORMATION ─────────────────────────────

EYE

EFFECT: No significant health hazards identified.

FIRST AID: Flush eyes with plenty of water.

PROTECTION: None required; however, use of eye protection is good industrial practice.

SKIN

EFFECT: Causes skin irritation. See Toxicology Section.

FIRST AID: Wash exposed skin with soap and water. Remove contaminated clothing and
              thoroughly clean and dry before reuse. Get medical attention if
              irritation develops.

PROTECTION: Do not get on skin or clothing. Wear protective clothing and gloves.

INHALATION

EFFECT: Can be harmful if high concentrations are inhaled. See Toxicology
              Section.

FIRST AID: If adverse effects occur, remove to uncontaminated area. Get medical
              attention.

PROTECTION: Avoid prolonged or repeated inhalation. Use with adequate ventilation.
              If ventilation is inadequate, use NIOSH/MSHA certified respirator which
              will protect against organic vapor/mist.

Figure 23.1. Continued

PANASOL AN-2K

PAGE 02 OF 04

_____ HEALTH HAZARD INFORMATION - CONTINUED _____

INGESTION

EFFECT: Harmful if aspirated into lungs. See Toxicology Section.

FIRST AID: If swallowed, do NOT induce vomiting. Get immediate medical attention.

_____ FIRE AND EXPLOSION INFORMATION _____

FLASHPOINT: 145°F, (63°C) ASTM D56

AUTOIGNITION TEMPERATURE: 910°F, (490°C)

EXTINGUISHING MEDIA: Agents approved for Class B hazards (e.g., dry chemical, carbon
                      dioxide, halogenated agents, foam, steam) and water fog.

UNUSUAL FIRE AND EXPLOSION HAZARDS: Combustible liquid.

PRECAUTIONS: Keep away from ignition sources (e.g., heat and open flames). Keep
              container closed.

_____ REACTIVITY INFORMATION _____

DANGEROUS REACTIONS: None identified.

HAZARDOUS DECOMPOSITION: None. Polymerization will not occur. Incomplete burning
                          can produce carbon monoxide, carbon dioxide, and other
                          harmful products.

STABILITY: Stable.

_____ CHEMICAL AND PHYSICAL PROPERTIES _____

BOILING POINT: 350°F TO   550°F, (177-288°C)

SOLUBILITY IN WATER: Negligible, below 0.1%.

SPECIFIC GRAVITY (WATER = 1):   0.93

VAPOR PRESSURE: 0.08 mmHg (20°C)

VISCOSITY: 15 cps @ 24°C.

Figure 23.1. Continued

PANASOL AN-2K

PAGE 03 OF 04

_____ STORAGE AND ENVIRONMENTAL PROTECTION _____

STORAGE REQUIREMENTS.   Store in combustible liquids storage area. Store away from
                        heat, ignition sources, and open flame in accordance with
                        applicable federal, state, or local regulations. Keep
                        container closed.

SPILLS AND LEAKS: Remove or shut off all sources of ignition. Remove mechanically or
                   contain on an absorbent material. Keep out of sewers and waterways.

WASTE DISPOSAL: Disposal must be in accordance with applicable federal, state, or
                 local regulations. Determine waste classification at time of
                 disposal. Conditions of use may render the spent product a hazardous
                 waste. Enclosed-controlled incineration is recommended unless
                 directed otherwise by applicable ordinances.

EMPTY CONTAINERS: The container for this product can present explosion or fire
                   hazards, even when emptied! To avoid risk of injury, do not cut,
                   puncture or weld on or near this container. Since the emptied
                   containers retain product residue, follow label warnings even after
                   container is emptied.

_____ TOXICOLOGICAL INFORMATION _____

EYE: Irritation score: 1.7/110 (rabbits).

SKIN: Irritation score: 1.5/8.0 (rabbits). Irritation score: 3.4/7.0 (4-day
       repeated patch test in human volunteers). No deaths or adverse effects
       occurred after a single dermal application of 2 g/kg in rabbits.

INGESTION: Acute oral LD50: 3,920 mg/kg (rats).

This product contains a catalytic reformer petroleum distillate. No deaths
occurred in rats exposed to distillate vapors at the maximum attainable vapor
concentration under the experimental conditions (1.67 g/m3) for six hours.
Signs of toxicity included red nasal and lacrimal discharge and dark red lung
foci. Rats exposed to distillate vapors at concentrations as high as 330 mg/m3
for 21 days or 110 mg/m3 for 90 days showed no significant adverse effects.

The distillate was practically non-toxic in rabbits via single dermal contact
and only slightly toxic via single ingestion in rats. In a 21-day rat oral
toxicity study at dose levels from 90 to 300 mg/kg, deaths in excess of
controls occurred only at the 3000 mg/kg level. The only adverse effect seen
in all other groups was gastrointestinal irritation.

In a 90-day study, the distillate was applied dermally to rats and mice at
doses ranging from 170 to 4500 mg/kg. Depression of the growth rates and
deaths occurred at both the 1500 and 4500 mg/kg dose levels in both species.
Dose-related irritation at the application site was observed, but no other
treatment-related effects were seen.

The distillate produced a weak skin tumor response in mice following repeated
application of high levels for life. The distillate was not washed off the
skin between doses. The dose levels and duration of exposure were very high
and do not reflect anticipated human exposure. We believe that this product
does not present a human health risk if the personal and industrial hygiene
practices recommended in this material safety data sheet are followed.

This product contains a cosolvent of a type which has been shown to produce
kidney damage in male rats following prolonged inhalation exposures. The
significance of these findings in terms of human health is uncertain at this

Figure 23.1. Continued

PANASOL AN-2K

PAGE 04 OF 04

_____ TOXICOLOGICAL INFORMATION - CONTINUED _____

time since the male rat seems uniquely prone to kidney damage following
exposures to a variety of hydrocarbons. Although we do not believe these
materials pose a serious human health risk, we recommend that users be cautious
and avoid prolonged breathing of vapors.

This product contains naphthalene. Inhalation of naphthalene vapors has been
reported to cause headache and nausea.

This product contains xylene. Overexposure to xylene can cause irritation,
narcosis, headache, fatigue, irritability, and gastrointestinal disturbances.
Some liver damage and lung inflammation were seen in chronic studies in guinea
pigs but not in rats.

In rat reproduction studies, xylenes were not teratogenic but were embryotoxic
when maternal toxicity was produced. In a mouse study, xylenes were found
teratogenic at doses approaching lethal levels.

Aspiration of this product into the lungs can cause chemical pneumonia and can
be fatal. Aspiration into the lungs can occur while vomiting after ingestion
of this product.

No component of this product present at levels greater than 0.1% is identified
as a carcinogen by NTP, IARC or OSHA.

_____ REGULATORY INFORMATION _____

OSHA HAZARD COMMUNICATION STANDARD: Combustible liquid. Irritant. Target organ
                                    effects.

DOT PROPER SHIPPING NAME (BULK, LAND): Combustible Liquid, N.O.S. (contains
                                       naphthalene and xylene), UN1993, RQ

_____ ISSUE INFORMATION _____

BY:

                                                         ISSUED: December 09, 1987
                                                      SUPERSEDES: February 03, 1987

- "Walk-throughs" or site surveys. The walk-through is the best method of finding hazards, since it allows the health service to search out and identify hazards before they affect workers. The search can be conducted periodically and systematically so that no major hazards will be missed.

Safety officers and occupational hygienists, health nurses, and physicians all are trained to conduct site surveys to detect health and safety hazards. While each professional is most knowledgeable in his or her own area of expertise, all should be alert to hazardous conditions and obvious dangers of any type. A safety officer inspecting the securing of compressed gas cylinders, for example, may notice that welders in the shop are producing great amounts of smoke and fumes that hang in the air but are not wearing respiratory protection. The officer should report these observations to the occupational hygienist, nurse, or physician so that appropriate action may be taken. Similarly, a nurse who observes workers using grinding tools without using eye protection should alert the safety officer.

Although site surveys often are conducted independently by members of the occupational health service, it is generally preferable to use a team approach with a representative of each occupational health specialty area. This approach is most appropriate when a worksite is visited for the first time or in connection with an investigation, and usually is called a "health hazard evaluation" (HHE). It has the advantage of minimizing disturbances to worksite operations; numerous visits over several days by assorted health or safety representatives can be very disruptive.

Before proceeding with an HHE, team members should collect some basic information on the workers at the plant. Form 23.1 specifies the types of information that should be sought. In order to discern patterns in work-related disorders, the team also should review injury and sickness absence records before entering the worksite.

The site visitors should have at least a basic knowledge of the operations carried out at the worksite. Although it is not necessary to know every detail of the work processes before setting out, participants should have sufficient understanding to be alert to the main potential hazards. There are many sources of information on worksite processes, some of which are included in the suggested library in Appendix 3. Sources of information specific to the plant include explanatory folders or brochures produced as part of the organization's public relations activity, engineering reports, interviews with site managers, and formal briefings by representative operational staff members. The information obtained should be recorded and kept by the occupational health service for future reference.

From data obtained in advance about the workforce and the work processes, the evaluation team should be able to anticipate the hazards likely to be encountered during the actual survey. Team members should check off mentally each of the four major hazard categories listed while inspecting the workplace. Common exposures are inventoried here in Table 23.1; Table 23.2 relates these common exposures to the industries in which they are likely to be encountered. These tables are not replacements for more detailed descriptions of the processes in the industry of concern, but may be helpful in anticipating some hazards in the absence of more comprehensive descriptions.

While on site, the visitor should comply with all applicable safety procedures. Certain personal items or grooming styles may be forbidden on the site for safety reasons. These may include matches, lighters, contact lenses, beards or moustaches, loose hair, nylon garments, metal boot cleats or studs, leather soles, normal or wire eyeglass frames,

Form 23.1. Information on Workers Needed Before a Site Survey is Conducted

Number of workers on site:	Male _____	Female _____
Age range of workers:	_____ to	_____ years.
Average age of workers:	_____ years.	
On-site Management:	(names) (positions)	(phone no.)
On-site health and safety representatives:	(names) (positions)	(phone no.)

coins, knives, firearms, jewelry, scarves, loose clothing, high-heeled shoes or boots, open-toed shoes, and running shoes. The visitor should always ask in advance whether restrictions exist, and obtain permission or submit to special arrangements required for an exception to the rules. The visitor also should use appropriate safety equipment during the walk-through, even if the equipment must be brought along. Some managers feel that using safety equipment may unduly alarm their employees, and some occupational health professionals avoid doing so for fear of looking foolish and losing the respect of workers. Even so, there is no reason to jeopardize the health of those entrusted with workers' well-being. Furthermore, by using personal protection, the visitor emphasizes the need for workers at risk to do the same.

An important part of the on-site survey is to confirm the availability of protective equipment to workers; the equipment provided should be appropriate, in good repair, easily accessible, and up-to-date. Table 23.3 presents a checklist of personal protection equipment that may be required.

Upon arriving at the site, the team immediately should report to the site manager and explain the intentions of the survey. This gives the manager the opportunity not only to clarify any questions about the workforce or its operations but also to advise the visitor of any deviations from normal work procedures that may be in effect at that particular time or of any areas that are closed or off-limits. If any areas are designated off-limits, the visitors should be informed of the reasons why and the implications for the thoroughness of the site survey.

During the first site survey, the evaluation team should be accompanied by a supervisor or a knowledgeable worker assigned by the supervisor. On subsequent visits, however, team members may wish to request permission to proceed on their own. Throughout the survey, team members should carry notebooks in which to jot down information, sketch floor plans, and note availability and use of protective equipment. Unless the worksite is excessively noisy, a cassette dictation recorder can be useful for making notes during the survey. A 35-mm reflex camera is handy for recording visual evidence of the working environment that can be used later for recall. Capturing environmental working conditions on film with available light, however, requires some degree of photographic skill and equipment that is capable of meeting the demands of suboptimal lighting conditions. Furthermore, explicit permission always must be obtained from management before taking a camera on-site—there may be safety restrictions on the use of flash photography or security bans on photographing certain industrial processes. The site surveyer should note the identity of the subject immediately after taking each shot, and label all slides or prints upon development to avoid the all too common problem of memory lapses.

Table 23.1. Inventory of Exposures to Common Hazards

A. *Aerosols, Irritants, and Gases*
   Carbon monoxide
   Ethylene oxide
   Formaldehyde
   Inert gases
   Hydrogen sulfide
   Nitrogen dioxide
   Ozone
   Phosgene
   Sewer gas
   Smoke
   Sulphur dioxide

B. *Biological Inhalants*
   Bacteria
   Fungi
   Molds
   Organic dusts
   Spores
   Viruses

C. *Corrosive Substances*
   Acids
   Alkalis
   Ammonia
   Chlorine
   Phenols

D. *Dyes and Stains*
   Aniline dyes
   Azo dyes
   Benzidine

E. *Inorganic Dusts and Powder*
   Asbestos
   Coal dust
   Fiberglass
   Silica
   Talc

F. *Insecticides and Herbicides*
   Carbamates
   Halogenated hydrocarbons
   Organophosphates
   Phenoxyherbicides
   Natural products

G. *Radiation*
   Infrared rays
   Laser beams
   Microwaves
   Radionuclides
   Ultraviolet light
   X-rays
   Yellowcake

H. *Metals and Metal Fumes*
   Aluminum
   Arsenic, arsine
   Beryllium
   Cadmium
   Chromium
   Cobalt
   Iron
   Lead
   Mercury
   Nickel
   Platinum salts

I. *Organic Dust*
   Cotton dust
   Poison oak

J. *Petrochemicals*
   Asphalt and tar
   Creosote
   PBB (polybrominated biphenyls)
   PCB (polychlorinated biphenyls)
   Petroleum distillates

K. *Physical Agents*
   Cold stress
   Heavy lifting
   Noise
   Thermal stress
   Vibration

L. *Plastic and Polymer Constituents*
   Acrylonitrile
   Aliphatic amines
   Epoxy resins
   Phthalates
   Styrene
   Toulene diisocyanate
   Vinyl chloride

M. *Welding Emissions*

N. *Solvents*
   Benzene
   n-Butanol
   Carbon disulfide
   Carbon tetrachloride
   Chloroform
   Glycol ethers (cellusolves)
   Ketones
   Methanol
   Perchlorethylene
   Toulene
   Trichlorethane
   Trichlorethylene

Table 23.2. Inventory of Industries and Occupations and Corresponding Exposures to Major Hazards

Industry/Occupation	Hazard Group
Agriculture/Farming/Pest control	A, B, F, K, M
Automobile/Aircraft mfg. and repair	A, C, E, H, K, M
Baking/Food handling	B, L, M
Boiler operations and cleaning	A, C, E, K
Carpentry/Woodworking/Lumber industry	B, I, J, K, N
Ceramics and masonry	E, H
Chemical industry, biotechnology, and users of chemicals	A–N
Construction/Demolition/Road work/Maintenance/Plastering	C, D, E, K, J, M, N
Dry cleaning/Laundry	D, K, N
Electricity/Electronics	A, C, E, H, J, N
Foundry work	A, C, E, H, K, M, N
Health care/Laboratory work/Dental work	A–E, G, J–L, N
Machinery/Grinding/Metalwork	A, C, H, K, M, N
Mining	A, E, G, K, M
Oil and gas/Petrochemical industry	A, C, G, J, K, N
Paper industry	E, H, N
Plastics manufacturing/Molding	E, J, L
Plumbing/Pipefitting/Shipfitting	A, C, E, H, K, M
Printing/Lithography	D, K, N
Sandblasting/Spray painting	A, E, H, K, N
Textile industry	A, D, K, I, N
Transportation maintenance (shipyard/dockyard)	A, C, E, H, J, K, N
Welding	A, E, H, M

The site survey should follow a logical sequence. The survey may follow a geographical orientation, with the team taking each building in turn. Whenever possible, however, the survey should follow the actual sequence of production, even if a particular process is of primary interest. Starting at the point where raw materials are brought onto the site or are stored for use, the walk-through should parallel the production process, observing each operation until the final finishing operation is carried out or the product leaves the site. The natural temptation is to head directly to the place where there is the greatest hazard. This tendency must be resisted if other significant hazards are not to be overlooked or missed due to time constraints or fatigue.

All hazards identified should be noted along with the engineering controls and protective equipment that may be present. The site visitor should not be afraid to be curious or to ask any questions that will clarify the procedures. When the visitor does not know the health effects of materials found in the workplace, the names and quantities of the materials should be recorded for later reference and investigation.

Besides observing, examining, and noting the condition of the protective equipment, the visitor should question workers about their methods of work and their use of protective equipment in actual practice. Asking the workers simple and direct questions about their opinions of the specific job hazards and their perceptions of the risks will illuminate their knowledge about the true potential effects of these hazards.

Workers expect answers from the plant nurse, hygienist, or physician. When asked, the visitor should not be reluctant to express an opinion based on expert knowledge;

Table 23.3. Inventory of Personal Protective Equipment

Head Protection:	Hardhat, bump cap, helmet, cloth cap, hairnet, hood.
Eye Protection:	Goggles (UV, infrared, clear), safety glasses, face-shield.
Respiratory Protection:	Dust mask, organic vapor mask, full-face cannister respirator, emergency compressed air bottle supply respirator, respirator spectacles.
Hearing Protection:	Earplugs, earmuffs, acoustic helmet.
Hand Protection:	Barrier cream, gloves, mitts, gauntlets.
Foot Protection:	Safety boots or shoes, instep protectors, cleats, insulated boots, grounded shoe covers, rubbers.
Body Protection:	Impervious suit, waterproof garment, apron, heatproof suit, flameproof/resistant garment, jacket, body armour, knee or elbow protection, wet suit.

otherwise he conveys the message that he considers current practices to be satisfactory, even when they are not. Furthermore, workers are reassured when a health professional takes an interest in their work and their personal health. The next meeting between the occupational health professional and the worker will benefit from the establishment of a relationship that allows for a better appreciation of the work and the hazards that are being faced.

Balancing the need for candor in answering questions is the need for discretion. The prospects for changing a harmful work procedure or eliminating a hazardous substance from a worksite should not be discussed with the individual worker when such matters are beyond the direct control of the visitor. Rather, the visitor should discuss findings first with the supervisor or manager of the operation to avoid embarrassment, misunderstandings, and long-term ill feelings toward the occupational health service.

Principal findings of the survey may be discussed with the site supervisor immediately following completion of the survey or may be conveyed later to the manager in a full report. In any event, before leaving the site, the visitor always should thank both the manager and the supervisor for the opportunity to visit and for all the assistance that has been given. Simple courtesies cement valuable relationships.

Monitoring Hazards

Hazards that can be sampled can be measured and compared to safe levels. If the results show the hazard level to be unsafe, appropriate action must be taken. Hazard monitoring is akin to having an early warning system that allows the service to detect and deal with a threat before the health of workers is affected.

Worksite monitoring is a technically complex pursuit, usually requiring the special knowledge and skills of an industrial hygienist. Laboratory analysis also calls for capabilities not normally possessed by medical or engineering laboratories. For the majority of smaller companies it is not economically feasible to have an in-house analytical laboratory or an industrial hygienist. In such situations these resources must be contracted from independent occupational hygiene consultation firms now available in many cities.

Permissible safe levels of significantly hazardous materials are regulated by national or provincial governments. The occupational health service must focus the attention of the employer on these regulated levels, the monitoring that is required to ensure compliance, and the necessity for reporting results.

Controlling Occupational Hazards

Only after workplace hazards are identified and evaluated can they be controlled. This three-part process is the responsibility of two specially trained occupational health professionals: occupational hygienists and safety engineers. Occupational hygienists deal mostly with problems of chemical exposure, ventilation, and plant processes. Larger companies generally have these professionals on staff; medium-sized firms sometimes retain them on a consulting basis. Small companies are frequently at a disadvantage in not having such expertise available. Engineers, on the other hand, are more common in medium and smaller-sized industries and deal mostly with physical hazards, fire control, and safe work practices.

Solving an occupational health problem at a reasonable cost usually involves knowledge and technical resources beyond the capacity of the physician. For one thing, the evaluation process requires experience with the particular industry and special monitoring instruments that test for the presence of appropriate chemical and physical hazards. For another, while some problems are simple to solve, many mandate extensive and costly changes in the plant structure and the manufacturing or production process. Selecting and designing the best solution to the problem can be a highly technical engineering challenge. Sometimes, the only solution is no solution—because of technical constraints in a complex work process or procedure, complete elimination of a particular hazard may be unfeasible. The objective then should be to isolate the hazard in order to prevent workers from coming into contact with it.

Table 23.4 summarizes the basic approaches to controlling occupational hazards: engineering controls, substitution, containment and isolation, personal protection, administrative controls, and behavioral controls. There are variations on these approaches and numerous "tricks of the trade," but working knowledge of these six basic approaches will help the physician understand what solutions may be proposed to a given occupational health problem. The optimal solution to a particular problem balances technical requirements with available resources and may involve a blend of several approaches.

Engineering Controls
The design of heavy equipment calls for mounting machinery on sound-absorbing pads so as to minimize noise and vibration. Such engineering controls are the preferred means of reducing occupational hazards because they minimize the chances of exposure due to accident or to individual oversight. But engineering controls can be very expensive, especially when they are added on, or "retrofitted," to older equipment; they usually

Table 23.4. Technical Approaches to Solving Occupational Health Problems

	Effectiveness	Cost	Reliability
Engineering Controls	High	High	High
Containment and Isolation	High	High	High
Substitution	High	Variable	Variable
Personal Protection	High	Moderate	Variable
Administrative Controls	Low	Low	Variable
Behavior Controls	Low	Low	Low

In individual cases, the effectiveness, cost, and reliability of a given solution compared to alternatives may vary greatly. These values are only the most likely characteristics in most situations.

are more effective and economical when built into the original design of the plant. Nevertheless, improper maintenance and operator neglect may cause a breakdown in the effectiveness of such controls.

Containment and Isolation

Complete automation is one way to isolate hazards; another is to contain the hazard by means of an appropriate barrier, such as a soundproof blanket over a noisy machine or a vent pipe to carry off a poisonous gas. Hazard containment has the advantage of allowing employees freedom to move about the workplace without encumbrance.

Containment may involve constructing a shell around a machine or placing a barrier between the source and the work area. Isolation may involve removing a particularly hazardous process to a location away from workers. Both are highly effective ways of dealing with many hazards. Chemical processes are usually tightly contained in an enclosed tank or reaction chamber. Sound-absorbing baffles or enclosures are commonly used to reduce noise exposure. As with engineering controls, however, the effectiveness of containment and isolation often depends on careful maintenance and is susceptible to carelessness. Care must also be taken that an isolated facility does not become an environmental hazard to the surrounding community, as in the case of secondary smelting operations where heavy metals are released.

If hazard containment or control is not possible (for example, if the noisy machine overheats if blanketed or the poisonous gas cannot be vented), the only alternative is worker containment. This can be done either by literally containing the workers themselves, for example in a soundproof control room, or by issuing personal protective clothing or equipment.

Substitution

Often, a hazard can be dealt with by substituting a less hazardous alternative. For example, the carcinogenic and relatively acutely toxic solvent trichlorethylene was replaced in the 1970s by trichlorethane, a much safer yet related compound. Asbestos insulation has been largely replaced by fibrous glass and other manmade mineral fibers. Unfortunately, acceptable substitutes are not always available at a reasonable cost, and even when substitutes are available, they often have not been subjected to the same rigorous evaluation as the materials they are supposed to replace. For example, manmade mineral fibers have not been as well evaluated for their cancer risk as has asbestos; recent reports suggest that the carcinogenic potential for manmade mineral fibers could be significant. The manufacture and use of these materials therefore should be carried out with the same precautions used for asbestos. Although substitution is very desirable and often effective, it is sometimes impossible, often impractical, and may still require engineering controls.

Personal Protection

Personal protection generally is considered less satisfactory than engineering controls in solving occupational health problems because the effectiveness of control devices depends on factors that are less easily controlled—the fit between a personal protective device (such as earplugs or a respirator) and the worker using it; the education and compliance of the worker; and the commitment of the employer in ensuring proper use of the device. Some hazards can be dealt with only by personal protection; in these cases, the occupational health service must ensure that it has selected the proper protective apparatus for the job and should make available a variety of alternative devices from which workers may choose. Nevertheless, the effectiveness of personal protection generally is affected by so many technical and behavioral variables that it should be avoided if engineering controls are possible and feasible.

Administrative Controls

Administrative controls are used primarily where cumulative exposure must be kept to permissible levels, as with noise and ionizing radiation. Workers are rotated among stations on a regular schedule to reduce the possibility of any one individual receiving an excessive exposure. Administrative controls are useful as added safety precautions but they are not a legitimate substitute for controlling the exposure itself. In acute emergency situations, usually involving radiation, they may be necessary as an extreme temporary measure until the problem is brought under control.

Behavioral Controls

Behavioral controls involve educating and motivating workers to minimize their exposure and practice safe work habits. They also may involve placing warning signs or signals. This approach is usually considered the least satisfactory because it depends on the individual worker's alertness, motivation, and comprehension and may be compromised easily by minor distractions, boredom, fatigue, passive-aggressive behavior, ill health, poor eyesight or hearing, misunderstanding, language barriers, and lack of personal motivation. Redesigning the job in order to avoid dangerous or awkward motions and exposure to hazards is a more effective form of behavioral control, especially when combined with engineering controls.

Further Reading

Clayton GD, Clayton FE (eds): Patty's Industrial Hygiene and Toxicology (ed 3). New York, John Wiley and Sons, 1982.

Doull J, Klausen C, Amdur M (eds): Casarett and Doull's Toxicology (ed 3). New York, MacMillan, 1980.

Finkel AJ: Hamilton and Hardy's Industrial Toxicology (ed 4). Littleton, Massachusetts, John Wright-PSG, 1982.

Guidotti TL, Goldsmith DF: Occupational cancer. Am Fam Physician 1986; 34:146–152.

Guidotti TL, Novak RE: Hearing conservation and occupational exposure to noise. Am Fam Physician 1983; 28(4):181–186.

Hatch LL, et al: Self-Evaluation of Occupational Safety and Health Programs. Washington DC, U.S. Government Printing Office, National Institute for Occupational Safety and Health Pub. No. DHEW (NIOSH) 78–187, 1978.

Identification and control of work-related diseases. Geneva, World Health Organization Technical Report Series No. 714, 1985.

Last JM (ed): Maxcy-Rosenau Public Health and Preventive Medicine (ed 11). New York, Appleton-Century-Crofts, 1980.

Occupational and Environmental Health Committee of the American Lung Association of San Diego and Imperial Counties: Taking the occupational history. Ann Intern Med 1983; 99:641–651.

Occupational Health/Safety Programs Accreditation Commission: Standards, Interpretations and Audit Criteria for Performance of Occupational Health Programs. Akron, Ohio, American Industrial Hygiene Association, 1979.

Olishifski JB (ed): Fundamentals of Industrial Hygiene (ed 2). Chicago, National Safety Council, 1979.

Parmeggiani L (ed): Encyclopaedia of Occupational Health and Safety (ed 3). Geneva, International Labour Organization, 1983.

Proctor NH, Hughes JP: Chemical Hazards of the Workplace. Philadelphia, J.B. Lippincott, 1978.

Rom WN (ed): Environmental and Occupational Medicine. Boston, Little Brown and Co, 1983.

Sax NI: Dangerous Properties of Industrial Materials (ed 6). New York, Van Nostrand, 1984.

U.S. National Institute for Occupational Safety and Health and Occupational Safety and Health Administration: Occupational Health Guidelines for Chemical Hazards. Washington, DC, U.S. Government Printing Office, 1981. DHHS (NIOSH) Publication No. 81–123.

24 INDUSTRIAL EMERGENCIES INVOLVING HAZARDOUS SUBSTANCES

Hazardous substances are compounds and mixtures that pose a threat to health and property because of their toxicity, flammability, explosive potential, radiation, or other dangerous properties. The public's attention tends to be drawn by the media to carcinogens, industrial waste, pesticides, and radiation hazards. However, innumerable compounds that do not fall into these categories also can threaten health and safety. Gasoline, for example, can explode with the destructive force of gunpowder. Although industrial emergencies involving hazardous substances take many forms and may be highly individual, the great majority seem to involve a relatively narrow range of hazardous substances, such as solvents, paints and coatings, pesticides, acids and alkalis, and metal solutions.

Advance Preparation

Many steps can be taken on the local level to prepare for a hazardous substances emergency and to reduce the likelihood of an incident occurring. This plan should include a frank and realistic assessment of the capabilities of local authorities in dealing with such problems. As part of the plan, responsible managers should inventory sites where an incident might occur and develop—and update regularly—a list of agencies and commercial firms available for backup and laboratory services.

Central to the plan is a system for communicating quickly with local physicians and health facilities, whether by telephone tree, telegram, or courier. The means chosen during the incident will depend on the urgency of the incident as it unfolds and the types of systems that already have been set up. Of equal importance is a means of disseminating accurate information to the public. This may include a rumor control committee composed of community representatives and public information agencies. The committee should be briefed regularly by the knowledgeable spokesperson representing the firm or agency and should be prepared to use a telephone hotline, reports to community groups, and regular press conferences to spread the word to the public.

Slight differences in opinion, interpretation, and understanding can come across as confusion, uncertainty, and rivalry. Therefore, it is particularly important to funnel all public information, whenever possible, through a single spokesperson.

Incident Management

The management of incidents involving hazardous substances and patients exposed to these substances does not necessarily depend on the specific hazard presented by the exposure. A specific exposure may not be identifiable nor an expected health outcome apparent. Many common exposures are nonspecific in their actions and are treated with supportive care. When an incident occurs in a community, the physician may be confronted with two groups to evaluate or manage: those with real signs of toxicity and those who only suspect exposure. Distinguishing between the two frequently is difficult. Very often individual patients are convinced that they have sustained a toxic exposure when it is very unlikely that exposure could have occurred.

A true hazardous substances emergency is best managed by a specialist with training in toxicology but such specialists are in short supply and may not be on the scene when an incident occurs. Table 24.1 provides a checklist of questions to be asked in the event a physician is called to assist in managing a hazardous substances incident. A careful, methodical approach and clear, concise statements to the authorities and to the public are in some ways more important than a detailed knowledge of the toxicology and safety hazards involved. It is important, however, to find out as much as possible before offering an opinion that is likely to affect the management of the situation. Therefore, when being interviewed by the press or when testifying at a public hearing, never guess—stick to the facts and well thought out opinions.

The physician involved in these types of emergency should follow a three-step process of incident management. Each step will go much more smoothly when the time comes if some investment in advance preparation has been made.

Step 1: Evaluate the Problem
As the incident unfolds, the physician in charge needs the most accurate information available. One good means of keeping track of information is an incident log, in which the physician can record in one place all pertinent information, with each entry dated, timed, and identified as to the source of the report. Preliminary data should allow the physician to estimate the magnitude of risk to the population and decide on the appropriate medical response: What hazardous substances are involved? What are their toxic and safety hazards? How many people now have been exposed and how many may be exposed in the near future? Among these people, are there likely to be any in the community who may be at exceptional risk (the very young, the very old, the ill and those susceptible to the effects of exposure as a result of a condition or illness, such as pregnancy or asthma)? The physician must be prepared to revise his or her opinions constantly.

Correct identification of the substances involved is important and requires technical expertise. The contents of drums should be sampled—labels on drums may be misleading because drums are often recycled. Only an occupational hygienist, using suitable

Table 24.1. Checklist for Physicians Involved in Industrial Emergencies Involving Hazardous Substances*

1. What toxic and hazardous substances have been identified?
   • What concentrations have been found in air, water, and soil?
   • What are the known health hazards at these concentrations?
   • What are the potential hazards of fire, explosion, or chemical interaction?
2. How many persons have been exposed and how many are likely to become exposed in the near future?
   • What groups in the exposed population are likely to be most susceptible to health effects?
   • How many cases of confirmed exposure are resulting in hospital admissions? Outpatient visits?
   • What clinical findings, if any, are being observed?
3. What technical resources are available on short notice to assist in evaluation and control?
4. What health and safety precautions should rescue and reentry workers be taking?
   • What environmental monitoring should be performed?
   • What protective equipment should workers use?
   • What is the maximum time workers should be allowed to spend at the location?
   • What health surveillance or health monitoring should be done after the emergency is over?
5. Is the community adequately handling the casualties?
   • What is the capacity of local hospitals, clinics, and physicians to absorb the additional caseload?
   • Should hospital disaster plans be mobilized?
   • Is intensive care of specialty services adequate or available where needed?
   • Are local physicians experienced and knowledgeable about medical aspects of this problem? If not, what is the best way to reach them quickly with the information they need?
6. Is this community covered by a controlled data repository (such as a tumor registry or population-based research study) that could be used to follow the exposed population in the future?

* This and subsequent tables in this chapter are adapted from: Managing incidents involving hazardous substances. Guidotti TL, American Journal of Preventive Medicine 1986; 2:148–154.

personal protective equipment, should take samples. After testing at the site to determine the basic properties of the chemicals, the samples should be securely and safely transported in sealed containers to a suitably equipped laboratory certified for this type of work. Unless there is a compelling reason to act, such as a fire or a rapid leak, it is usually more prudent to let the material sit undisturbed than to act hastily before it is identified and appropriate precautions can be taken. The process of analyzing, evaluating, and cleaning up a hazardous substances site, already expensive on a routine basis, can become extremely expensive on an emergency basis. There are few commercial firms specializing in these operations and they may have to travel long distances if the incident occurs away from an urban or industrial center. If circumstances force action before the material is identified, the only prudent move is to assume the worst, unless one has exceptionally strong circumstantial evidence that the material is not highly toxic.

Once a material is identified, the hazard potential must be determined. Users of any hazardous material are required to keep on file a Material Safety Data Sheet (MSDS) prepared by the manufacturer. MSDSs usually give reasonable information on the safety hazard of chemical formulations, but they almost always have incomplete descriptions of a compound's toxic effects. Since many chemical formulations are proprietary mixtures, the MSDS may fail to identify all components of a product or their proportions. Table 24.2 lists hotline numbers for determining quickly the hazard or toxicity of substances that may be involved in an emergency incident.

Determining the number of residents and employees at risk requires only a general estimate at this point. Not everyone in the community actually will be exposed to the substance; for purposes of planning the medical response, the physician must concentrate on the characteristics of the persons who may come into contact with the material. Knowledge of the community at risk allows one to alert local health providers in advance and to warn susceptible individuals of the need to take protective measures.

Step 2: Contain the Problem

The next step in the emergency response process is to control the situation and minimize the potential for exposure.

Where sealed drums have been discovered at an illegal or abandoned dumpsite, for example, the affected area should be cordoned off with barricades that restrict access to everyone except authorized personnel. Later, a company licensed to haul commercial hazardous materials can be hired to perform an initial evaluation and to remove the waste to an approved disposal site.

More complex situations require good coordination with police, fire, and public health authorities. Fire departments are best equipped to handle safety hazards but often need advice and assistance when dealing with toxic materials. Very difficult situations, such as fires that involve multiple toxic substances either known and unknown, pose serious threats to public safety personnel and may require a medical presence on site.

Protecting workers engaged in clean-up and control activities at the site is an important responsibility for the medical officer. Workers should be guided by a site work plan that includes proper security and emergency provisions; be equipped with suitable protective gear, back-up personnel, and emergency telecommunications from the site; and follow proper decontamination procedures.

Another important aspect of containing the problem is squelching public overreaction. Any incident provokes rumors and misinformation that must be controlled in order to avoid panic or misguided interference in public safety measures. While large-scale population evacuations are very rare, stressful, costly, and may create additional safety problems, in extreme situations evacuation may be unavoidable. In these cases, medical assistance stations may be needed.

Step 3: Manage the Health Effects

Medical emergencies involving hazardous substances are less common than ambiguous exposure situations—those in which a person is believed to have been exposed to a toxic substance and requires an appropriate medical evaluation. When the substance in question is known, an appropriate medical surveillance evaluation can be derived from information in many of the references given at the end of this book. The most

Table 24.2. Telephone Numbers for Emergency Information on Toxicology

1. National Response Center, U.S. Coast Guard (24 hour)

   800 424-8802   Used in USA only

   202 267-2675   To be used in Washington DC or from outside the USA

   Provides emergency information and response to a chemical spill or release in U.S. coastal or inland waters.

2. CHEMTREC, Chemical Manufacturers Association (24 hour)

   800 424-9300   Used in USA only

   202 483-7616   To be used in Washington DC or for outside the USA (call collect)

   Provides emergency information on spills and chemical emergencies involving the transportation of hazardous materials.

3. RCRA, Superfund Industry Assistance Hotline, U.S. Environmental Protection Agency

   800 424-9346   Used in USA only

   202 382-3000   From Canada, agency would take caller's number and return call toll-free

   Provides information on toxic wastes, dump sites, and the Resource Conservation and Recovery Act.

4. CANUTECH, Transport Canada (24 hour, collect)

   613 996-666   Used in Canada only

   Provides information of a first-aid nature for fires or spills; can provide LD_{50} and other toxicological information from Material Safety Data Sheets.

5. National Pesticide Telecommunications Network (24 hour), U.S. Environmental Protection Agency and Texas Tech University

   800 858-7378   Used in USA only

   806 743-3091   In Texas or from outside USA

   Provides information on toxic potential, proper use, effects, and appropriate disposal and clean-up of pesticides. Does not handle emergency calls.

6. Asbestos Hotline, U.S. Environmental Protection Agency (9:00 a.m.–5:00 p.m. EST)

   800 334-8571   Used in USA only

   Provides information and referral to testing laboratories for issues related to asbestos.

appropriate medical monitoring evaluation may be difficult to determine, however, when the substance is not known or involves a complex mixture.

Lacking a positive identification of the substance, the clinician first should consider the possibility of acute effects to those organ systems most commonly involved in toxic injury: the respiratory, renal, hepatic, dermatologic, and nervous systems. Many incidents involve multiple exposures and/or substances that have multiple effects. Therefore, it is good practice to provide a basic comprehensive evaluation even when a patient presents with a specific clinical complaint. Tables 24.3 and 24.4 outline a comprehensive clinical evaluation strategy for patients presenting with a history of exposure in such circumstances.

When the effects of the incident go beyond the boundaries of the plant, causing injuries or illnesses to be sustained in the community, occupational health professionals

Table 24.3. A Comprehensive Medical Monitoring Evaluation for Persons
Suspected of Toxic Exposure

1. Complete medical history, emphasizing:
   • Current medication
   • Allergies
   • Skin disorders, chronic and acute
   • Respiratory disease, chronic
   • Renal disease, chronic and acute
   • Cancer
   • Pregnancy
   • Estimate of alcohol consumption and timing of last consumption (to assist in
     interpreting liver function tests)
2. Complete physical examination, emphasizing:
   • Skin (irritation, dermatitis)
   • Lungs (bronchitis and bronchospasm)
   • Liver (evidence of early chemical hepatitis)
   • Neurological examination (evidence of peripheral or central neurotoxicity)
   • Pregnancy
3. Laboratory studies:
   • Urinalysis, chemical and microscopic
   • Serum creatinine
   • Liver function tests: SGOT, SGPT, bilirubin
   • Chest film
   • Pulmonary function tests
   • Blood cholinesterase, if organophosphate pesticides may be involved
   • Pregnancy test, if a reproductive hazard may be involved

should furnish local health care providers with regular and accurate bulletins on the
extent of the problem and suggest appropriate management of incident-related cases.
In major incidents, it is very useful to establish a central registry of exposed individuals. This registry can be an invaluable resource for future epidemiologic studies, can
establish eligibility for disability benefits at some future date, and can prove intent in
case of any subsequent legal action.

A major industrial emergency often has serious mental health consequences. Unlike
natural disasters, such as earthquakes and hurricanes, manmade disasters are very difficult for communities to cope with psychologically. Natural disasters, as devastating
as they may be at the time, can knit communities together and are associated with relatively low frequencies of mental health problems among survivors. Manmade disasters,
including industrial incidents, often take a higher social toll for the number of victims
actually involved. They frequently cause divisive speculations on who bears the blame —
and financial responsibility — for the incident, and may create a sense that those affected
are "contaminated," especially when the incident has involved toxic exposures. The
lengthy political and legal maneuvering that usually follows almost always leads to suspicions among the general population that the victims are exploiting the situation. The
victims, meanwhile, exhibit great concern over their future health, often expressed as
questions regarding their risk of cancer or birth defects. They often feel alienated from
their former friends and neighbors, who may come to believe that any action taken
against the interests of the responsible company could lead to economic loss for the

Table 24.4. Interpretation of Tests for Persons Evaluated for Exposure to Toxic Substances

Type of Toxic Response	Test[1]	Common Confounding Factors	Follow-up Tests
Dermatitis	Physical Exam	Any cause of rash	Physical examination[3]
Respiratory injury[2]	Chest film Pulmonary	Acute and chronic respiratory disease	Chest film[4] Pulmonary function tests[4] Bronchoprovocation challenge
Hepatotoxicity	Liver function tests	Hepatitis of any cause, alcohol consumption	Repeat tests
Nephrotoxicity	Urinalysis Serum creatinine	Chronic or acute renal disease	Urinalysis[3] Serum creatinine[3]
Neurotoxicity	Neurological exam	(Many)	Neurological exam[3]
Carcinogenicity	(None)	(Many)	Reporting system[5]
Reproductive	Fetal auscultation	(Many)	Pregnancy

1. Perform on second or third day after exposure.
2. Significant respiratory injury is usually associated with symptoms at the time of exposure or shortly thereafter.
3. Repeat in one or two weeks if screen is normal, but patient's exposure documented.
4. Repeat in one or two months if screen is normal, but patient's exposure documented.
5. There is no sure way to predict individual risk of cancer; latency period after exposure is measured in decades.

community as a whole. Furthermore, litigation tends to be prolonged and bitter in such incidents, magnifying the divisive effects. In such situations, counselling and preventive mental health interventions are very valuable.

Further Reading

Gist R, Stolz SB: Mental health promotion and the media. American Psychologist 1982; pp. 1136–1139.

Green BL: Assessing levels of psychological impairment following disaster: Consideration of actual and methodological approaches. Journal of Nervous and Mental Disorders 1982; 170:544–552.

Guidotti TL: Managing incidents involving hazardous substances. Am J Prev Med 1986; 2:148–154.

Guidotti TL: San Diego County's Community Right-to-Know Ordinance: Case study of a local approach to hazardous substances control. J Pub Health Policy 1984; 5:396–409.

Highland JH (ed): Hazardous Waste Disposal: Assessing the Problem. Ann Arbor, Ann Arbor Science and the Society for Occupational and Environmental Health, 1982.

Irey NS: Environmental emergencies—their characteristics and variations. Military Medicine 1985; (4):191–199.

Logue JN, Melick ME, Hansen H: Research issues and directions in the epidemiology of health effects of disasters. Epidemiology Review 1981; 3:140–162.

Maxwell C: Hospital organizational response to the nuclear accident at Three Mile Island: Implications for future-oriented disaster planning. Am J Pub Health 1982; 72:275–279.

Miller RW: Areawide chemical contamination: Lessons from case histories. JAMA 1981; 245:1548–1551.

National Institute for Occupational Safety and Health: NIOSH Work Bulletin: Hazardous Waste Sites and Hazardous Substance Emergencies. Cincinnati, DHHS (NIOSH) Publication No. 83–100, 1982.

National Response Team of the National Oil and Hazardous Substances Contingency Plan: Hazardous Materials Emergency Planning Guide. Washington DC, U.S. Environmental Protection Agency, NRT-1, March 1987.

Office of Technology Assessment, U.S. Congress: Technologies and Management Strategies for Hazardous Waste Control. Washington, DC, US Government Printing Office (GPO ffl052-003-00901-3), 1983.

Reggiani G: Medical problems raised by the TCDD contamination in Seveso, Italy. Arch Toxicol 1978; 40:161–168.

Reko K: The psychosocial impact of environmental disasters. Bull Environ Contamination and Toxicology 1984; 33:655–661.

Rutherford WH, de Boer J: The definition and classification of disasters. Injury 1983; 15:10–12.

Sanner Ph, Wolcott BW: Stress reactions among participants in mass casualty simulations. Ann Emerg Med 1983; 12:426–428.

Seta JA, Sundin DS: Trends of a decade: A perspective on occupational hazard surveillance, 1970–1983. MMWR 1984; 34(2SS):15SS-24SS.

Singer TJ: An introduction to disaster: Some considerations of a psychological nature. Aviat Space Environ Med 1982; 53:245–250.

Smith JS Jr, Fisher JH: Three Mile Island: The silent disaster. JAMA 1981; 245:16561659.

Wilkinson CB: Aftermath of a disaster: The collapse of the Hyatt Regency Hotel skywalks. Am J Psychiat 1983; 140:1134–1139.

Zaki MH, Moran D, Harris D: Pesticides in groundwater: The aldicarb story in Suffolk County, N.Y. Am J Pub Health 1982; 72:1391–1395.

25 ALCOHOL AND DRUG TESTING

For decades, alcohol abuse has been recognized as a serious problem for industry. Only recently has such recognition been extended to drug abuse. To the employer, the symptoms—or results, as it were—are similar: lowered productivity, increased absenteeism, endangered security, and increased accident rates. The Research Triangle Institute of North Carolina has estimated the cost of drug abuse to the U.S. economy in 1983 at $60 billion, triple the amount for 1980. Since 1975, more than 50 train accidents have been attributed to drug- or alcohol-impaired workers. In Canada, according to the Canadian Council of Safety Associations, substance abusers have triple the absenteeism and tardiness rates of other workers and double the number of accidents considered normal for the type of work they are doing.

In response to these problems, growing numbers of companies in North America have introduced employee drug testing programs. Currently, about half of the Fortune 500 companies screen job applicants for drug use. Some companies, with little or no planning, have introduced mandatory drug testing of the entire workforce. Unfortunately, the results of these efforts often have been as bad as or worse than the situation they were intended to correct. The outcomes of testing programs have included expensive and lengthy legal battles, acrimonious labor-management conflicts, and disastrous declines in worker morale and productivity. Many firms now are taking a long second look at the matter of drug testing and are approaching the issue with greater caution.

Testing Pros and Cons

The fundamental question concerning testing conducted at the workplace for alcohol and drug abuse is whether it is effective in reducing the problems created by substance abuse. Studies carried out by the U.S. Army and Navy and by companies that have tested their employees for alcohol and drug use show that a carefully planned testing program is associated with significant reductions in on-the-job use of drugs and with corresponding improvements in performance. Whether drug testing acts as a deterrent, causes reduction of drug use, or simply weeds out drug users remains uncertain, however. Although the theory may appear plausible, the evidence available to date has not proven that employee drug testing can make the workplace safer and more secure.

Polls conducted following President Reagan's September 1986 "declaration of war" on drugs showed widespread support in the United States for mandatory drug testing in the workplace. However, many organizations and informed parties, including labor unions, are opposed to mandatory testing. As a matter of policy, for example, the American Medical Association does not endorse mandatory drug screening. The chief objections to drug testing are as follows:

- Mandatory drug testing conflicts with civil liberties.
- Drug testing is authoritarian in nature and the inconsistencies that occur in test results inevitably will lead to labor-management unrest.
- The most accurate and reliable test methods are not used because employers find them too expensive.
- There is little or no regulation of the quality of laboratory analyses.
- There is insufficient evidence linking drug use to worksite accidents.
- Worker drug testing has more to do with morality than with safety. This explains why employers do not require their employees to take tests for alcohol although alcohol use can be most clearly correlated with accidents and is the most commonly used drug in North America.
- Although positive test results may indicate use of a drug, they give no measure of impairment.

Clearly, companies that choose to test employees for substance abuse need to develop programs that address their problems effectively without causing undue disruption or more trouble than benefit. Input should be sought from all quarters. Employers with unionized workforces, especially, must seek labor support for drug testing early in planning, since most bargaining contracts fail to include mention of drug testing. Company management, labor leaders, employees, the occupational health service, and legislative authorities each have a role to play in developing a workable drug testing program. Outlined in this chapter are the many factors that must be considered in developing an alcohol and drug testing program. Included here also are guidelines for planning an anti-drug program.

The Rationale for Drug Screening

There are a number of reasons why an employer might want to test workers for drugs. Although any one employer may posit a variety of reasons, all may be categorized into two groups: those that have a moral or altruistic basis and those that have a pragmatic or operational basis. A moralistic viewpoint may underlie, and to some degree shape, the approach used in a drug testing program initiated for operational reasons. It is, however, important that these two reasons be quite clearly identified in order to avoid misunderstandings and misapplication of screening.

Drug testing programs undertaken for either reason may be intended to solve an ongoing problem (reactive program) or to guard against a problem that otherwise might occur (preventive program). Reactive programs, if successful, may be perpetuated as preventive programs.

Based on their reason and intent, drug testing programs, then, may be characterized as follows:

- *Practical-Preventive.* Drug use in the local community is high and the employer wants to guard against accidents or poor productivity.
- *Practical-Reactive.* Drug use is known to be associated with or is suspected as a cause of unacceptably high accident rates, increases in workplace thefts, or a hike in absence and drop in productivity.
- *Moral-Preventive.* The employer has a strong aversion to drugs and wants to deter or prevent their use at the place of business.
- *Moral-Reactive.* The employer feels an obligation to identify and assist workers who have a drug dependency.

These examples illustrate the many motivations that underlie drug testing programs. In practice, drug testing always should be undertaken primarily for clearly defined operational reasons. The moral aspects should be of secondary importance in a drug screening program, serving a strictly supportive role, if the employer is to avoid serious problems when screening workers for drug abuse.

The reasons an employer chooses to institute a drug testing program will dictate who should carry out the tests, which workers will be tested, and how the testing will be done. For example, if drug use testing is done to counter theft at work rather than for health and safety reasons, it should be conducted by security personnel. The type and timing of tests done for this purpose and the selection of workers for testing will differ greatly from testing done for health or safety reasons. The reporting of test results and the subsequent disposition of workers found to have positive results also will differ depending on whether testing is done for security or for health or safety reasons.

It is important for the occupational health service to dissociate itself completely from security checks and disciplinary action in order to maintain its credibility with workers. If the service becomes linked with security in the minds of workers, it no longer will be viewed as an objective resource to which the worker can bring personal health problems in confidence.

In establishing a rationale for undertaking drug testing, the employer should realize that drug testing alone will not reveal whether an individual is addicted to a drug or will suffer future functional impairment or even if his use of drugs will worsen. Furthermore, studies have found no simple correlation between casual off-job use of drugs and safety on the job.

Assuming that the drug test used is valid and specific (see Chapter 20), the results may reveal that a specific drug has been used, but it cannot say why. There are several relatively "benign" reasons why an individual may take an addictive drug: as an act of rebellion, out of curiosity, for pleasure, as a means of identifying with the "counterculture" or an alternative lifestyle, or for a quasi-religious experience. True drug abuse, however, always indicates the presence of a significant underlying condition – such as anxiety, depression, chronic feelings of inadequacy, uncontrollable resentment, or anger – or social disruption that may not yet be overt. These are not simple matters that can be made clear by drug testing alone. The wise employer will avoid trying to solve the drug-related problems of society as a whole through drug testing at the workplace.

Determining Testing Subjects

The reason for introducing a drug testing program determines which workers will be selected for testing. This selection is constrained by a number of ethical and legal obligations and by technical limitations to drug testing. The employer also must consider the possible consequences to workforce morale should drug testing be applied in a manner that employees consider unjust. Far from improving or maintaining productivity, a poorly applied drug testing program could have the opposite effect.

The possible options for selecting workers for testing include:

- All employees, without exception.
- Workers directly involved in "hazardous" operations or who are at greater than average risk of injury.
- Operators of equipment that, if improperly used, could endanger the health or safety of co-workers or the public.
- All applicants for employment, without exception.
- Applicants who apply for "hazardous" jobs.
- Applicants who apply for jobs that, if improperly carried out, could endanger the health or safety of co-workers or the public.
- Workers involved in a workplace accident that is under investigation.
- Workers who show deficits in work performance and who are suspected of using drugs.
- Workers suspected of workplace theft.
- Workers suspected of dealing drugs at work.
- Applicants who apply for jobs that, if improperly done, could have grave financial or legal consequences for the company or that could seriously damage its reputation.

The list may be summarized in four categories: all current employees, selected current employees, all work applicants, and selected work applicants. (It should be noted that the discussion here is concerned only with those options on the list that focus on health issues. Occupational health personnel should not be involved in drug testing activities in which neither health nor safety are the prime considerations.)

Testing all employees or all job applicants, without exception, is arbitrary, non-discriminatory, and not likely to be cost-effective. Such a "shotgun" approach is not tied to actual workplace hazards or performance requirements; occasional and moderate use of alcohol and some drugs away from the workplace has no noticeable effect on performance in many jobs, so the improvement in productivity may be minimal. Unless skillfully handled, such a comprehensive program runs the risk of being perceived by workers simply as the employer's moral crusade. It has the effect of announcing to job applicants, in particular, that the company doesn't want drug users as employees because it disapproves of drug use.

Selecting for drug testing workers who could endanger themselves, their co-workers, or the public by working under the influence of drugs or alcohol has the advantage of concentrating efforts where they are likely to be most useful. Selective testing lacks the moral overtone presented by universal testing and accommodates the important principle that mandatory worker health examinations should be specifically related to the hazards of the job.

Preplacement screening of applicants for hazardous jobs may have a deterrent effect by discouraging drug abuse, but this theory has never been proven. Putting applicants on notice that they must agree to submit to periodic drug testing while employed would seem sufficient to turn away many drug users.

Studies on the association between drug and alcohol abuse and industrial accidents are inconsistent. The publicity surrounding spectacular disasters in which workers were intoxicated convey the impression that drug or alcohol use is invariably associated with workplace accidents. However, some studies have reported surprisingly low correlations. Nonetheless, in communities where drug or alcohol abuse is thought to be prevalent, it would be wise for an employer to test workers who have been involved in a workplace accident that is to be investigated.

Workers whose performance is below reasonable expectations and who are suspected of being alcohol or drug abusers should be referred for medical assessment. (See Chapter 18.) The occupational health service can then advise whether drug testing is appropriate, on the basis of its evaluation of the worker.

Often, the first signs of drug abuse are social or occupational disruption—a personality change; unusual irritability or mood swings; inexplicable work absences; problems with the law, family, or friends; or decreased attention to safety and work productivity. Drugs usually have one effect during the "high" and another during withdrawal. Pathological use of alcohol and other drugs is characterized by at least one of the following: intoxication throughout the day, inability to stop using the substance, repeated failed attempts to control its use, a daily need for the substance, or continual use despite serious resulting illness. Table 25.1 presents clinical features of the abuse patterns of common drugs; physical dependence may be recognized by withdrawal signs. Alcohol abuse is still by far the most widespread type of drug disorder, but unfortunately there are still no reliable predictors as to who will become an alcoholic or repeated abuser of alcohol.

Legal and Ethical Issues

Workplace drug testing of employees has spawned a plethora of unresolved legal issues. Throughout the United States, employers are confronted by threats of litigation or court battles from disappointed job applicants or disgruntled employees who have been subjected to drug testing. Situated between the employer and the workers, the occupational health practitioner tries to balance the interests of both. (See Chapter 18.)

Employers find themselves in a double bind. Occupational Safety and Health Administration regulations and state or provincial laws require them to maintain a healthy and safe workplace. At the same time, guarantees of individual rights and freedoms impede attempts to forestall drug use by employees outside the workplace.

Workers may feel that the employer has discriminated against them or has invaded their privacy through mandatory drug testing. From this perspective, they have no recourses other than the courts if they are fired or denied a job denied because of a drug test. In the absence of specific laws, worker opposition to drug testing rests on basic principles, including the rights to privacy of the person, to freedom from unreasonable search and seizure, to due process of the law, and to equal protection under the law. It is clear that the individual's right to privacy is not absolute; state

Table 25.1. Specific Drugs of Abuse

Drug Class	Drug Names	Effects of Dependence	Effects of Withdrawal	Effects of Overdose
Barbiturates, sedatives, and hypnotics	Phenobarbitol Diazepines Meprobamate Methaqualone Chloral hydrate Glutethimide	May produce physical and psychological dependence. Tolerance occurs.	Life-threatening seizures may occur.	Coma and death
Opioids and similarly acting non-opioids	Morphine Heroin Meperidine Hydromorphone Methadone Codeine Propoxyphene Pentazocine	Physical dependence.	May be incapacitating but no seizures occur.	Coma and death
Stimulants	Amphetamine Phenteramine Phenmetrazine Phenylpro-panolamine Methylphenidate	Produce pro-found psycholog-ical dependence. Tolerance occurs.	Depression last-ing months.	Manic State
Cocaine	Cocaine	Extremely addic-tive. Casual use not possible.	Depression.	Coma and death
Hallucinogens	LSD Mescaline Psylocybin Pencyclidine (PCP)	Chronic use is unusual. Toler-ance develops.	Flashbacks may occur.	Depersonaliza-tion, delusions of superhuman powers. Paranoia.
Marijuana	Cannabis THC	Psychological dependence.		
Alcohol	Ethanol	Physical and psychological dependence.	Hallucinations. Seizures may occur.	Coma and death

interests, for example, can override it. Nonetheless, there are laws in some states that support privacy by prohibiting employers from asking whether a worker or job applicant has ever been arrested on a drug-related charge.

Legislative Protections

Managers should be aware of legislation that applies to the employment of drug abusers. In the United States, the Rehabilitation Act of 1973 prohibits employment discrimination against the handicapped, including drug abusers who are able to do their jobs. It applies to federal employers and to workers whose employers receive federal grants, federal contracts, or federal revenue-sharing funds. (See Chapter 19.) However, a 1978 amendment recognizes the employer's right to deny employment on the basis of alcohol or drug use in certain circumstances. An alcohol or drug abuser whose use of these

Table 25.2. Characteristics of Screening Tests for Drugs in Urine

Test	Analytic Method	Advantages of Method	Disadvantages of Method	Detectable drugs	Relative Cost
Color (Spot) Test	Sample response to color reagents	Simple. Immediate Results can be read by eye.	Poor specificity (many false positives) Poor sensitivity (misses many true positives).	Most types	Cheap
*TLC	Interpretation of migratory pattern and colors of treated sample.	Adulteration of sample not possible.	Requires sample preparation. Hard copy of results difficult to obtain. Poor specificity (many false positives).	Most types** except cannabinoids, PCP and hallucinogens	Moderate
RIA	Radioactively labelled sample is compared as an antigen with non-labelled drug.	Gives quantitative result.	Only one drug can be tested for at a time. Sensitive to tampered sample (produces false negatives). Drugs cross-react (produce false positives and false negatives).	Opiates, barbiturates, amphetamines, cocaine, PCP, cannabis and LSD.	Equipment cost is high.
*EMIT	Non-radioactive comparison of enzyme activity.	Rapid. Semi-quantitative. May cross-react with some drugs.	Sensitive to tampered sample (produces false negatives).	Opiates, barbiturates, amphetamines, cocaine, PCP, cannabis, benzodiazepine, methaqualone and methadone	Equipment cost is low. Reagents are costly.
FPIA	Measures fluorescence pattern of treated sample.	Rapid. Easy to do. Quantitative results. Highly sensitive.	Sensitive to tampered sample.		Expensive

TLC — Thin-layer Chromatography
RIA — Radioimmunoassay
EMIT — Enzyme-multiplied Immunoassay
FPIA — Fluorescence Pattern Immunoassay

 * Most commonly used methods.

 ** TLC test can detect the following drugs 3–12 hours after use: opiates, pentazocine and cocaine. It can detect amphetamines, benzodiazepines, barbiturates, methodone and propoxyphene for 24 hours after use.

substances currently presents a direct threat to the property or safety of others can be denied employment. On the other hand, individuals who have their addiction under control remain protected under the Act. All 50 states and the District of Columbia prohibit discrimination in employment on the basis of handicap. Some of these laws specifically include alcohol and drug abusers.

Drug testing results must be kept in the worker's occupational medical file and are considered confidential by the courts. The Drug Abuse Offense and Treatment Act of 1972 (P.L. 92-255, Title 21), applies to U.S. federal facilities, agencies, and federally funded facilities. The Act requires a worker's written consent for release of personal information contained in the employment medical records, except in emergencies. Even in emergencies, an attempt must first be made to obtain a court order to release the information. The Act also prohibits the use of worker medical records to verify that a worker is taking part in a rehabilitation program or to deny the worker employment.

Workers have sued their employers successfully in some states for unlawful invasion of privacy after mandatory drug testing, even though the workers signed consent forms when they were hired. Nevertheless, courts have generally found drug testing not to be an unwarranted invasion of privacy when carried out in a reasonable, confidential, and nondiscriminatory manner for legitimate business reasons. They have also found refusal by workers to undergo testing to be legitimate grounds for termination or other disciplinary measures by the employer.

The Fourth Amendment of the U.S. Constitution guarantees protection against unreasonable search and seizure. While courts consider blood and urine sampling to be searches, they have also acknowledged the legitimate interests of employers. A wise employer would avoid random testing of workers until a warning is given that testing will be started soon. The employer also should document the evidence that workers showed signs suggesting drug use sufficient to justify the test. The courts have held that U.S. employers have a broad legal right to investigate suspected violations of their rules, and that workers have a duty to cooperate in these investigations. (There are, however, alternatives to drug testing that may be considered preferable by the employer. These are discussed later in this chapter.)

Equal protection under the law is guaranteed in the United States under the Fourteenth Amendment to the Constitution. Employers can reject job applicants who fail a job-related examination of any kind, as long as all applicants are examined in the same way. If only selected applicants are tested for drug use, the onus is on the employer to present valid reasons why some are tested and others are not. Under U.S. federal and some state employment discrimination laws, drug and alcohol addictions are considered to be handicaps. Employers who are subject to these laws cannot refuse to hire, and may not fire or even discriminate against, drug or alcohol dependent workers, provided that they can do their job with "reasonable accommodation" on the part of the employer. (See Chapter 18.)

Canadian law is similar to U.S. law on drug testing in the workplace in its general intent, but derives from the Canadian Charter of Rights and Freedoms, the Canada Labour Code, the Canadian Human Rights Code, provincial human rights codes, and collective agreements between labor and management. The Canadian Charter of Rights and Freedoms is similar to the U.S. Bill of Rights. Section 8 of the Charter, like the Fourth Amendment to the U.S. Constitution, guarantees the right to protection against unreasonable search and seizure. A demand by an employer for a urine or blood sample for drug testing, without grounds for suspecting abuse, might be interpreted as a contravention. Section 11c of the Charter protects individuals against self-incrimination. An involuntary drug test may be construed as contravening this section. The Charter was only enacted in 1981, and at the time of writing few cases pertinent to drug testing have been tested in court. Federal and provincial human rights codes have been in place longer and provide more in the way of legal precedent, although the Charter is the higher law.

In Canada, the federal and provincial human rights codes are administered by appointed commissions, which operate independently of the normal court system. These codes consider drug and alcohol addictions to be physical or mental disabilities and specifically prohibit employers from discriminating against disabled workers or job applicants. Employers are not allowed to dismiss or refuse to hire a disabled worker unless the employer can clearly show that the disability has a detrimental effect on job performance or safety. Positive drug test results must be used to direct workers to rehabilitation. In addition, samples obtained for testing for particular drugs must not be used for the detection of other substances unless they, too, are specifically applicable to job performance or safety. If challenged, the employer must provide scientific or expert evidence to support the need for such tests.

The Canadian Human Rights Commission has prepared guidelines for federally regulated employers who want to test their employees and job applicants for drug use:

- The employer must show that the drug being tested may have a detrimental effect on the worker's ability to concentrate, operate equipment, and perform tasks efficiently and safely, and may increase absenteeism, accident rates, or turnover of staff.
- The employer must have reasonable grounds, based on objective evidence, that drug use is a problem in the workplace and that it reduces performance or safety.
- The drug test must be used only to screen for the targeted drug or its metabolite and the test used must be recognized and valid.
- If the test result is positive, the employer must make reasonable accommodation for the worker.

Ethical Considerations

These legal guidelines are further complicated by ethical considerations. These include the customary ethics of business practice and the codes of professional ethics of the medical, nursing, and laboratory personnel who carry out their drug testing program. The American Occupational Medical Association (AOMA, now organized into the American College of Occupational Medicine) produced a set of ethical guidelines for physicians who are involved in drug testing. Unfortunately, these guidelines are not very helpful and may destabilize the delicate balance the physician must maintain between the employer and the employed. The AOMA guidelines use imprecise terminology, such as "reasonable business necessity" (which is offered as a legitimate ethical basis for drug screening), and advise an inherent contradiction by recommending that the employer obtain employee consent for mandatory screening.

What course of action should be taken by an employer who receives a positive drug test result on an employee? A panel of lawyers, business people, and labor representatives at a 1986 workshop sponsored by the U.S. National Institute on Drug Abuse agreed that the employer should provide the worker with an opportunity to enter a drug education or, if appropriate, drug rehabilitation program; alternative employment (if available); and consideration for full reinstatement upon successful completion of the rehabilitation program.

Legal Challenges

Although important legal issues in testing workers for drug use remain in dispute, employers clearly face potential liability in the following circumstances:

- Negligence in the collection or handling of blood or urine samples.
- Improper disclosure of positive test results.
- Testing or testing procedures that fail to comply with collective bargaining agreements.
- Failure of the employer to take action to maintain workplace safety in the face of positive test results.

Negligence in the collection of samples or in sample handling is particularly touchy. It can result in legal action against the employer if it damages a worker's reputation or livelihood. Negligence also can create distrust of the program among workers as well as lower employee morale. Recommendations for handling samples are described below with the technical aspects of drug testing.

In summary, drug testing is legal under certain conditions, but the employer must plan the program with care in order to minimize the likelihood of a legal challenge. Complete protection from lawsuits initiated by employees or job applicants cannot be expected until there is further guidance from the courts and more precedents are established under case law. An employer who contemplates introducing drug testing into his workplace should obtain expert legal counsel. In the final analysis, the employer must weigh the legal risks of drug testing against the likelihood of improving worker performance and safety.

Limitations of Testing

The technical achievements of drug testing are clouded by important elements of uncertainty. Without other evidence, a single test for any drug cannot justify the diagnosis of addiction. Such diagnosis should be left to the physician, who will take into account not only the laboratory findings but also the results of a physical examination and information on the behavioral characteristics of the individual.

The results of drug testing can have profound effects on the lives of the individuals tested. The tests used must be reliable and must withstand rigorous examination in court. In practical terms, this means that the tests must accurately identify the drug or drugs tested for, must quantify the amount of drug present, and must be supported by documentary evidence of an unbroken "chain of custody"—the sequence of obtaining, handling, and transporting the sample to a secure laboratory. All steps in the chain should be documented, accounted for, and secured so that no possibility exists of unobserved tampering with the sample. Table 25.2 describes the common screening techniques used for drug detection.

Predictive Value of Drug Tests

The same principles that underlie screening tests in health monitoring and surveillance (see Chapter 20) apply to drug testing. The following example illustrates the application of these concepts to drug testing.

An employer uses a test that has a sensitivity of 99 percent, i.e., it will pick up

99 out of every 100 samples that contain the drug. It will also miss 1 out of every 100 positive samples. The same test has a specificity of 90 percent—for every 100 samples identified as containing the drug, only 90 actually do. The test is applied to 10,000 workers, of whom 100 are in fact using the drug. Of the 100 users, 99 would be correctly identified by the test (99 percent sensitivity), but 990 of the 9,900 nonusers would test incorrectly as positive (90 percent specificity). The predictive value of the test here is 99/990 x 10 percent; 90 percent of the positive results would be false! In such a situation, this test would be worse than useless because it would incriminate the innocent 10 times more often than it fingered the guilty.

If the same test is applied to another population of 10,000 workers in which there are 1,000 drug users (a tenfold greater prevalence), the predictive value of the test is 52 percent (48 percent of the positive results are false). The predictive value of a drug test increases with the proportion of drug users in the population tested. The fewer the number of drug users in the tested population, the poorer the predictive value of the drug test and the more likely the employer is to face serious dilemmas in interpreting and confirming the results.

This example illustrates two important aspects of drug testing: avoid testing where no problem exists and schedule confirmatory testing of workers whose screening tests are found to be positive. In the first example, the test showed that one worker in 10 was using drugs, when in fact only one in 100 was actually a user. In the second example, one in 10 workers was identified as using drugs, but half of these were innocent workers incorrectly identified. An employer basing disciplinary action on the basis of the tests alone in either of these situations would be courting legal disaster. For this reason, drug testing must always be confirmed when a positive result has been obtained. An initial screening test should be used only to detect the presence of the drug, and must be followed by a more precise and quantitative confirmatory test using a different analytical method. Some of the confirmatory tests for drug identification are described in Table 25.3.

Defining the "Positive" Result
Whether a test will be reported or accepted as positive or negative depends on the test's sensitivity and the specific use of the drug by the subject. The more sensitive the test, the greater the proportion of positive samples that will be detected. Since most tests are quantitative in nature (that is, they measure the concentration of the drug in the sample), the definition of "positive" depends not only on the test's absolute sensitivity but also on the cutoff point established as the maximum level acceptable. For some drugs, such as heroin or cocaine, the employer will usually establish a cutoff level of zero. For alcohol, however, the employer may be willing to accept blood levels of up to the legal level of impaired driving, somewhere in the range of 50 to 85 mg/dl.

Further complicating selection of an appropriate cutoff level is the need to consider the length of time that may have elapsed since the drug was last used. Drugs and their metabolites may remain in the body for varying lengths of time. Some drugs, such as marijuana, leave traces for several weeks after use. By contrast, cocaine derivatives remain detectable in body fluids for only one to three days. Table 25.4, reproduced by courtesy of the AMA Council on Scientific Affairs, presents the time limit for detecting drugs in urine samples and the smallest concentration of each that can be reliably detected. Variables such as these create problems in analysis; a detectable level in some

Table 25.3. Characteristics of Confirmatory Tests for Drugs in Urine

Test	Analytic Method	Advantages of Method	Disadvantages of Method	Detectable drugs	Relative Cost
GC	Comparison of sample component peaks with standards.	Extremely sensitive. Most commonly used. Very specific. Quantitative. Sample adulteration can be detected.	Slow. Only one sample can be run at a time.	Hypnotics opiates, sedatives and alkaloids.	Equipment cost is high.
GC/MS	Same as GC but uses MS as the detector.	Extremely sensitive. Very specific. Quantitative. Sample adulteration can be detected.	Slow. Only one sample can be run at a time.	All	Extremely expensive equipment needed.
HPLC	UV spectrum of sample is compared with standards.	Good sensitivity. High specificity	Slow. Only one sample can be run at a time.	All	Equipment cost is high.

GC — Gas chromatography
GC/MS — Gas Chromatography/Mass Spectrometry
HPLC — High Performance Liquid Chromatography

situations may reflect drug use confined to the worker's leisure time and may have no effect on work performance.

Drug dose and frequency of drug use also are important as determinants of a positive result. The higher the dose used, the more likely it is that the drug will be detected and the test will be called positive. Similarly, the more frequently a drug is used, the more likely it is to be detected in testing a given subject.

False positive results can be avoided by using a screening test that has good specificity, having the specimen analyzed by a laboratory with high standards, and using an appropriate confirmatory test. False positive test results are usually a result of human error or cross-reactivity. Cross-reactivity, the phenomenon in which substances other than the drug in question produce a positive result to the test, are more common in preliminary or screening tests than in the confirmatory tests. The physician must be sure that the substance detected by the test is, in fact, a drug and not an innocent contaminant or a prescribed medication that happens to cross-react in the test. Table 25.5 lists medications that may cross-react, causing false positive tests.

One common way to avoid false positives is to establish a cutoff level that identifies workers who have used a drug within a certain time period before the sample was taken. Results above that concentration arbitrarily would be called positive. The cutoff level for marijuana should always be set well above levels resulting from passive inhalation of secondhand smoke. Otherwise, there is too great a risk of falsely implicating

Table 25.4. Approximate Duration of Detectability of Selected Drugs in Urine

Drug	Detectability	Sensitivity
Amphetamine	48 hours	0.5 μg/mL
Metamphetamine	48 hours	0.5 μg/mL
Barbiturates		
Short-acting	24 hours	
Hexobarbital		1.0 μg/mL
Pentobarbital		0.5 μg/mL
Secobarbital		0.5 μg/mL
Thiamylal		1.0 μg/mL
Intermediate-acting	48–72 hours	1.0 μg/mL
Amobarbital		1.5 μg/mL
Aprobarbital		1.5 μg/mL
Butabarbital		0.5 μg/mL
Butalbital		1.5 μg/mL
Long-acting	+7 days	
Barbital		5.0 μg/mL
Phenobarbital		1.0 μg/mL
Benzodiazepine	3 days[1]	1.0 μg/mL
Benzoylecogonine		0.5 μg/mL
Ecogonine methyl ester (Cocaine metabolites)	2–3 days	1.0 μg/mL
Methadone	±3 days	0.5 μg/mL
EDDP (metabolite of methadone)		0.5 μg/mL
Codeine	48 hours	0.5 μg/mL
Morphine		1.0 μg/mL
Propoxyphene	6–48 hours	0.5 μg/mL
Norpropoxyphene		1.5 μg/mL
Cannabinoids	3 days[2]	
(11-nor-9-tetrahydro-	5 days[3]	20 μg/mL
cannabinol-9-	10 days[4]	
carboxylic acid)	21 days[5]	
Methaqualone ±7 days	1.0 μg/mL	
Phenocyclidine	±8 days	0.5 μg/mL

Note: Interpretation of the duration of detectability must take into account many variables, such as drug metabolism and half-life, subject's physical condition, fluid balance and state of hydration, route and frequency of ingestion. *These are general guidelines only.*

1. therapeutic doses
2. single use
3. moderate smoker (4 times/week)
4. heavy smoker (smoking daily)
5. chronic heavy smoker

Table 25.5. Potentially Cross-Reactive Prescription and Nonprescription Medications in Radioimmunoassay of Enzyme-Multiplied Immunoassay Tests*

Amphetamines	Diethylpropion
	Dopamine
	Ephedrine
	Fenfluramine
	p-Hydroxyamphetamine
	Isoxuprine
	1-Methamphetamine
	Methylphenidate
	Nylidrin
	Phentermine
	Phenylephrine
	Phenylpropanolamine
	Propylhexedrine
	Pseudoephedrine
Opiates	Chlorpromazine
	Codeine
	Dextromethorphan
	Diphenoxylate
	Hydromorphone
	Meperidine
	Oxycodone
	d-Propoxyphene
Phencyclidine	Chlorpromazine
	Dextromethorphan
	Diphenylhydramine
	Doxylamine
	Meperidine
	Thioridazine

* From Baselt Rc: Urine drug screening by immunoassay: Interpretation of results, in Baselt RC (ed): Advances in Analytical Toxicology, Biomedical Publications, 1984, as quoted in: AMA Council on Scientific Affairs, Scientific Issues on Drug Testing, JAMA 257:22 June 1987.

someone who was merely present when marijuana was smoked. (This obviously is not a problem for drugs that are injected or ingested.) The cutoff level might be set to detect applicants who used marijuana less than three to four weeks before being sampled.

Laboratories interpretating the results of drug test generally will use either their own reference value or the limits of detection of their method. If more than one laboratory is used, or an employer switches from one to another, samples containing the same concentration of a drug may be reported as positive by one and as negative by the other. The employer, in consultation with the laboratory and occupational health professionals, should establish a cutoff level for testing in order to be consistent.

Test results are very limited in what they can tell about the worker's use of drugs.

Detection of drugs in a single test cannot determine whether the worker has used the drug repeatedly, intermittently, or just once. There is no reliable test to determine whether a worker is actually addicted to a particular substance. A negative test result does not mean that the worker has never used the drug being tested for, or any other drug, only that he or she is unlikely to have recently used the drug in question or had used it recently, but in a dose so low that the test was below the cutoff. Alternatively, the sample may have been collected too late.

No drug test can prove that a worker's behavior was adversely affected at the time the sample was collected. The only drug in which quantitative test results correlate clearly with behavior is alcohol — an "expired-air" test may be used for screening and a blood test for confirmation. It is now generally accepted that a blood alcohol level of 50 mg/dl (11 mmol/l) may cause sufficient loss of coordination and judgment to create a hazard when driving. Some investigators suggest that impairment due to alcohol often begins at a blood alcohol level of 35 mg/dl (7.25 mmol/l). In terms of alcohol intake, two bottles of beer consumed within one hour provides the average person with over 35 mg/dl of alcohol in his blood. Three bottles in the same hour results in a blood alcohol level of over 50 mg/dl. A worker weighing 67.5 kg (150 lbs) can usually oxidize and eliminate 10 ml of alcohol per hour, roughly decreasing the blood alcohol level by about 15 mg/dl per hour.

Problems of Sample Tampering

Without a chain of custody, it is impossible to be sure that a urine sample has not been tampered with by an unscrupulous or fearful employee. Some of the ways that urine samples can be surreptitiously invalidated include:

- Releasing chemicals, such as salt or detergent, from under the fingernails into the sample to neutralize the drug residues or to make them unreactive.
- Punching a pinhole in the bottom of the sample container, so that the urine leaks out during shipping.
- Substituting or switching samples or their identification labels. Drug-free urine can now be purchased on the street for such purposes.
- Diluting the sample with water, either by directly introducing it into the sample or by drinking large quantities of water and voiding frequently prior to the collection of the sample.

Suspicions about the validity of urine samples have led to overreaction by some employers and charges of invasion of privacy by outraged workers; short of observing the worker urinating, which is not generally recommended, the occupational health care professional may not always know that a given sample is valid.

A chain of custody must be established for every sample that is obtained for drug testing. Any sample may end up as the basis for a legal action and as crucial evidence in court. An intact or "unbroken" chain of custody establishes that the original sample provided by the worker is the same as that analyzed by the laboratory. The National Institute on Drug Abuse (NIDA) has published details on security, documentation, and transmittal procedures for drug urine specimens in its 1986 Research Monograph 73, "Urine Testing for Drugs of Abuse."

The laboratory that will carry out the analysis also must be chosen with care. The laboratory's services to the employer consist of:

- Ensuring that the chain of custody is not compromised;

- Conducting the analysis;
- Reporting the results in a standardized and interpretable way;
- Ensuring that the analysis is accurate and reliable; and
- Documenting each specimen as to the type and amount, when and from whom it was received, who performed the analysis, and the analytic method used.

NIDA has developed standards for proficiency testing and the accreditation of laboratories that review the credentials, training, and experience of laboratory personnel and assess the use of in-lab and external quality control procedures. In North America, the Centers for Disease Control and the College of American Pathologists are accrediting agencies.

Alternatives to Drug Testing

Alcohol and drug testing may not be worth the effort, but an employer need not simply ignore the problem, hoping it will die. Where drugs are a potential threat, several options can be used singly or in combination, with or without drug testing. These include worker observation, drug searches, monitoring of work performance itself to detect drug use, employee-oriented drug education program, and an addiction rehabilitation policy. The last three options may be part of a more comprehensive Employee Assistance Program (EAP), and are discussed in Chapter 26. The first two are examined in detail below.

Observation and Investigation

One "hard line" approach to eradicating drugs from the workplace is the use of worker observation to detect drug-related activity. U.S. employers have a broad legal right to investigate suspected violations of their workplace rules and regulations. The courts have supported this right and the duty of employees to cooperate with such investigations. In the course of carrying out investigations, some employers use lie-detector devices. The use of these instruments is controversial, however; there are serious questions concerning their reliability as well as charges that they constitute an invasion of privacy. Federal law and laws in half of the U.S. states prohibit or limit the use of lie-detector tests as a condition of employment and the type of questions workers may be asked. The federal law is the Employee Polygraph Protection Act of 1988 (P.L. 100-347).

Alternatives used by employers for security purposes include electronic eavesdropping and closed circuit video observation in such places as washrooms, lounges, and lunch and locker rooms. These techniques are more commonly employed to deter and detect theft or to monitor productivity, but are tempting to those who mistakenly see them as a quick solution to the drug abuse problem. The U.S. Federal Omnibus Crime Control and Safe Streets Act (1968) and laws in about half of the states restrict the employer's right to use electronic eavesdropping devices. Visual observation is generally permissible, but cameras cannot be used in locations where workers have a reasonable expectation of privacy.

Some employers conduct drug searches of their workers, often as employees enter the worksite. As with worker observation, searches usually originate as measures to deter material theft. In general, the employer may not search in places where workers have a reasonable expectation of privacy. In order to search workers' lockers without the worker present, the employer must supply and thereby own the locks and must distribute a clear statement in advance that the lockers may be searched at any time. The employer can also require workers to open their lockers, tool kits, or vehicles to examine their contents. Labor arbitrators generally have interpreted an employee's refusal to undergo a reasonable search at the worksite as an act of insubordination.

Employers should realize that programs of random drug testing, lie-detection, electronic eavesdropping, video observation, or searches indicate to employees that management considers them unworthy of trust. Well motivated workers who are drug and alcohol free are bound to feel resentment toward any employer displaying this attitude. Workers will object to having to prove that they do not use drugs and will consider such programs as violations of their rights. A small number will probably quit. Some of these may be drug users who want to avoid being tested but many will be drug-free workers who simply cannot tolerate working under constant suspicion.

Most workers, however, are likely to stay on, unable to risk looking for another job, angry at themselves for not standing up for their beliefs, and feeling guilty for not quitting and resentful toward the employer. Over time, such feelings will subside gradually, only to be stirred up by random drug tests or searches. Employers creating this type of atmosphere should anticipate lowered morale and sliding performance in many subtle ways. Employers who treat their workers as trustworthy people who want to do a good job, on the other hand, usually will see their expectations bear fruit.

Planning an Anti-Drug Program

Developing an anti-drug program is not a simple procedure, as demonstrated by the outline in Figure 25.1. All planning should be based on up-to-date information about alcohol and drug abuse in general and specific data from health and rehabilitation agencies on education and treatment resources in the local community.

Planning will normally be undertaken because of suspicion or evidence that drug abuse is a problem *at the company worksite*. A preliminary assessment of whether or not drug abuse is a problem may be obtained from reports of on-site accidents, sickness absence rates for suspected drug abusers, and the first-hand opinions of occupational health professionals and company managers and supervisors. A survey of employees may be conducted by using anonymous questionnaires or anonymous drug testing. The latter measures can be particularly useful if the workers are willing to participate on a voluntary basis—but they will not do so unless they are convinced that the questionnaire and drug testing will be absolutely anonymous and that no disciplinary action of any kind will occur.

Where there is no indication of problems and employees' work performance does not appear to be affected, the only action appropriate for the company is to offer some form of drug education. Consideration should be given to such preventive measures to forestall problems. Furthermore, this idyllic condition may not last, and management should regularly review the situation.

If drug abuse does seem to be causing security or health and safety problems,

Figure 25.1. Steps in Planning a Company Anti-Drug Program

1.
Obtain background knowledge of
drugs and drug and alcohol abuse

2.
Determine whether drug abuse is
a problem at the workplace

3.1	3.2	3.3
Yes	Yes	No
Security	Health and Safety	Not a problem
problem	problem	at present
4.1	4.2	
Evaluate	Evaluate	
with security	with medical and EAP	
advisors and	advisors and labor	
labor representatives	representatives	
5.1	5.2	
Revise current	Revise or develop new	
security procedures	drug abuse policy and	
	procedures	
6.1	6.2	
Obtain	Obtain	
Resources	Resources	

7.
Announce and disseminate
new policy and procedures

8.1	8.2	8.3
Educate and	Apply policy and	Consider introduction
train employees	review situation	of preventive education
	periodically	program

existing policy and procedures should be critically reviewed. Where security is affected, advisers should include security staff and labor representatives; where health and safety are main concerns, medical and EAP consultants should be consulted. In unionized workplaces, the implications of amending the bargaining agreement will have to be considered before new policy or procedures are introduced. Applicable laws and regulations should be examined with regard to cooperation with law enforcement agencies, permissible techniques for detecting drug abuse, and reasonable accommodation for drug users undergoing rehabilitation. Once agreement is reached that new policies or procedures on drug use are required, the difficult task of revision or formulation can begin.

Drug testing procedures must be designed so that they do not embarrass or affront the dignity of employees. The employer has a responsibility to maintain strict confidentiality and to observe the rights of privacy of employees. The drug testing policy should include a statement to the effect that:

All information obtained in the course of examinations, rehabilitation and treatment of employees with drug abuse problems shall be protected as confidential health information. No data concerning the information or participation in any rehabilitation program shall be made part of the employee's personnel file or will be provided to any other party without the direct written consent of the employee except as required by law or by established company policy in connection with the adjudication of that employee's rights.

The preceding statement was developed by NIDA.

Information regarding a former employee's drug or alcohol abuse problem should never be communicated to prospective employers, only a description of poor performance as documented in the employee's record. Results of drug testing should always be communicated by the analytical laboratory directly to the physician or nurse providing occupational health services, not to the employer. The occupational health professional should keep the report confidential—the results should be treated as private health information and the assessment handled like a fitness-to-work evaluation. (See Chapter 18.) The drug test results should not be made available to law enforcement agencies nor company security personnel unless a crime is suspected or the information is subpoenaed.

Drug testing of employees is best done when an EAP exists to serve employees in an organization. If an EAP does not already exist, a drug testing program should imply a commitment to establish one. To do otherwise is to abandon the philosophy of helping the worker overcome the problem.

Before drug testing is seriously considered, the employer should establish a drug policy based on company needs. The statement of policy should explain that the rationale for the policy and the employer's expectations are firmly intended to protect the health and safety of the employee at the workplace or to safeguard the employer's need to protect property. Corporate executives should not be omitted from coverage under the policy.

The policy should include clear statements of the rules that can be enforced by the employer (in, of course, a consistent and fair manner). These rules must cover at least the following:

• The use and possession of drugs or alcohol on company premises;
• The selling or provision of drugs or alcohol on company premises;
• The consequences of arriving at work or working while under the influence of drugs or alcohol;
• The company's policy on searching an employee's person and personal possessions;
• The names of prohibited substances; and
• The penalties for violating the rules.

All contracts let by the company should include the policy so that all individuals on company worksites are subject to the same procedures as apply to company employees.

After the company policy and procedures have been developed in detail, the costs to implement the program—expenses associated with occupational health personnel or security staff, the laboratory, and EAP or drug rehabilitation personnel—must be considered. The anticipated costs of employee testing and counselling, the possible expenses of litigation, and the detrimental effects on employee-management relations also must be assessed.

When the policy and procedures are complete, a decision to proceed should be followed by an announcement of the drug policy and the drug testing program. The announcement must be absolutely clear and must reach every employee in the organization. The announcement should give detailed information on testing. Workers will want to know:

- Who is going to be tested, how they will be tested, when, how often, and where?
- Who is going to analyze the samples?
- Which drugs will be tested for?
- Who will get the results?

They will also want to know the rules about drug use and possession at work and the consequences for employees who are found in violation or refuse to be tested. They will want to know their rights and means of appeal and the options – or requirements – for treatment and rehabilitation. Employees should be given the opportunity to ask questions without disclosing their identity, and replies should be made promptly. Careful and painstaking attention to this part of the process will go a long way toward obtaining the cooperation of employees.

An important factor in the success of the program is the education and training of supervisory personnel. The program requires the cooperation of supervisors in confronting and referring workers for assessment and assisting in their rehabilitation. Supervisors should follow uniform disciplinary guidelines, basing their actions firmly on unsatisfactory performance or documented violations of rules, making no exceptions. Workers in violation of the drug policy should be told of their options so that they may choose between rehabilitation and discipline. Suspected violations should be investigated following standardized procedures that aim for proof. Suspected drug users should be suspended during such investigations. By being as fair as possible, the employer can keep labor-management relations on an even keel.

The policy and procedures should be reviewed regularly in the light of changing drug use patterns. This review should involve operational supervisors, security staff, occupational health and safety staff, and employee representatives. Although the basic policy on drug use is unlikely to require frequent changes, the specific substances tested for may need to be reconsidered and specific procedures may require revision from time to time.

Further Reading

AMA Council on Scientific Affairs: Issues in employee drug testing. JAMA 1987; 258:2089–2096.

AMA Council on Scientific Affairs: Scientific issues in drug testing. JAMA 1987; 257:3110–3114.

Angarola RT: Drug detection programs in industry. PharmChem Newsletter, Jul–Aug 1984; 13(4):1–11.

Castro J: Battling the enemy within: Companies fight to drive illegal drugs out of the workplace. Time, 17 Mar 1986, pp. 40–54.

Chamberlain RT: Drug screening in the workplace: Medicolegal implications. American Association for Clinical Chemistry TDM-T June 1986; 7(12):1–7.

Cowell JWF: Drug and alcohol testing: Playing with fire. OHS Canada 1987; 3(5):120.

Diagnostic and Statistical Manual of Mental Disorders (ed 3 revised): Washington DC, American Psychiatric Association, 1986.

Employee-Related Drug Screening: A Public Health and Safety Perspective. Toronto, The Ontario Addiction Research Foundation, April 1987.

Fishbein GW (ed): Drugs in the workplace: What to do about it? Occupational Health & Safety Letter, 22 Aug 1985; 15(16):1.

Geidt TE: Drug and alcohol abuse in the workplace: Balancing employer and employee rights. Employee Relations Law Journal 1985; 11(2):181–205.

Gordon J: Drug testing as a productivity booster? Training, 22 Mar 1987, pp. 21–34.

Hawks RL, Chiang CN (eds): Urine Testing for Drugs of Abuse. Rockville, Maryland, National Institute on Drug Abuse, Research Monograph 73, 1986.

Schachter V, Geidt TE: Cracking Down on Drugs. Across the Board, November 1985, pp. 28–37.

Walser AH, et al.: Statement of the Committee on Ethical Practice in Occupational Medicine: Drug screening in the workplace: Ethical guidelines. J Occup Med 1986; 28(12):1240–41.

Walsh JM, Gust SW (eds): Consensus Summary: Interdisciplinary Approaches to the Problem of Drug Abuse in the Workplace. Rockville, Maryland, National Institute on Drug Abuse DHHS Pub. No. (ADM) 86-1477, 1986.

Walsh JM, Hawks RL: Employee Drug Screening: Detection of Drug Use by Urinalysis. Rockville, Maryland, National Institute on Drug Abuse DHHS Pub. No. (ADM) 86-1442, 1986.

Wells V, Halperin W, Thun M: The estimated predictive value of screening for illicit drugs in the workplace. Am J Pub Health 1988; 78:817–819.

26 EMPLOYEE ASSISTANCE PROGRAMS

In any group of people, a certain number have personal problems that interfere with their work, attitude, and enjoyment of life. These problems do not develop overnight; they are frequently deeply rooted in the individual's psychology and past experience. If such problems are identified early, before they cause the worker to be dismissed from the job, an enlightened employer can intervene to help the worker and in so doing avoid the loss of a valuable employee who may have many productive years ahead.

Employee assistance programs (EAPs) are employer-sponsored counselling services that assist employees with personal problems. EAPs commonly focus on alcohol and drug abuse and behavioral disturbances due to stress, referring employees for treatment, giving them support, helping to motivate them to complete treatment, and assisting in their rehabilitation. Some so-called "broad brush" programs also recognize family, financial, and legal problems as frequent sources of stress and provide additional special services in these areas. Employee assistance programs, like health promotion programs, are concerned primarily with the "wellness" of individual workers, and the activities of both programs may overlap when both exist in the same organization. The emphasis in EAPs, however, tends more toward the resolution of socially oriented problems.

Programs designed to help employees who have personal problems that interfere with their work performance and enjoyment of life have been around since the 1940s, when alcohol abuse began to be recognized as a treatable illness. At that time, a few corporations, such as Eastman Kodak, E.I. Dupont de Nemours, and Consolidated Edison, set up medically oriented assistance programs run by their medical departments. It was not until the 1950s, when the American Medical Association sanctioned the concept that alcohol abuse was a treatable medical condition, that the foundation for modern EAPs was established. Since then EAPs have emerged in various forms and been called by various names, although they are still by no means universally available or accepted.

Program Design

The design and implementation of an EAP depend upon the perceptions and attitudes of the various stakeholders, the nature of the industry, the characteristics of the community, the background of professional consultants, and the availability of local agencies to receive referrals. If an EAP is to succeed, key players—including management, the union or other employee representatives, the occupational health service, and the human resources or personnel department—must participate in its design and implementation. Outside consultants knowledgeable in the design of EAPs also may be involved.

The program itself may be administered and delivered by the occupational health team, by the human resources department, or by an EAP counsellor working as an employee of the company or as a consultant. Each of these arrangements has strengths and weaknesses. Regardless of the situation, there are underlying principles that must be in place if the program is to succeed. The underlying principles of the EAP include recognition that alcohol and drug abuse and stress-related behavioral disturbances are legitimate, treatable illnesses and that the program is not to be used as a substitute for usual disciplinary procedures or to compromise rules, regulations, or binding agreements. These principles must be articulated in a company policy that is known and understood by all employees. A complete EAP policy should outline these underlying principles, describe the program content, identify the key players, describe their roles and responsibilities, and specify the program's relationship to other employment policies. (A sample EAP policy appears as Exhibit 26.1.)

Program Operation

A complete EAP provides for education and training as well as counselling, treatment, and rehabilitation. In the educational sessions, employees receive information on how to avoid or to cope with alcohol, drugs, and stress, and how the overall program works. Supervisor training encourages the supervisor not to speculate on the meaning of a person's behavioral problem but rather to watch for and react to early signs of trouble—irritability, tardiness, absenteeism, sloppy work habits, and any unusual changes in behavior on the part of the worker. Supervisors are taught to refer workers who may be exhibiting these symptoms to the EAP before the problem leads to failing job performance.

Employees who are experiencing difficulties also may enter the program through self-referral. In self-referral, the employee, for whatever reason, has decided to get help before work performance has deteriorated to the point where it is necessary for a supervisor to become involved. In the directed situation, job performance has already deteriorated such that, if improvement does not occur, discipline or dismissal is possible.

For the EAP to work effectively, the underlying principle of confidentiality must be in place. In the case of the voluntary self-referral, not only must the details of the problem be kept in confidence but also the fact of the referral itself.

In the case of a directed referral, the fitness-to-work procedure described in

Chapter 18 should be followed. This procedure ensures confidentiality for the worker, while at the same time giving the supervisor and others who are involved sufficient information to manage the employment situation. The fitness-to-work procedure should be followed whether the case is being handled by an occupational health physician or nurse or an EAP counsellor. The employer monitors the progress of the employee and guarantees return to the same job or one involving similar work.

Most EAPs do not attempt to provide ongoing in-house counselling, treatment, or rehabilitation. Rather, they provide the necessary framework for case identification, management, and follow-up, and provide liaison with community treatment and resources for rehabilitation.

EAPs should be widely advertised, but in a nonthreatening way. The employee falling deeply into alcohol abuse has considerable powers of denial and usually will resist an accusatory tone. Appeals to responsibility to one's family, indirect references to "troubles," and such visual images as a picture of an empty bottle seem to be more effective than the direct approach. All publicity regarding the EAP should emphasize strict confidentiality and professionalism and provide an outside phone number so that the employee can call from a private phone. Table 26.1 is a well established questionnaire used successfully by Rohr Industries, an aerospace corporation based in Chula Vista, California, to assist employees with problems related to alcohol abuse. It was distributed widely, with an invitation to call the firm's EAP if the worker answered yes to any question.

The location of the EAP offices is another important consideration. The entrance should be easily accessible but discreet, so that a visit is not conspicuous. Often the EAP office is placed out of sight of the waiting room in the occupational health service or in an office building a few blocks away.

The counsellor is the key to an effective EAP. Alcohol rehabilitation counsellors have a special rapport with alcohol abusers and many themselves have had and overcome drinking problems. Increasingly, psychologists and counsellors specially trained in EAP services and management are becoming available. Whatever the credentials of the counsellor, an employee must feel at ease and confident in his or her presence. For this reason the demeanor and attitude of the counsellor is critical, as is the counsellor's ability to relate to workers of different ages and social classes.

For programs based on referral to community agencies, the counsellor should be familiar with the resources available in the local area, their suitability for different people and situations, their fees, criteria for enrollment, and treatment approaches. Not every treatment center is suitable for every worker. Some people respond to intensive residential programs away from home and work; others do better in a visiting setting, such as Alcoholics Anonymous. Sometimes referral to a special counsellor is required; the EAP counsellor should have on hand a roster of practicing professionals in the area and extensive knowledge about the ones used.

The EAP counsellor closely monitors the progress of the worker through treatment (and after returning to work if time off is required), thereby reinforcing treatment and increasing the likelihood of successful recovery. By providing assistance before a worker's performance deteriorates to the point of dismissal, the EAP preserves an important part of the worker's life. In many cases the worker's family has been so negatively affected that the job remains the only point of stability in a chaotic life. By stepping in before the worker's job performance goes the way of his or her family life, the EAP

Table 26.1. Questionnaire Used by Workers to Evaluate Their Own Drinking Habits (Courtesy of the Rohr Corporation)

"Drinking . . . 20 Important Questions"

The most frustrating aspect of alcohol use, abuse, and alcoholism is the inability of the drinker to accept the fact that alcohol can, and often does, result in serious problems for the drinker. The primary characteristic of alcoholism itself is denial that problems exist in spite of evidence to the contrary. The 20 questions below are designed to assist drinkers to objectively examine their own use of alcohol.

	Yes	No
1. Has anyone suggested you quit or cut back on drinking?	☐	☐
2. Has drinking affected your reputation?	☐	☐
3. Have you made promises to control your drinking and then broken them?	☐	☐
4. Have you ever changed your drink or drinking pattern in an effort to reduce your alcohol consumption?	☐	☐
5. Have you ever gotten into financial, legal, or marital difficulties because of drinking?	☐	☐
6. Have you lost time from work because of drinking?	☐	☐
7. Have you ever "sneaked" or "gulped" drinks?	☐	☐
8. On occasion, do you feel uncomfortable if alcohol is not available?	☐	☐
9. Do you continue drinking when friends or family suggest you've had enough?	☐	☐
10. Have you ever felt guilty or ashamed about your drinking or what you did while drinking?	☐	☐
11. Has your efficiency decreased as a result of drinking?	☐	☐
12. When drinking, do you neglect to eat properly?	☐	☐
13. Do you drink alone?	☐	☐
14. Do you drink more than usual when under pressure, angry, or depressed?	☐	☐
15. Are you able to drink more now without feeling it, compared to when you first began to drink regularly?	☐	☐
16. Have you lost interest in other activities or noticed a decrease in your ambition as a result of drinking?	☐	☐
17. Have you had "shakes" or tremors following heavy drinking or after not drinking for a period of time?	☐	☐
18. Do you want a drink at a particular time each day?	☐	☐
19. Do you go on and off "the wagon"?	☐	☐
20. Is drinking jeopardizing your job?	☐	☐

Answering yes to one or more of the above questions does not necessarily imply a drinking problem. However, three or more yes answers suggest that you should more closely evaluate your use of alcohol.

---

gives the worker a foundation from which to work toward recovery. Both employer and employee gain as the employee's job performance returns to normal.

EAP services do not have to be very costly, particularly when health insurance covers the treatment programs. Many employers assume rehabilitation costs for key or long-term employees if reimbursement under the health plan is not complete. Essential to program effectiveness, however, is sufficient staffing so that a counsellor can spend adequate time with the worker, manage the caseload without difficulty, and stay abreast of new developments in treatment and community resources.

Help in developing an EAP, with an emphasis on controlling alcohol abuse, may be obtained from the Association of Labor-Management Administrators and Consultants on Alcoholism in Arlington, Virginia. In the future, it is likely that EAP programs will combine with health promotion programs to form an integrated wellness program that seeks to provide a full range of lifestyle guidance and support.

Exhibit 26.1. Policy on Employee Assistance Program
(The following is an example of a corporate policy on employee assistance that may serve as a model for management.)

Purpose
   To outline the company's approach for assisting employees with alcohol, drug, or stress-related problems.

Policy
   1. The company recognizes that inappropriate alcohol and drug use and stress-induced emotional disturbances can result in health and behavioral problems.
   2. Alcohol, drug, and stress-related health problems will be considered and handled as would any illness that may affect job performance. Treatment will be included within the scope of sickness income benefits.
   3. The Employee Assistance Program encompasses education, treatment, and rehabilitation.

Scope
   This policy applies to all operations, subsidiary, and affiliate companies.

General Procedures
   1. Voluntary Self-Referral
      Employees who believe they have a health problem that is affecting or could affect work performance may voluntarily seek confidential assistance through the company occupational health service. In this circumstance, no other member of management or any other employee will be informed of the referral unless authorized by the employee or where the employee's life or the lives of others are in imminent danger.
   2. Employer-Initiated Referral
      • Suggested Referral: Employees who may have a health problem that is beginning to affect their work performance adversely may be advised to seek a confidential evaluation by the company occupational health service.
      • Directed Referral: Employees whose work performance has deteriorated to an unacceptable level apparently because of health reasons will be required to undergo an evaluation by the occupational health service. Following the confidential evaluation by the company occupational health service, the employee may be required to obtain rehabilitative counselling, treatment, or assistance to resolve the problem. Employees who refuse to accept a confidential evaluation or to follow recommended treatment will be referred back to their supervisor to follow normal procedures for dealing with deteriorating work performance. Employees will not be disciplined for refusing a referral to the company occupational health service, nor will acceptance of a referral necessarily replace disciplinary action. (Continued)

Exhibit 26.1. Continued

3. Costs incurred for services not normally covered by the company benefit plan may be assumed by the department at its discretion. Otherwise, the costs will be the responsibility of the employee.

Responsibilities
1. Supervisor
   • The supervisor responsible will establish work performance standards, identify unsatisfactory or deteriorating work performance, and set guidelines for improving performance.
   • Employer-Suggested Referral: If work performance is beginning to deteriorate, the supervisor will discuss performance factors with the employee. The factors discussed will be those contributing to the quality and quantity of the work performed and may include attendance, punctuality, attitude, behavior, and dependability. No attempt should be made to diagnose or discuss a health problem, but if health reasons are given or suspected as the cause of deteriorating work performance, the supervisor should suggest that the employee seek an evaluation from the company occupational health service.
   • Employer-Directed Referral: If work performance is unacceptable and health reasons are given as or suspected to be the cause, the supervisor will direct the employee to seek assistance from the company occupational health service. The directed referral immediately precedes any formal disciplinary process.
2. Employee: Employees have a responsibility to maintain their own good mental and physical health insofar as possible and a satisfactory standard of work performance. Employees also have a responsibility to seek assistance and participate in appropriate treatment programs when health conditions are affecting or could affect adversely their personal well-being or work performance.
3. Human Resources: The Human Resources department will provide consultation to supervisors and employees on the various options available when dealing with deteriorating work performance.
4. Occupational Health Service
   • Voluntary Self-Referral: The occupational health service staff will evaluate the employee's situation and, where appropriate, coordinate treatment and/or rehabilitation. Except under defined situations (where the employee's life or the lives of others are in imminent danger), the fact that the employee sought help will never be revealed to any other employee or member of the company.
   • Employer-Initiated Referral (Suggested or Directed): The occupational health service staff will objectively evaluate relevant information and determine fitness to work, and may arrange referral to an appropriate internal resource or community agency. Following the health evaluation, the Fitness-to-Work Record procedure will be used. (See Chapter 18.) The occupational health service staff will coordinate the treatment and/or rehabilitation plans between the company and any outside health professionals and will maintain complete confidentiality of health information.
   • Consultation: The occupational health services staff will be readily available to interpret policy, procedures, and practices to management, employees, and other health professionals involved in treatment and/or rehabilitation.
   • Education and Training: The occupational health service staff will develop and assist in the delivery of educational material and training programs for management and employees.

(Continued)

Exhibit 26.1. Continued

Exceptions

Departures from this policy must be approved in advance by the senior corporate officer responsible for occupational health and safety or by the company medical director.

Further Reading

Cowell JWF: Drug and alcohol testing: Playing with fire. OHS Canada 1987 3(5):12.

Dickerson OB, Kaminer AJ (eds): The troubled employee. Occupational Medicine: State of the Art Reviews 1986; 1(4):541–682.

Gaeta E, Lynn R, Grey L: AT&T looks at program evaluation. EAP Digest, May 1–June 1982; 2(4):22–31.

McClellan K: The consortium approach to EAP services. EAP Digest, January/February 1982; (2):33–35.

27   HEALTH PROMOTION

In recent years, an increasing number of employers of all sizes and types have introduced health promotion programs for their workers. Health promotion programs, like employee assistance programs, are not obligatory activities for an occupational health service but they are proving to be useful and popular. They focus on enhancing the health of workers who are already well by emphasizing lifestyle and wellness strategies. They are entirely voluntary; participation should never be a condition of employment.

Health promotion programs usually incorporate several health-related activities. They may be based at an employer's location or at a community facility. Some are run directly by the employer, but many of the most successful programs are sponsored through employee recreation associations. Although the management of such programs has become highly specialized and professional, an employer can begin by offering small-scale programs or by paying for memberships in local health clubs. Health promotion programs can be expanded in phases with the addition of new activities, and can be shared among employers.

Components of Health Promotion Programs

Health promotion programs typically blend three approaches to employee health: health education, preventive medicine, and physical fitness. Table 27.1 presents the typical components of these types of programs:

- *The health education component* is concerned with teaching employees the essentials of a healthy lifestyle, such as good health habits, sound nutrition, and the consequences of smoking, alcohol, and drug misuse. However, simply providing information is not enough; lectures on health seldom change attitudes and the straightforward approach that may be appropriate for educating a patient as to necessary lifestyle changes may not be as successful with employees who are well. Beyond the informative aspect of health education, attention must be given to the

Table 27.1. Typical Components of a Health Promotion Program*

Health Education

Cancer prevention	Common minor illnesses
Heart disease	Cardiopulmonary resuscitation
Mental health	Diabetes
Nutrition	Allergies
Stress	Family health
Substance abuse	Automotive safety
Smoking	Occupational hazards
Travel health	Sexually transmitted diseases
Back care (prophylactic)	Health fairs

Preventive Medicine

Screening Activities	*Intervention Activities*
Hypertension screening	Smoking cessation
Diabetes screening	Dietary interventions
Cardiovascular risk factors	Back care (rehabilitation)
Pulmonary function testing	Weight control
Weight monitoring	Stress reduction
Breast cancer	Prescriptive exercise regimes
Stool occult blood	Referral to physician

Physical Conditioning

Aerobic activities	Fitness center
Strength and stretch	Sports medicine

* Adapted from: Guidotti TL. Occupational Medicine: AAFP Home Study Self-Assessment Monograph 65. Kansas City, American Academy of Family Physicians, 1984.

psychological principles that motivate people to comply with sound health practices or to take unnecessary risks that jeopardize their health. The design of a health education component within a workplace health promotion program should take into account the characteristics of the workers as a group (age, sex, class, education, health status, language, etc.); the most important health problems in the community as perceived by the workers; the most important health problems actually present in the community; and the goals for changing health-related behavior.

- *The preventive medicine component* is typically limited to screening for common disorders and risk factors and to intervention activities that supplement, but do not substitute for, personal health care. The twin emphases of health promotion programs are primary prevention—helping to reduce the incidence of disease in the working population—and secondary prevention— the early detection of disease and referral for care. Programs usually stress lowering cholesterol levels and improving cardiovascular fitness; reducing risk factors for later health problems is more easily accomplished in an integrated health promotion program. In these types of programs, the workers are treated as a group. Every effort is made to build a team spirit, to provide feedback and constant encouragement, and to create a support network, thereby making compliance easier than if the worker were acting alone.

- *Physical fitness* is an important part of most health promotion programs. Participation in fitness activities and sports programs is fun and builds morale among workers. It also provides a regularly scheduled opportunity for conditioning and exercise with the benefits of encouragement and the sense of belonging to a group, both of which motivate compliance with the program. Workplace fitness programs should not be oriented to athletes; persons of normal strength and coordination should be able to set reasonable goals within the program and attain them.

The health promotion activities offered in a program vary with the employee population and setting. Most programs begin with a fitness component, screening for cardiovascular risk factors, and a health education activity emphasizing smoking cessation and common health problems. Many employers also sponsor voluntary health evaluations for employees as part of the health promotion program. The employer pays for a periodic health evaluation, up to a maximum dollar amount and within prescribed intervals of time. These examinations should not be confused with fitness-to-work evaluations (see Chapter 18). The clinical opinion formed by the physician regarding the worker's participation in sports or cardiovascular fitness exercises does not affect the worker's employment status: no fitness-to-work judgment is made and the outcome of the examination is strictly confidential. Furthermore, these examinations do not have to be performed in the occupational health service or by an occupational health professional, although they are best conducted by physicians who are experienced in preventive medicine. The content of the examination should be based on the worker's age, lifestyle, past health status, family history, and risk factors for subsequent disease. The frequency of the examination is a clinical judgment that takes into account the worker's age, condition, and interest in achieving better health. (Aspects of these evaluations are discussed in greater detail in Chapter 20.)

Program Benefits and Principles

Health promotion programs in industry can be extremely rewarding for both employees and employers. In general, these programs appear to succeed in encouraging good health habits and improving fitness among employees. Whether they actually reduce illness rates and increase productivity is not certain, although likely. Studies are now confirming that employees who take charge of their health by eating well, exercising regularly, learning to cope with life stresses, eliminating smoking and drug use, using alcohol in moderation, and following common sense in everyday activities, are likely to live longer and healthier lives. They appear to have fewer days of illness, suffer fewer injuries, and lead more productive lives. Employers support these programs because they contribute to employees' well-being and provide economic rewards as well.

Furthermore, these programs clearly do improve employee morale and promote positive attitudes. Program sponsorship is a tangible gesture of interest by the employer in the well-being of the employee; participation in the program helps create bonds linking employees, their co-workers, and the employer.

Even in the face of such benefits, however, health promotion programs are not universally accepted. Workers are sometimes cautious about participating in such programs when working conditions are otherwise unsatisfactory. Some employers wonder whether supporting them is an effective use of company resources. Unions often view these programs as a diversion intended to gain the support of workers without making concessions on fundamental issues such as wages, hours, working conditions, and autonomy on the job. While occupational health professionals understand their importance for the worker's personal health and are generally supportive of health promotion programs, too often support for them comes at the expense of programs designed to ensure worker health and safety on the job.

Program success seems to hinge on eight critical principles:

- Employees should want and trust the program.
- Employees should participate in the creation of the program and be able to influence its evolution.
- Employers should believe that the program is making a measurable contribution to the well-being of the workforce and to the economics of the organization.
- The program should be effectively integrated with the employee health assistance program (emphasizing alcohol and drug abuse and stress-related problems).
- The program should be effectively integrated with and make use of available community resources.
- The program should focus on individual responsibility.
- The program should be suitable for the employee population (age, sex, class, education, health, language) and the type of industry (size, type, location).
- The program should be evaluated on a regular basis, with new ideas and concepts continually introduced and old or unpopular ideas quickly discarded. (Evaluation is an essential part of program management—employee needs and interests should always be taken into consideration before introducing new activities, and programs that are unpopular or poorly attended should be phased out.)

If the employer expects to measure the economic impact of the program, such indices as absence rates, turnover rates, health insurance costs, accident rates, and other measures of employee productivity should be chosen and documented before the program begins. If the budget allows, it is advantageous to contract with an outside research agency (whether a private firm or a university) to conduct an independent objective analysis of the program's impact. The general strategy for evaluation is oulined in Chapter 14.

Program Goals and Objectives

The aim of a health promotion program is to influence the health attitudes of individual employees so that they will make everyday decisions that foster more positive and healthy lifestyles. Before a program is launched, the employees may be polled to determine their level of knowledge and attitude towards wellness and their current level of physical activity. It is useful to open this line of communication at the beginning in order to gauge which programs have a likelihood of success. The preliminary poll also will provide a baseline against which program results can be measured.

Employers should clearly state the objectives of the program to all potential participants. Program objectives might include:

- Enhancing the health of workers, not only by preventing disease but also by helping them to achieve new levels of fitness and well-being.

- Encouraging workers to adopt and maintain more physically active lifestyles or proper eating habits that optimize nutrition and weight.
- Helping workers cope better with ordinary and unexpected life stresses.
- Encouraging workers to stop smoking—and helping them do so—and to eliminate or at least decrease substantial alcohol and drug abuse.
- Educating workers about common diseases and how to prevent or minimize their impact.
- Training workers in cardiopulmonary resuscitation (CPR) and first aid skills.

Program Elements

Table 27.1 lists typical components of a health promotion program. Common elements of these components are:

- *Physical fitness*, which focuses on aerobic exercise, muscle power, endurance, and joint flexibility. Individual and group programs may be modified to suit gender and age groups. All physical activity programs should be supervised, either directly or indirectly, by qualified fitness counsellors, and every participant should have a medical clearance before entering the program. The screening can be as simple as a questionnaire administered by a fitness counsellor or as elaborate as a full and detailed examination by a physician. Activities also should incorporate regular tests that measure the progress of each participant and provide encouragement to continue. The program should be adaptable to accommodate the physically handicapped whenever possible. Successful physical fitness programs range from state-of-the-art, company-owned fitness facilities to the reimbursement of membership fees in private or public clubs in the community.
- *Nutrition and weight control activities*, which provide individual nutrition or weight counselling or classes on current knowledge and information regarding sound nutrition and weight control. Special attention is usually placed on dietary cardiovascular risk factors, diabetes, and obesity. Counselling and teaching preferably should be provided by a qualified nutritionist, but where this is not possible, the program should be based on the authoritative advice of recognized nutritional experts as presented in available pamphlets and bulletins.
- *Stress management*, which focuses on helping employees cope with both ordinary, day-to-day stress and unusual stressful events. The program should not attempt to provide in-depth counselling or psychotherapy, as this is more appropriately dealt with by an employee assistance program. Care must be exercised in choosing qualified resource persons for this area; all too often, persons with questionable credentials present themselves as experts. Certified psychologists tend to be the best qualified and most credible for such programs. Short one- or two-hour group sessions that are cheerful and informative can be very effective in teaching techniques to reduce stress. The sessions can be further enhanced by individual questionnaires to help participants determine the levels of stress they are experiencing. Longer sessions, lasting one to three days in a "retreat" format, are useful but require a considerable commitment of time and resources and must be organized and led by a properly qualified professional. These stress management retreats or

seminars are often incorporated into management training programs for executives.

- *Smoking cessation activities*, which use various techniques, ranging from individual counselling to group sessions and special aversion methods, to help workers stop smoking. Sometimes this element is so successful that it is responsible for changing an organization from mostly smokers to mostly non-smokers. When the reconstituted company then issues a no-smoking policy, it places considerable stress on those who cannot quit.

- *Alcohol and drug abuse programs*, which function as the preventive link to the employee assistance program. As alcohol and drug consumption progresses from casual use through misuse to regular abuse, so do the types and intensity of the intervention strategies needed to deal with the problem. The health promotion component provides information to enhance self-awareness through a variety of media, including films, videos, demonstrations, and printed material. Frequently, community resource agencies are brought into the program to give demonstrations of their services. The goal of these programs is to inform employees about the nature of alcohol and drugs so that casual use is kept under control and abuse is prevented.

- *Health education activities*, which often are surprisingly popular. Employees learn about common medical problems and how to keep themselves and their families healthy. The information provided covers basic human biology, detection of health problems, prevention of diseases, and control of chronic disorders. Although different topics appeal to different individuals and groups, depending on their experiences and concerns, topics that are consistently of interest are cancer (in all its forms), heart disease, back and other musculoskeletal problems, sports medicine, diabetes, AIDS, and mental disorders. The information session, or special event such as a health fair, provides a useful—and fun—forum for demonstrating and actually conducting screening tests for hypertension, diabetes, and other conditions easily detectable in a clinic setting.

- *CPR and first-aid training* dovetail nicely with an employee safety training program. Many health authorities believe that everyone should know CPR and at least basic first aid in order to create a first line of emergency care in the community. The workplace is an excellent place to help realize this goal. Over the years, most large workplaces have had employees who sustained heart attacks while at work. After such an incident, other workers are usually highly motivated to learn CPR. If all workers had these skills, the benefits to the workers and the employer would be quite considerable.

Issues in Health Promotion

Health promotion is a new strategy for improving the health of all people. It has adopted many of the techniques of preventive medicine and health education but has also developed its own unique approaches based on behavior modification and the concept of shared individual and community responsibility for health. The workplace has been a particularly effective and profitable avenue for introducing health promotion.

The concepts of health promotion have had a major impact on society in a very short time. Health promotion is both riding and adding momentum to a wave of interest and enthusiasm for health and fitness in society at large. However, while it is indisputably very constructive, the fitness movement does have its drawbacks. It tends to put a great deal of pressure on those who do not choose to participate or who do not conform to idealized standards of weight or physical activity. Health promotion may encourage a certain tendency to "blame the victim," by assuming that the individual is responsible for all health problems that develop as a result of his or her lifestyle, even if the choices were made years before when society had different norms. It tends to encourage fanatical participation, rather than moderation and adaptation to individual needs, and the adoption of fads, some of which may later prove to be of questionable usefulness. Professionals in the field of health promotion are well aware of these tendencies and do their best to minimize them in the programs they run.

For the occupational health professional, the major issue is whether a health promotion program will complement or compete with efforts to advance occupational health and safety and the control of hazards in the workplace. At times, management may see health promotion as a new and exciting development and occupational health and safety as mundane or old hat. The budget for health promotion activities may come at the expense of funding for control of workplace hazards. This is obviously not in the best interests of the worker nor, ultimately, the employer. For this reason, it is important that the occupational health service keep management informed of the contribution it is making in hazard control and specify how this contribution differs from the benefits that may be expected from a health promotion program. Whenever possible, it is desirable for the two programs to be linked and to be mutually supportive. Conflict and competition for resources is detrimental to both.

Further Reading

Aberlin T, Brezezinski ZJ, Carstairs VDL (eds): Measurement in Health Promotion and Protection. Copenhagen, World Health Organization, Regional Publications: European Series No. 22.

Berwick DM: Screening in Health Fairs: A Critical Review of Benefits, Risks, and Costs. Washington, U.S. Office of Disease Prevention and Health Promotion, 1985.

Chen MS, Jones RM: Establishing priorities in the wellness program. Occup Health Safety 1982; 51:6–7, 36.

Chenowith D: Fitness program evaluation: Results with muscle. Occup Health Safety 1983; 52:14–17, 40–42.

Chenowith D: Health promotion: Benefits vs. costs. Occup Health Safety 1983; 52:37–41.

Dedmon RE, et al: Employees as health educators: A reality at Kimberly-Clark. Occup Health Safety 1980; 49:18–24.

Guidotti TL: Health promotion in perspective. Can J Pub Health 1988, in press.

Leatt P, et al: Seven year follow-up of employee fitness program. Can J Pub Health 1988; 79:20–25.

Nast PF, McDonald L: Planning the employee fitness program. Occup Health Safety 1981; 50:27–29.

O'Donnell MP, Ainsworth TH: Health Promotion in the Workplace. New York, John Wiley and Sons, 1984.

Parkinson RS et al: Managing Health Promotion in the Workplace: Guidelines for Implementation and Evaluation. Palo Alto, California, Maryfield Publishing, 1982.

Shephard RJ: Employee health and fitness: The state of the art. Prev Med 1983; 12:644–653.

U.S. Office of Disease Prevention and Health Promotion: Disease Prevention and Health Promotion: The Facts. Palo Alto, California, Bull Publishing, 1988.

U.S. Office of Disease Prevention and Health Promotion: A National Survey of Worksite Health Promotion Activities: A Summary. Silver Spring, Maryland, ODPHP National Health Information Center, 1987.

Worksite Health Promotion: A Bibliography of Selected Resources. Washington, Office of Disease Prevention and Health Promotion, U.S. Public Health Service, 1986.

APPENDICES

APPENDIX 1

An Occupational Health Audit

This occupational health audit is adaptable to working units in many different types of organizations. The audit is presented as a questionnaire divided into sections, each with a series of questions and associated measures. The measures have been kept simple and qualitative. No two areas of a plant are in the same situation and no two employers are the same. Where a rating is less than satisfactory, corrective action must be initiated.

	Inade-quate	Needs Improvement	Satis-factory
1.0 *Occupational Health and Safety Policy*			
1.1 The policy enjoys wide acceptance and publicity throughout the organization:			
1.1.1 A written statement affirms the employer's commitment to protecting the health and safety of all persons affected by their operations.			
1.1.2 Senior management of the company endorse the policy.			
1.1.3 Officers of the company publicly support these principles and require their managers to follow them.			
1.1.4 All legislated occupational health and safety standards are considered to be the minimum standards acceptable and will be exceeded where possible.			
1.1.5 The policy is accessible, posted, and distributed to all employees throughout the organization.			

(Continued)

	Inade-quate	Needs Improvement	Satis-factory

1.1.6 The policy is regularly reviewed and updated in order to reflect changes in legislated and company requirements.

1.1.7 Each aspect of health, safety and hygiene is covered.

1.1.8 Employee accountability meets the employer's standards for all operations.

1.2 The policy is compatible and consistent with corporate policy in other areas.

2.0 *Occupational Health and Safety Administration*

2.1 There is a clearly defined administrative program to manage health and safety:

2.1.1 This is a clearly defined role for each level of management in administration.

2.1.2 There is a clearly defined role for the health and safety professionals responsible for the area.

2.1.3 There is a clearly defined expectation for action to resolve health and safety issues.

2.1.4 There is a clearly established preference for proactive, preventive programs.

2.1.5 There is a clear understanding among all levels of management and by safety professionals of the priorities of the program and the expectations placed on them for its successful implementation.

2.1.6 Qualified resource personnel are available in:

2.1.6.1 safety.

2.1.6.2 occupational hygiene.

2.1.6.3 occupational medicine.

2.1.6.4 occupational health nursing.

2.2 There are clearly defined:

2.2.1 safe work practices.

2.2.2 workplace standards.

2.2.3 personal protective equipment standards.

2.3 There is a written procedure requiring proper incident/accident investigation that clearly defines the role and duties of all personnel involved.

2.4 There is a written, clearly established procedure for reporting and recording data on all incidents/accidents, conforming at a minimum to OSHA requirements.

2.5 There is a well established program to communicate current health and safety issues to employees that includes the following:

(Continued)

	Inade-quate	Needs Improvement	Satis-factory

2.5.1 Regular health and safety meetings of management, supervisors, and local health and safety specialists.

2.5.2 Regular health and safety meetings involving all employees.

2.5.3 Regular health and safety inspections.

2.5.4 Written communication of incident/accident investigation reports to all personnel with responsibilities that may be affected.

2.5.5 Films, bulletins, posters, and other posted information to maintain health and safety awareness.

2.5.6 Communication to employees of known or potential hazards associated with the workplace and their possible effects.

2.6 Each area within the plant location has a coordinated annual health and safety program that includes:

2.6.1 Clearly defined goals established by operating management in consultation with company health and safety personnel.

2.6.2 An identified plan to achieve the goals.

2.6.3 There are regular and thorough reviews involving management and health and safety specialists to examine performance and to adjust the plan as necessary.

2.6.4 There are written objectives for each health and safety specialist specifying how their activities support the goals established by the operating components of the employer.

2.7 There is a written plan to handle all levels of emergency incidents, including:

2.7.1 Identification of potential emergencies.

2.7.2 Identification of personnel assigned to handle an emergency and their responsibilities in the event of an incident.

2.7.3 Identification and organization of resources available to manage emergencies.

2.7.4 Practice sessions to ensure readiness in the event of an incident.

2.8 Regular health and safety inspections are performed and documented by:

2.8.1 Supervisors.

2.8.2 Health and safety specialists.

2.9 Local health, safety and work procedures are reviewed regularly to ensure:

2.9.1 Compliance with current internal and legislated standards.

(Continued)

	Inade-quate	Needs Improvement	Satis-factory

2.9.2 Suitability for use in the workplace.

2.9.3 Availability and familiarity in the workplace.

2.10 Management and the local safety specialist are involved in the review.

2.11 All action items are identified and resolved.

3.0 *Site Management*

Site managers are required to:

3.1 Consider occupational health and safety as a normal part of business that must be planned for, organized, controlled, and measured.

3.2 Understand their responsibilities related to health and safety.

3.3 Ensure that their employees know their responsibilities related to health and safety, and hold them accountable.

3.4 Ensure that procedures/instructions are established and followed regarding:

3.4.1 Health and safety practices.

3.4.2 Job/work practices.

3.4.3 Enforcement of health, safety, and work regulations.

3.4.4 Accident investigation.

3.4.5 Workplace hazard control.

3.4.6 Exposure to health hazards.

3.5 Require that training is provided to ensure that all employees are properly trained to perform their work safely.

3.6 Receive training and demonstrate competence in:

3.6.1 Management's responsibility for occupational health and safety, as expressed in company policy and legislation.

3.6.2 Basic principles of hazard recognition and accident prevention.

3.6.3 Basic principles of occupational hygiene.

3.7 Actively participate in the health and safety program by:

3.7.1 Holding regular recorded meetings to discuss health and safety issues and performance with:

3.7.1.1 their manager/supervisor.

3.7.1.2 safety personnel.

3.7.1.3 hygiene personnel.

3.7.2 Participating in safety tours.

3.7.3 Requiring regular reports on health and safety problems and their resolution.

(Continued)

	Inade-quate	Needs Improvement	Satis-factory

3.7.4 Ensuring that adequate resources are put in place to support the health and safety activities.

3.7.5 Reviewing all accident, injury, and occupational illness reports and ensuring that proper corrective action is implemented.

4.0 *Foremen/Supervisors*

The foremen/supervisors:

4.1 Maintain records of the health and safety performance of the workers in their area.

4.2 Include health and safety as a regular part of their daily activities, and encourage a positive, safe attitude on the part of employees.

4.3 Ensure that their employees are trained in and follow health and safety practices associated with their job. Only competent employees or employees under the direct supervision of a competent employee are permitted to perform a hazardous task.

4.4 Have the necessary training in the areas of:

    4.4.1 Supervisory responsibilities related to health and safety.

    4.4.2 Accident prevention techniques.

    4.4.3 Hazard recognition and control.

    4.4.4 Occupational hygiene.

    4.4.5 Accident investigation.

    4.4.6 First aid and cardiopulmonary resuscitation.

    4.4.7 Local emergency procedures.

4.5 Ensure that the written procedures that apply to any job involving work of a hazardous nature are available to and are reviewed with the employees involved.

4.6 Perform regular health and safety inspections in their area, and record the results and any corrective action required.

4.7 Work with the local health and safety specialists to ensure that proper safe work practices and procedures are established for the area.

4.8 Ensure that the facilities for which they are responsible are maintained in a safe and healthy condition.

5.0 *Joint Employee-Manpower Health and Safety Committee*

5.1 A committee exists in accordance with:

    5.1.1 Employee-management agreement.

    5.1.2 Legislation.

    5.1.3 Other (specify).

5.2 The committee meets regularly and follows an agenda.

(Continued)

	Inade-quate	Needs Improvement	Satis-factory

5.3   There is representation from the following:

    5.3.1 Senior management.

    5.3.2 Operations engineering.

    5.3.3 Facilities engineering.

    5.3.4 Employees.

5.4   The committee performs regular health and safety inspections in the area.

5.5   There is a training program to ensure that the members have sufficient knowledge of health and safety matters to function effectively.

5.6   The committee issues minutes of the meetings on a regular basis.

5.7   The minutes are action-oriented, identifying tasks to be done.

5.8   There is a positive and timely response to the action items by operational personnel.

5.9   The committee is perceived as effective by both the employees and management.

5.10   The committee reviews all incident/accident reports.

6.0 *Training Program*

6.1   A standard training format has been established to provide the health and safety training required for the preparation of:

    6.1.1 Supervisors.

    6.1.2 Employees.

6.2   A standard training program is in place to ensure that all operators are properly trained or supervised before they operate any of the facilities or equipment.

6.3   Employees' assigned responsibilities are directly dependent on the training that has been successfully completed.

6.4   All new employees are given a health and safety orientation covering the following:

    6.4.1 Job hazards.

    6.4.2 Health hazards.

    6.4.3 Use of protective equipment.

    6.4.4 Proper work procedures.

    6.4.5 Work restrictions.

    6.4.6 Health and safety regulations.

    6.4.7 Hazard reporting.

    6.4.8 First aid resources.

6.5   All new employees are closely supervised until they are capable of working without risk of injury.

(Continued)

	Inade-quate	Needs Improvement	Satis-factory

6.6 Are all employees aware of:

    6.6.1 Potential and existing hazards to their health and safety.

    6.6.2 Proper work procedures.

    6.6.3 Proper use and limitations of protective equipment.

    6.6.4 Health and safety regulations.

    6.6.5 Special skills necessary to perform their job safely.

6.7 There are sufficient numbers of people qualified in:

    6.7.1 First Aid.

    6.7.2 Cardiopulmonary resuscitation.

    6.7.3 Fire fighting.

    6.7.4 Use of respiratory protection.

    6.7.5 Special hazard awareness.

    6.7.6 Special hazard detection.

    6.7.7 Hazardous chemical control and use.

    6.7.8 Incident/accident investigation.

    6.7.9 Other (specify).

6.8 All the training programs offered meet current company and legislated standards.

6.9 The training program includes:

    6.9.1 Permanent records of all health, safety, and job training courses completed by each employee.

    6.9.2 A periodic review to ensure that the required level of expertise is maintained.

7.0 *Incident/Accident Handling*

7.1 All incidents/accidents are suitably investigated in order to determine the following:

    7.1.1 A clear understanding of what occurred and all factors contributing to the incident.

    7.1.2 The direct causes of the accident.

    7.1.3 The basic causes that allowed the incident/accident to occur.

    7.1.4 The proper short- and long-term corrective action.

7.2 There is a written procedure for recording and reporting the incident/accident and communicating findings to:

    7.2.1 Employer officials.

    7.2.2 Required government authorities.

    7.2.3 Supervisors.

7.3 The investigation involves all appropriate levels of management, supervisors, and health and safety professionals.

(Continued)

	Inade-quate	Needs Improvement	Satis-factory
7.4 There is a clearly defined procedure to ensure that options for corrective actions are reviewed by management and appropriate action is taken to resolve the problems identified.			
7.5 All types of incidents/accidents are covered, including the following:			
7.5.1 Personal injury.			
7.5.2 Occupational illness.			
7.5.3 Property damage.			
7.5.4 Vehicle accidents.			
7.5.5 Near miss (incidents/accidents that are narrowly avoided).			
7.5.6 Transportation incidents.			
7.6 The following incidents are discussed with all employees:			
7.6.1 Personal injury.			
7.6.2 Property damage.			
7.6.3 Vehicle accidents.			
7.6.4 Transportation incidents.			
8.0 *Occupational Health and Safety Specialist*			
8.1 At least one employee is assigned to management with responsibility for coordinating health and safety programs.			
8.2 The duties, responsibilities, and relationships of the health and safety specialists are clearly described and known to workers.			
8.3 The people assigned to health and safety duties are adequate in number and skills to fulfill their responsibilities in all areas, including the following:			
8.3.1 Safety.			
8.3.2 Occupational hygiene.			
8.3.3 Emergency response.			
8.3.4 Transportation of hazardous materials.			
8.4 The specialists are provided with adequate opportunities to maintain and to improve their qualifications by attending seminars and courses.			
8.5 There are adequate facilities and equipment to support the specialists in their duties including the following:			
8.5.1 Office and records storage.			
8.5.2 Meeting room facilities.			
8.5.3 Audiovisual materials.			
8.5.4 Specialized equipment (including emergency supplies).			
8.6 The facilities and equipment are regularly maintained.			

(Continued)

	Inade-quate	Needs Improvement	Satis-factory

8.7 The specialists are required to submit regularly monthly reports on their activities.

8.8 The specialists are required to prepare an annual plan, in cooperation with management, to coordinate the management of their programs.

9.0 *Facilities and Equipment*

9.1 A visual inspection of the facilities finds that it is free of significant problems in:

    9.1.1 Housekeeping.

    9.1.2 Adequate work areas and access paths.

    9.1.3 Material and chemical storage.

    9.1.4 Ventilation.

    9.1.5 Provision of guardrails and handrails.

    9.1.6 Machine tools and equipment guards and protective devices.

    9.1.7 Roadways and walkways.

    9.1.8 Lighting.

    9.1.9 Facilities and equipment maintenance.

9.2 Access to areas with significant health and safety hazard is restricted to employees with training and a reason to be in the area.

9.3 Waste material is properly collected and disposed of.

9.4 The fire protection systems are adequate in the following ways:

    9.4.1 Suited to the facility and equipment therein.

    9.4.2 Properly located.

    9.4.3 Properly maintained (with maintenance recorded).

9.5 All hazardous confined spaces are properly identified and controlled.

9.6 Adequate first aid facilities are provided.

9.7 There is a suitable program to ensure proper maintenance in the following areas:

    9.7.1 Regular maintenance checks are made to ensure that all equipment is kept in good condition.

    9.7.2 All work is performed only by competent and trained personnel.

    9.7.3 Proper locking and tagging procedures are used to isolate all hazards during maintenance work.

    9.7.4 Written maintenance records are kept in accordance with policy and legislated regulations.

(Continued)

	Inade-quate	Needs Improvement	Satis-factory

9.7.5 Critical failures, or processes that have the potential for significant hazard in the event of failure, are identified and corrected.

9.8 When facilities are modified or expanded, procedures are in place to ensure that:

9.8.1 All plans are reviewed by a qualified health and safety specialist.

9.8.2 Government authorities are notified as required by the employer's policy and by law.

9.8.3 All construction work is observed and managed in accordance with the employer's policy, legal regulations, and the following:

9.8.3.1 health and safety policies of the contractor.

9.8.3.2 adherence by the contractor to the employer's policies, legal regulations, and accepted practices.

9.8.3.3 construction and material quality standards.

9.8.3.4 standing with the workers' compensation board.

9.9 A process analysis (or the equivalent) has been completed to identify possible hazardous areas that could endanger workers.

10. Safety Programs and Procedures

10.1 Published guidelines on safe work practices are available to all employees.

10.2 Management regulates personnel who perform work that requires specialized knowledge, training, or licensing.

10.3 There is a work control system to identify and control hazardous situations through a system of safe work permits.

10.4 There is a program to ensure that mobile equipment is in a safe condition when purchased, is properly maintained, and is operated only by competent, authorized operators.

10.5 There is a program to ensure that hoisting and lifting equipment is in a safe condition when purchased, is properly maintained, and is operated only by competent, authorized operators.

10.6 There is a written record of all inspection and maintenance work done on mobile and lifting equipment.

10.7 There are programs to ensure the following:

(Continued)

	Inade-quate	Needs Improvement	Satis-factory

10.7.1   Vehicles used on company business are maintained in safe condition and are operated in a safe manner and in accordance with all laws.

10.7.2   Only properly licensed employees may operate a motor vehicle on company business.

10.7.3   Vehicles requiring a licensed operator other than a holder of a Class 5 license (or equivalent) are operated only by a properly licensed operator.

10.8   There is a complete written procedure for locking, tagging, and blocking equipment that ensures that the equipment is in a state of "zero energy" (i.e., will not roll, snap, spring, or discharge) before and during the time it is worked on.

10.9   There are written standards covering the storage and use of flammable materials that include the following:

10.9.1   Proper ventilation.

10.9.2   Proper storage cabinets or rooms.

10.9.3   Suitable fire extinguishing equipment, which is checked regularly and is readily available.

10.9.4   Separation of potentially reactive materials.

10.9.5   Proper grounding of containers.

10.9.6   Limits on the quantities of flammable materials kept in work areas.

10.9.7   Control of ignition sources close to flammable materials in work and storage areas.

10.10   Maintenance employees and others as needed are trained in proper procedures of performing elevated work, including the following:

10.10.1   Proper use of ladders and scaffolds.

10.10.2   Proper use of personal protective equipment.

10.11   Work on electrical equipment is controlled to ensure that:

10.11.1   Only qualified competent personnel perform the work.

10.11.2   Proper locking and tagging procedures are followed.

10.12   All excavation and trenching work is controlled to ensure that:

(Continued)

	Inade-quate	Needs Improvement	Satis-factory

10.12.1   All excavations are properly prepared prior to entry by any personnel.

10.12.2   All buried hazards and cables are identified and safely exposed by hand digging.

10.12.3   All trenches are properly shored according to sound work practices and legislation.

10.13   Written procedures are followed to ensure that the opening of pipes, sumps, valves, tanks, and cisterns during maintenance is properly controlled and done only by competent personnel.

11. *Occupational Hygiene Program*

11.1   A program is in place to identify all existing and potential chemical, physical, and biological hazards, including the following:

11.1.1   Identification of hazards associated with raw materials and their location.

11.1.2   Identification of hazards associated with process chemicals and additives and their location.

11.1.3   Identification of process by-products and their locations.

11.1.4   Identification of equipment and activities that can give rise to such physical hazards as heat, noise, and radiation.

11.1.5   Assessment of the potential exposure in the event of a process failure, or a system breakdown.

11.1.6   Assessment of all new processes, equipment and process chemicals to determine potential hazard.

11.2   There is a program in place to identify all chemical products used or stored at the facility that includes the following elements:

11.2.1   A complete written inventory of all chemicals and their location.

11.2.2   A standardized format for Material Safety Data Sheets (MSDS) that meets all legislated requirements.

11.2.3   A review of the accuracy and completeness of all MSDS performed by qualified personnel.

11.2.4   A process for updating the chemical inventory list on a regular planned basis.

11.2.5   Sufficient distribution of MSDS to ensure that all employees have access to them.

(Continued)

	Inade-quate	Needs Improvement	Satis-factory

11.2.6 An on-going evaluation of new chemical products during their initial research and later industrial development to identify any health and safety concerns before the products are used within the company.

11.2.7 An ongoing evaluation of new chemical products throughout the process by which they are developed for industrial and commercial use that aims at identifying all health and safety concerns.

11.3 A program is in place to identify hazards associated with final products. This program includes the following elements:

11.3.1 Identification of all components of the products and a review of their potential hazard.

11.3.2 Identification of potential product contaminants that could be hazardous or that could increase the hazard of the product.

11.3.3 Preparation and provision of accurate MSDS to customers.

11.3.4 Documentation, including the date of issue, for the distribution to customers of MSDS for the product.

11.3.5 Testing of equipment for physical hazards (noise, vibration, heat, radiation).

11.4 A program is in place to ensure that any known or potential carcinogens and other hazardous substances have been identified and controlled.

11.5 A program is in place to evaluate exposure to health hazards and includes the following elements:

11.5.1 Regularly monitoring of potential employee exposures under operational conditions.

11.5.2 Testing and analysis by qualified specialists.

11.5.3 Comparison of all readings to recognized standards in order to evaluate the need for control.

11.5.4 Recognized monitoring and analytical methods.

11.5.5 A suitable procedure for verification of and follow-up on problems.

11.5.6 Equipment calibration and maintenance.

11.6 A hazard control program is in place that includes the following:

11.6.1 Engineering, administration, and personal protective controls, as appropriate.

(Continued)

	Inade-quate	Needs Improvement	Satis-factory
11.6.2 A control strategy that considers the following responses, in order of preference:			
11.6.2.1 elimination and/or replacement of the hazardous substance.			
11.6.2.2 engineering controls to minimize or eliminate the exposure potential.			
11.6.2.3 administrative controls to protect employees from exposure.			
11.6.2.4 use of suitable personal protective equipment to protect employees from overexposure.			
11.7 A follow-up program is in place to ensure that the controls that have been implemented are effective and maintained.			
11.8 A training program is in place to ensure that employees are made aware of all health hazards and the proper procedures associated with them. This program includes a MSDS retrieval and interpretation exercise to assist in dealing with all hazardous materials.			
11.9 There is a hearing conservation program to control exposure to harmful noise levels that includes the following:			
11.9.1 Noise measurements.			
11.9.2 Employee hearing tests (baseline and periodic).			
11.9.3 Employee training.			
11.9.4 Suitable controls.			
11.10 A complete program is in place to control entry into confined spaces, in accordance with the employer's policy and legislated standards.			
11.11 The required "Codes of Practice" are all in place.			
12. Transportation of Hazardous Materials			
12.1 The requirements of legislation are considered to be the minimum standard and are to be improved upon if possible.			
12.2 The facility is registered as a shipper/manufacturer of hazardous materials, as required by law.			
12.3 An emergency response plan has been filed with government authorities.			
12.4 There is a complete listing of all regulated goods used at the facility.			
12.5 There is a training program in place in accordance with legislated requirements.			
12.6 There is a program in place to monitor changes in legislation.			

(Continued)

	Inade-quate	Needs Improvement	Satis-factory

12.7 Regulated wastes generated by the facility are identified and monitored.

12.8 Copies of all bills of lading are stored in one place and available for review.

12.9 Copies of all federal and state or provincial inspection reports are easily available for review.

12.10 This facility has participated in an audit on the handling of hazardous materials.

12.11 A program is in place to ensure proper placarding (signage on the vehicle) of vehicles transporting hazardous materials.

13. *Personal Protective Equipment*

13.1 A written program is in place to control the selection, use, and maintenance of personal protective equipment.

13.2 The selection of personal protective equipment available to workers at the worksite takes into consideration the following:

    13.2.1 Nature of the specific hazards.

    13.2.2 Employee fitting and fit testing for use of respirators (as applicable).

    13.2.3 Employee training.

13.3 The selection available includes all necessary personal protective equipment to protect employees adequately from all hazards in the workplace (foot, head, face, eye, skin, respiratory, hearing, fall protection, etc.) and gives them a choice wherever possible.

13.4 Personal protective equipment is made available to all employees in accordance with the employer's policy and legislated standards for employee protection.

13.5 The supervisors, in consultation with health and safety personnel, specify which type of personal protective equipment is required by their workers on all jobs.

13.6 Prior to the specification or purchase of any personal protective equipment, a qualified occupational health or safety professional reviews and approves the purchase order so as to ensure that the final selection of equipment is in accordance with recognized standards and operational requirements.

13.7 Supervisors actively promote and require the use of personal protective equipment by their workers, and use the appropriate equipment themselves.

(Continued)

	Inade-quate	Needs Improvement	Satis-factory

13.8 Supervisors make sure that all workers understand the need for proper use of the personal protective equipment and the limitations on their effectiveness.

14. *Occupational Health Service Policy and Procedures*

    14.1 The medical staff has direct access to the general manager of the plant.

    14.2 Regular staff meetings are held. (Identify the frequency and the date of the last meeting.)

    14.3 Staff members have job descriptions that are current.

    14.4 Staff members work from annual goals/objectives. (Identify the person responsible for setting goals.)

    14.5 Staff members are given the opportunity to attend professional courses, conferences, and seminars.

    14.6 There is a detailed policy and procedure manual.

    14.7 The manual reflects corporate policy regarding occupational health and safety.

    14.8 The manual includes statements on the following:

        14.8.1 Individual staff responsibilities.

        14.8.2 Control and dispensing of medication.

        14.8.3 Use of special equipment.

        14.8.4 Authorization for medical procedures.

        14.8.5 Liaison with health resources in the community.

        14.8.6 Services on weekends and after normal hours.

        14.8.7 Communications with hygiene and safety departments, where applicable.

        14.8.8 Communications with management.

        14.8.9 Transportation of sick and injured.

        14.8.10 Emergency care policy and procedures.

        14.8.11 Sickness absence investigations.

        14.8.12 Long-term disability procedures.

        14.8.13 Work appointments procedures.

        14.8.14 Recordkeeping procedures.

        14.8.15 Retention time for records.

        14.8.16 Staff meetings.

        14.8.17 Laboratory procedures.

        14.8.18 Objectives and procedures for health programs.

        14.8.19 In-house safety procedures.

        14.8.20 Procedures concerning investigations of incidents/accidents.

    14.9 The manual includes the following:

(Continued)

		Inade- quate	Needs Improvement	Satis- factory

14.9.1   Disaster plan outlining the appropriate response of the occupational health services.

14.9.2   Use of record and requisition forms.

14.9.3   Contracts for hospital and emergency services.

14.10   The manual is reviewed regularly by all parties responsible. (Specify date of last review.)

14.11   The occupational health service meets regulatory requirements in the following areas:

14.11.1   Hearing conservation.

14.11.2   Examination of vehicle operators.

14.11.3   Workers' compensation reports.

14.12   The most significant illness and injury problems arising in the workplace (specify) have been identified and discussed by the responsible supervisor:

14.12.1   The physician.

14.12.2   The head nurse.

14.12.3   Supervisors.

14.12.4   Employee representatives.

14.13   The most frequent occupational injuries and illnesses in the workplace have been addressed by effective programs or controls.

14.14   The principal health and safety hazards presented by this workplace are known to all service personnel and are frequently discussed.

14.15   The health staff has a mechanism in place for becoming aware of and knowledgeble about changes in hazards and conditions in the workplace. These include:

14.15.1   MSDS.

14.15.2   Site visits (regularly and as needed).

14.15.3   Review of clinical records (regularly and as needed).

14.15.4   Worker complaints.

14.15.5   Union complaints.

14.15.6   Hygiene notifications.

14.15.7   Management consultations.

14.15.8   Special studies conducted on the workplace.

14.15.9   Other (list).

14.16   The physician and nurse have become familiar with the processes, materials, and products found in the workplace.

14.17   The physician and nurse make regular and frequent site visits.

(Continued)

	Inade-quate	Needs Improvement	Satis-factory

15. *Health Service Programs and Activities*

Evaluations of services provided have demonstrated satisfactory performance of the following:

15.1   Acute injury and illness management.

15.2   Fitness-to-work evaluations:

    15.2.1 Preplacement examination.

    15.2.2 Return-to-work examination.

    15.2.3 Job transfer.

    15.2.4 Continuing education.

    15.2.5 Changes in health conditions.

    15.2.6 Changes in working conditions.

    15.2.7 Performance-initiated examination.

    15.2.8 Voluntary periodic health evaluation.

15.3   Health surveillance.

15.4   Health monitoring.

15.5   Assessments of fitness to wear respirators.

15.6   Audiograms.

15.7   Immunizations.

15.8   Ongoing therapy/checks.

15.9   Stress reduction.

15.10 Low back care and prevention of back injury.

15.11 Smoking cessation.

15.12 Physical fitness.

15.13 Dietary consultation and nutrition.

15.14 Workplace rehabilitation.

15.15 Employee assistance.

15.16 Site health surveys and health hazard evaluations.

15.17 Health and safety committee.

15.18 Worker health training.

15.19 Management health training.

15.20 Collection of illness/trauma data.

15.21 Analysis of illness/trauma data.

15.22 Reporting results of analysis to management.

15.23 Incident/accident investigation.

15.24 First-aid training.

15.25 Workers' compensation reporting and referral.

16. *Health Service Resources Facilities*

The location, main components, and age of the occupational health service facilities are appropriate to the service's use and function.

16.1   The facilities are accessible to workers.

16.2   The facilities are accessible to the handicapped.

(Continued)

	Inade-quate	Needs Improvement	Satis-factory

16.3 The facilities ensure the privacy of workers who come for care.

16.4 The facilities are quiet.

16.5 The facilities are well maintained and clean.

16.6 Equipment is properly maintained and, if applicable, calibrated, including the following:

    16.6.1 Diagnostic and treatment equipment.

    16.6.2 Training equipment.

    16.6.3 Administrative and office equipment.

16.7 Information resources are available and include the following:

    16.7.1 Medical and nursing texts.

    16.7.2 Occupational health newsletters.

    16.7.3 Occupational health journals.

    16.7.4 Occupational health regulations.

    16.7.5 MSDS.

    16.7.6 First aid manuals.

17. *Records and Forms*

17.1 Access to confidential records is controlled in a satisfactory manner.

17.2 Occupational history records are maintained for each worker.

17.3 Hazard exposure records are maintained for each worker.

17.4 Consultation and treatment records are maintained for each worker.

17.5 Periodic health evaluation records are maintained for each worker.

17.6 Medical records are separated so that confidential and non-confidential information are not mixed.

17.7 A satisfactory flagging system is in operation for special cases and for scheduled evaluations.

17.8 Biological monitoring records are maintained.

17.9 Immunization records are maintained.

17.10 Forms for authorization for release of information are used as needed.

17.11 Fitness-for-work certificates are used.

17.12 Site-survey reports are maintained.

17.13 A daily log (visit record) is kept.

17.14 Minutes of meetings are retained.

17.15 A record of equipment maintenance and calibration is kept.

17.16 Records are kept of equipment, supplies, and inventories.

(Continued)

	Inade-quate	Needs Improvement	Satis-factory
17.17 Drug dispensing records are kept.			
17.18 Records are kept of equipment loans (such as crutches, canes, splints).			

APPENDIX 2

Sources of Information for Managing Occupational Health Problems

Hot Lines

Canadian Centre for Occupational Safety and Health.
> Provides literature searches and data summaries on toxic substances; may not be suitable on an urgent basis (416 523-2981).

Canutech, Transport Canada, Dangerous Goods Branch.
> Provides information and assistance on transportation incidents in Canada; call collect (613 992-4624).

Job Accommodation Network.
> Provides information and suggestions on accommodating disabled persons in the workplace; 8:00 a.m.–8:00 p.m. EST Monday through Thursday,   8:00 a.m.–5:00 p.m. EST Friday (800 526-7234, 800 526-4698 in West Virginia).

National Council on Alcoholism.
> Provides general information and refers inquiries to local affiliates (800 NCA-CALL).

National Safety Council.
> Provides information on safety and accident prevention (800 621-7619, 312 527-4800 in Illinois).

NIDA Hotline.
> Provides information on employee assistance and drug abuse treatment for managers; 9:00 a.m.–8:00 p.m. EST Monday through Friday (800 843-4971).

ODPHP National Health Information Center
> Central source of health-related information by the U.S. Office of Disease Prevention and Health Promotion; 9:00 a.m.–5:00 p.m. EST (800 336-4797, 202 429-9091 in the District of Columbia).

Toxicology Information Response Center, Oak Ridge National Laboratory.
> Provides information on hazardous substances to physicians, lawyers, and other users on a fee-for-service basis (615 576-1743).

U.S. Office of Substance Abuse Prevention.
   Provides information to industry on drug abuse prevention, 8:15 a.m.-4:45 p.m.
EST (800 638-2045, 301 443-6500 in Maryland).

Reference Works (* indicates excellent resources for the physician's shelf)

   Clayton GD, Clayton FE (eds): Patty's Industrial Hygiene and Toxicology ed 3. New
York, John Wiley and Sons, 1982, in three volumes. An exceedingly detailed compen-
dium describing industrial processes and hazards, available in reference libraries and
in the offices of many large corporations and consulting services.
   Doull J, Klausen C, Amdur M (eds): Casarett and Doull's Toxicology, ed 3. New
York, MacMillan, 1980. A useful textbook and reference book in toxicology.
   Finkel AJ: Hamilton and Hardy's Industrial Toxicology, ed 4. Littleton, Massachusetts, John Wright-PSG, 1982. A standard reference in toxicology.
   Last JM (ed): Maxcy-Rosenau Public Health and Preventive Medicine, ed 11. New
York, Appleton-Century-Crofts, 1980.* Excellent reference for public health and policy
aspects of toxic substances; useful first reference in a toxic exposure emergency but
incomplete.
   McCunney RJ (ed): Handbook of Occupational Medicine. Boston, Little, Brown,
1988.* Convenient and authoritative source emphasizing management of common problems and situations.
   Olishifski JB (ed): Fundamentals of Industrial Hygiene, ed 2. Chicago, National
Safety Council, 1979.* An excellent reference in industrial hygiene easily understood
by the non-engineer; extensive bibliographies and a supplement on toxic substances
make this a convenient source in an emergency.
   Parmeggiani L (ed): Encyclopaedia of Occupational Health and Safety, ed 3. Geneva,
International Labour Organization, 1983.* A comprehensive source of information on
occupational health that is also a useful guide in hazardous materials incidents.
   Proctor NH, Hughes JP, Fischman ML: Chemical Hazards of the Workplace (ed 2).
Philadelphia, J.B. Lippincott, 1988.* Strongly recommended; an excellent and convenient
source of information.
   Rom WN (ed): Environmental and Occupational Medicine. Boston, Little Brown
and Co., 1983.* A superb, comprehensive reference in occupational and environmental
medicine.
   Sax NI: Dangerous Properties of Industrial Materials (ed 6). New York, Van Nos-
trand, 1984.* An invaluable, comprehensive, and definitive reference.
   U.S. National Institute for Occupational Safety and Health, Occupational Safety
and Health Administration. Occupational Health Guidelines for Chemical Hazards.
Washington DC, U.S. Government Printing Office, 1981. DHHS (NIOSH) Publication
No. 81-123. Useful and inexpensive, but cannot be used alone; guidelines for many common and important hazards are omitted because of U.S. federal standards review.

Local Resources
Company libraries. Local employers may maintain working libraries.
Computer search services through medical libraries.
Fire departments. Most large fire departments have the information systems and equip-
   ment required to deal with common hazards that involve fire, explosion, or acciden-
   tal chemical release and should be notified in any event.

Law libraries. Because of the need for references on forensic toxicology, law libraries often have useful collections.

Medical schools. Important to evaluate the practical experience of faculty providing the information.

Poison control centers. Most lack in-depth expertise on occupational exposures and are not well equipped to deal with large-scale incidents.

State or provincial agencies. (e.g., the Medical Toxicological Information Program in Alberta maintains a phone number during working hours, 403 427-6724).

University programs in occupational and environmental health, toxicology, industrial hygiene, or chemistry. Health and safety offices of large research universities or laboratories often have extensive knowledge of and experience in managing chemical hazards.

APPENDIX 3

Recommended Occupational Medicine Clinic Library

Adams RM: Occupational Skin Disease. New York, Grune and Stratton, 1982.

Brady GS, Clausen HR: Materials Handbook (ed 12). New York, McGraw-Hill, 1986.

Cailliet R: Low Back Pain Syndrome. Philadelphia, F.A. Davis, 1981.

Chiazze L, Lundin FE, Watkins D: Methods and Issues in Occupational and Environmental Epidemiology. Ann Arbor, Ann Arbor Sciences, 1983.

Daugaard J: Symptoms and Signs in Occupational Disease: A Practical Guide. Copenhagen, Munksgaard (distributed in U.S. by Year Book Medical Publishers), 1978.

Doull J, Klaassen CD, Amdur MO (eds): Casarett and Doull's Toxicology: The Basic Science of Poisons. New York, Macmillan, 1980.

Eastman Kodak Co: Ergonomic Design for People at Work. Belmont, CA, Lifetime Learning Publications, 1983.

Engelberg AL (ed): Guides to the Evaluation of Permanent Impairment. Chicago, AMA, 1988.

Finkel AJ: Hamilton and Hardy's Industrial Toxicology. Boston, John Wright—PSG, Inc., 1983.

Fries JF, Ehrlich GE (eds): Prognosis: Contemporary Outcomes of Disease. Menlo Park, CA, Addison-Wesley, 1981.

International Labor Office. Encyclopaedia of Occupational Health and Safety. Geneva, ILO, 1983.

Key MM, et al (eds): Occupational Diseases: A Guide to Their Recognition. NIOSH Pub. No. 77-181, 1977.

Kusnetz S, Hutchison MK (eds): A Guide to the Work-Relatedness of Disease. NIOSH Pub. No. 79-116, 1979.

LaDou J (ed.): Occupational Health Law: A Guide for Industry. New York, Marcel Dekker, 1981.

Last JM: A Dictionary of Epidemiology. New York, Oxford University Press, 1983.

Lauwerys RR: Industrial Chemical Exposure: Guidelines for Biological Monitoring. Davis, CA, Biomedical Publications, 1983.

Levy B, Wegman D: Occupational Health. Boston, Little Brown, 1983.

Lewy R: Preventive Primary Medicine: Reducing the Major Causes of Mortality. Boston, Little Brown, 1980.

McCunney RJ (ed): Handbook of Occupational Medicine. Boston, Little Brown, 1988.

Monson RR: Occupational Epidemiology. Boca Raton, FL, CRC Press, 1980.

NIOSH: Registry of Toxic Effects of Chemical Substances. (Obtain microfiche version in latest edition. Last printed version was 1980 and is now outdated.)

NIOSH: Occupational Health Guidelines for Chemical Hazards. NIOSH Pub. No. 81-123, 1981.

NIOSH, OSHA: Pocket Guide to Chemical Hazards. NIOSH Pub. No. 78-210, 1978.

Olishifski JB (ed): Fundamentals of Industrial Hygiene. Chicago, National Safety Council, 1981.

Oskamp S: Applied Social Psychology. Englewood Cliffs, NJ, Prentice-Hall, 1984.

Parkes WR: Occupational Lung Disorders. Boston, Butterworths, 1982.

Proctor NH, Hughes JP, Fischman ML: Chemical Hazards of the Workplace. Philadelphia, J.B. Lippincott, 1988.

Rom WN (ed): Environmental and Occupational Medicine. Boston, Little Brown, 1983.

Schilling RSF (ed): Occupational Health Practice. London, Butterworths, 1981.

Schottenfeld D, Fraumeni JF (eds): Cancer Epidemiology and Prevention. Philadelphia, W.B. Saunders, 1982.

U.S. Office of the Surgeon General: Healthy People: The Surgeon General's Report on Health Promotion and Disease Prevention. Public Health Service Pub. No. 79-55071, 1979.

Periodicals
American Industrial Hygiene Association Journal
American Journal of Industrial Medicine
Business and Health (Washington Business Group on Health)
Journal of Occupational Medicine
Occupational Health and Safety
Occupational health legislation reporting system
Other publications appropriate to the industry
Patient education publications

Data Bases
CCINFO disc. Canadian Centre for Occupational Health and Safety. A serially updated information service providing 250,000 pages of information on compact disc, in English and French, incorporating reference, technical, standards, and directory material.

APPENDIX 4

Survey on Occupational Health Services

Part I. Please indicate your opinion of the importance of each occupational medicine service by circling the number that corresponds most closely; please indicate the way in which each service is handled in your company by checking the box which applies.

Please circle one: This service is:
1 = not useful,
2 = helpful,
3 = desirable,
4 = important,
5 = essential.

Occupational Medicine Services

Treatment of on-the-job injuries	1 2 3 4 5
Safety inspections to prevent on- the-job injuries	1 2 3 4 5
Treatment of job-related illnesses	1 2 3 4 5
Periodic health-hazard evaluations to prevent job-related illnesses	1 2 3 4 5
Engineering and industrial hygiene services to identify and correct hazardous conditions	1 2 3 4 5
Reporting of job-related injuries and illness to government agencies (required by law)	1 2 3 4 5
Consultation with plant management on an on-going basis to correct problems as they appear	1 2 3 4 5
Preplacement physical examinations to determine fitness for work	1 2 3 4 5
Regular oversight of workers' health problems to detect problems early	1 2 3 4 5
Referral to outside specialists when needed	1 2 3 4 5
Comprehensive diagnosis and treatment in all specialties at one location	1 2 3 4 5
Supervision, training, and continuing education of your in-plant staff (nurses, safety officers)	1 2 3 4 5
Maintenance of health records for all employees in one place	1 2 3 4 5

Annual physical examinations for executives and essential personnel   1 2 3 4 5
Health promotion programs to keep essential personnel fit and healthy   1 2 3 4 5
Examination to determine impairment for injured employees   1 2 3 4 5
Rehabilitation therapy and treatment to minimize disability   1 2 3 4 5
Consultation with management to determine needs and to design occupational
  health services tailored to your company's needs   1 2 3 4 5
Consultation and visits to control liability and insurance costs by reducing risks
  to employees   1 2 3 4 5

Special Programs
  Worker education about safety   1 2 3 4 5
  Worker education about health hazards from hazardous substances (toxic
    chemicals)   1 2 3 4 5
  Health promotion for workers (physical fitness and disease prevention)   1 2 3 4 5
  Noise control and hearing conservation   1 2 3 4 5
  Alcohol abuse detection, diagnosis, treatment   1 2 3 4 5
  Drug abuse detection, diagnosis, treatment   1 2 3 4 5
  Mental health counselling for employees   1 2 3 4 5
  Stress reduction programs for employees   1 2 3 4 5
  Screening programs to detect early diseases as an *employee benefit*
    (not preplacement examination)   1 2 3 4 5

Part II. Please circle the answer which comes closest to your opinion or the policy of your company.

Question 1. Do you have an in-house health service?   Yes   No
            (If you have answered No, please go to Question 2.)
            a. Is it staffed by a physician?   Yes   No
            b. If so, is the physician full- or part-time?   Full   Part
            c. Is your service staffed by a registered nurse?   Yes   No
            d. Is your service staffed by a licensed nurse practitioner?   Yes   No

Question 2. Do you use an outside medical service?   Yes   No
            (If you have answered No, please go to Part III.)
            a. Does this service have a full range of specialists?   Yes   No
            b. Does this service have industrial hygiene and engineering
               services available?   Yes   No
            c. Is this service convenient for your workers?   Yes   No
            d. Are you satisfied with this service?   Yes   No
            e. Please write in what occupational medicine services you
               obtained last year from an outside medical organization:

Part III. Please circle the numbers which best represent your opinion or the policy of your company.

Question. What characteristics would you look for in selecting a medical organization to handle your employees' occupational medicine problems? Please rate each characteristic by importance. It would be helpful if you could also rate your present service on the scale indicated.

Characteristic in Selection

	How important is this characteristic?	How do you rate your present service?
	This characteristic is: 1 = not important, 2 = of minor importance, 3 = desirable, 4 = important, 5 = essential.	Our present service would be rated: 1 = poor, 2 = unacceptable, 3 = good, 4 = very good, 5 = superior.
High quality of medical care	1 2 3 4 5	1 2 3 4 5
Respectful and interested attitude toward your employees	1 2 3 4 5	1 2 3 4 5
Availability of all services in one location	1 2 3 4 5	1 2 3 4 5
Conscious effort to contain costs	1 2 3 4 5	1 2 3 4 5
Reputations of the physicians involved	1 2 3 4 5	1 2 3 4 5
Positive, friendly attitude	1 2 3 4 5	1 2 3 4 5
Interest in solving problems facing the employer	1 2 3 4 5	1 2 3 4 5
Convenient, accessible location for employees	1 2 3 4 5	1 2 3 4 5
Other: (Please write in) _____	1 2 3 4 5	1 2 3 4 5

Part IV. Please use this space to comment on responses to any of the questions above or to offer your options. We very much would like to hear your views on occupational medicine services.

Would you like to receive a report on the findings of this survey? If so, please supply your name and address below:

Name _____

Title _____

Company _____

Mailing Address _____

_____

Industry or product line _____